RESOUNDING
THE IMMUNE POW

"This book is a captivating synthe[...]
Dreher delights in both science and the soul. He has given us a
book that is inspiring and utterly trustworthy. I feel healthier
having read it!"   —Larry Dossey, M.D., author of *Healing Words*

"Henry Dreher has taken the discourse in mind-body health to
a new level. At the same time, he has expertly transformed a
wealth of research and clinical experience into an exciting and
practical book."
                    —Martin L. Rossman, M.D., author of *Healing Yourself*

"A wonderfully useful book; a generous, thoughtful overview of
the clinical implications of immunology research and a superb
guide to using these research findings to improve immune
functioning."   —James S. Gordon, M.D., director,
                            Center for Mind-Body Medicine

"Skillfully weaves together findings from psychology, immunology,
and medicine into a readable and useful guide to health
promotion and disease prevention."
                    —Steven E. Locke, M.D., Assistant Professor,
                        Harvard Medical School; director of medical student
                        education in psychiatry, Beth Israel Hospital, Boston;
                        co-author, *The Healer Within*

HENRY DREHER is a leading writer in the fields of health and med-
icine, specializing in cancer, mind-body science, and complemen-
tary medicine. He is the co-author of *The Type C Connection: The
Mind-Body Link to Cancer and Your Health* (Plume) and the author of
Your Defense Against Cancer. Formerly staff writer for the Cancer
Research Institute, he is a regular contributor to *Natural Health* and
Advances: The Journal of Mind-Body Health.

HENRY DREHER

THE IMMUNE POWER PERSONALITY

7 Traits You Can Develop to Stay Healthy

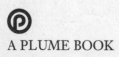

A PLUME BOOK

For Stephanie, Ira, Jesse,
and Molly Krotick

PLUME
Published by the Penguin Group
Penguin Books USA Inc., 375 Hudson Street, New York, New York 10014, U.S.A.
Penguin Books Ltd, 27 Wrights Lane, London W8 5TZ, England
Penguin Books Australia Ltd, Ringwood, Victoria, Australia
Penguin Books Canada Ltd, 10 Alcorn Avenue, Toronto, Ontario, Canada M4V 3B2
Penguin Books (N.Z.) Ltd, 182–190 Wairau Road, Auckland 10, New Zealand

Penguin Books Ltd, Registered Offices: Harmondsworth, Middlesex, England

Published by Plume, an imprint of Dutton Signet,
a division of Penguin Books USA Inc.
Previously published in a Dutton edition.

First Plume Printing, May, 1996
10 9 8 7 6 5 4 3 2 1

Figure from L. D. Jamner, G. E. Schwartz, and H. Leigh. "The Relationship Between Repressive and Defensive Coping Styles and Monocyte, Eosinophile, and Serum Glucose Levels: Support for the Opioid Peptide Hypothesis of Repression." *Psychosomatic Medicine*, 50, page 570, 1988. Reprinted by permission from Williams and Wilkins.

Figure from J. B. Jemmott, C. Hellman, et al. "Motivational Syndromes Associated with Natural Killer Cell Activity." *Journal of Behavioral Medicine*, 31, 1, page 59, 1990. Reprinted with permission of Plenum Publishing and Dr. John B. Jemmott, III.

Figure adapted from J. B. Jemmott, et al. "Academic Stress, Power Motivation, and Decrease in Salivary Immunoglobulin A Secretion Rate." Reprinted with permission of Dr. John B. Jemmott, III.

Figures from H. Andrews. "Helping and Health: The Relationship Between Volunteer Activity and Health-Related Outcomes." Reprinted with permission from *Advances: The Journal of Mind-Body Health*, 7, 1, page 29, 1990.

Table from P. W. Linville. "Self-Complexity as a Cognitive Buffer Against Stress-Related Illness and Depression." *Journal of Personality and Social Psychology*, 52, 4, page 667, 1987. Reprinted with permission of Dr. Patricia W. Linville.

Questionnaire from Suzanne Ouellette Kobasa. "How Much Stress Can You Survive?" *American Health* (September 1984). © Suzanne Ouellette Kobasa, 1984. Reprinted with permission of the publisher.

Ⓟ REGISTERED TRADEMARK—MARCA REGISTRADA

The Library of Congress has catalogued the Dutton edition as follows:

Dreher, Henry.
   The immune power personality : 7 traits you can develop to stay healthy / Henry Dreher.
      p.   cm.
   Includes bibliographical references
   ISBN 0-525-93838-9 (hc.)
   ISBN 0-452-27546-6 (pbk.)
   1. Psychoneuroimmunology.   2. Mind and body.   I. Title.
QP356.47.D74   1995
613—dc20   94–37484
                                                        CIP

Printed in the United States of America

Original hardcover design by Steven N. Stathakis

BOOKS ARE AVAILABLE AT QUANTITY DISCOUNTS WHEN USED TO PROMOTE PRODUCTS OR SERVICES. FOR INFORMATION PLEASE WRITE TO PREMIUM MARKETING DIVISION, PENGUIN BOOKS USA INC., 375 HUDSON STREET, NEW YORK, NEW YORK 10014.

CONTENTS

Acknowledgments   ix
Introduction   1

1 Deeper into the Mind-Body Connection   12
2 The ACE Factor: Attend, Connect, Express   48
3 The Capacity to Confide   96
4 Hardiness: Commitment, Control, and Challenge 125
5 Assertiveness: The Hub of the Wheel   168
6 The Power of Love vs. the Love of Power   211
7 Healthy Helping: The Trait of Altruism   255
8 Self-Complexity: The Healthy Hydra   288

Appendix Following the Program: The Author's Experience
          and Immune Test Results   324
          References   329
          Index   357

ACKNOWLEDGMENTS

I wish to thank, first and foremost, the seven researchers whose work is this book's primary subject and inspiration. Each one of them was forthcoming and unstintingly helpful.

Gary Schwartz has been insufficiently recognized as a pioneering investigator in mind-body science; he is one of those few individuals whose vision has helped to shape the field. In our meetings, his incisive mind, his humor, and his compassion shone through. I thank him for his warm support of my endeavors.

James Pennebaker has two qualities that, combined, are the stuff of greatness in scientific endeavors: ingenuity and sheer boldness. He also has a keen critical intelligence and a terrific wit. I am extremely grateful for his support of this project and my work in general.

Suzanne Ouellette helped to fashion the concept of health-promoting traits, and she has brought complexity, compassion, and an authentic philosophic underpinning to mind-body research. She was a pleasure to interview, and I greatly appreciate her cooperation for this project.

George Solomon is a visionary whose early work formed the basis for psychoneuroimmunology. He has bridged so many specialties in the medical sciences that no term could possibly be concocted for a field that would represent his vision—it would have far too many syllables and no one could remember let alone pronounce it. And Solomon's science has always been infused with compassion. He has also had the stubborn will and energy to endure despite many obstacles. I thank him for his support of my work, and his friendship.

David McClelland has devoted much of the last fifteen years to the mind-body field, and his contributions have been enormous. I am grateful to him for the generous time he took to share his work and insights. I am also grateful for the spirit of compassion and care he has brought to the field.

Allan Luks deserves great credit for bringing attention to the health benefits of helping. Through sheer tenacity, he has helped to stimulate and disseminate an important body of work. I greatly appreciate the support he has given me for this project.

Patricia Linville's contributions to mind-body research have yet to be fully recognized, but she has brought an imaginative perspective to the field and backed it with hard-nosed science. I thank her for taking so much time for our interviews, and for the clarity and eloquence with which she described her work and ideas.

I also wish to thank individuals who have collaborated with these seven researchers, or whose work has paralleled theirs, all of whom have helped me with this project: Warren Berland, Herbert Benson, Matthew Budd, Jon Kabat-Zinn, Steve Keller, Anne Krantz, James McKay, Salvadore Maddi, Martin Rossman, Lydia Temoshok, and Joel Weinberger.

I am grateful to those individuals with medical conditions who have benefited from treatments that enhance Immune Power traits, all of whom gave generously of their time: Howard Paris, Nancy Horniak, Judy Weintraub, David Kriser, Marty Carls, and Kelly Forsberg-Said.

My transcriber, Therese Brown, has not only done an extraordinary job, she has been a source of support throughout this project. I thank her for her skills, patience, and kindness.

ACKNOWLEDGMENTS

Certain family members and friends gave me their unstinting support during the course of this project, and I wholeheartedly thank them all: Marion Beckenstein, Daniel Chiel, Diane Dreher, Marcy Klapper, and Barbara Miller.

Barbara Gess, a charter member of the three-person committee that passes on all my project ideas, gave an immediate enthusiastic thumbs up on this one, for which I am most grateful. Special thanks also to Tom Rawls, who helped to stimulate the idea for this book in one of our many enjoyable conversations, and who gave me important opportunities to write on subjects I cared about.

I wish to thank the people at Dutton Signet—particularly Carole DeSanti, Arnold Dolin, and Elaine Koster—for believing in this project from the very start.

I thank my agent, Chris Tomasino, for her wisdom, patience, integrity, and friendship. She helped me inordinately during every phase of this project.

As always, my wife, Deborah Chiel, has been heroic in her support of my work. I cannot thank her enough for her thoughtful criticisms, her willingness to stick with me through difficult patches, and her steadfast belief in me.

I am grateful to the late Michael Callen for providing inspiration for this book. Although I only met Michael a few times, I was moved by his work, his ideas, his presence. For people suffering with any life-threatening disease, Michael transmitted a message of hope and compassion: Let us bring a new dimension to medicine, one in which surgery, drugs, and diets are complemented by our own fighting spirit, that inner reserve of resilience and energy with a healing potential yet to be imagined.

INTRODUCTION

The 1990s have seen the dawning of a new model for promoting health and preventing disease. This model accepts that genes, environmental pollutants, disease agents, and diet are all factors in the genesis of illness. But it also accepts the role of the mind, both in illness and in health. As the mind-body field blossoms, we are learning that psychological factors influence the immune system, the body's network of defense and healing. Thus, *the mind can contribute to our risk and our recovery from almost any disease.*

Discoveries by today's mind-body scientists are compelling us to replace outmoded ideas about stress and health. Stress has been a buzzword since the 1960s, when our culture began disseminating the notion that external pressures and upsetting events are key psychological factors in illness. Recent investigations have altered that view. They reveal that stress is an inevitable and sometimes even positive force in our lives. The pivotal psychological factor in illness is not stress but rather *how we cope with stress.* And how we cope depends, in large part, on our *personalities.*

A small band of scientists on the cutting edge of mind-body research has identified personality traits that enable us to cope effectively with the emotional wear and tear of daily existence. These traits represent facets of our psychological makeup that protect us from *internal distress* caused by *external stress*. By buffering us from the harmful effects of stress, healthy traits keep us strong in mind and body.

Over the past ten years, I have written exclusively about the burgeoning fields of mind-body science and medicine. In the course of my investigations, I have identified a group of seven researchers, each of whom has uncovered a particular personality trait associated with psychological and physical well-being. Since each trait has been directly or indirectly linked to a vigorous immune system, I call them Immune Power traits. This book is about Immune Power traits, the research that has uncovered them, and the strategies each one of us can employ to become an Immune Power Personality. These strategies offer new hope that our own psychological resources can be activated to prevent and to heal diseases affecting every organ and system of the body.

What is an Immune Power Personality? The research I have explored suggests an individual who is able to find joy and meaning, even health, when life offers up its most difficult challenges. The Immune Power Personality handles stressful events not with denial but with acceptance, flexibility, and a willingness to learn and grow. These characteristics prevent the individual from breaking down emotionally and physically in the midst of life crises. Psychologists have long documented the role of healthy traits in maintaining a healthy state of mind. Now mind-body scientists are demonstrating the role of healthy traits in maintaining a healthy state of body.

In each chapter of this book, I follow the searches of one investigator who has defined and studied one Immune Power trait. Here are the traits and the researchers who identified them:

- **The ACE Factor: Attend, Connect, Express:** University of Arizona psychologist Gary E. Schwartz, Ph.D., has shown that people who are tuned to mind-body signals of discomfort, pain, fatigue, distress, sadness, anger, and pleasure cope better psychologically and have a better immune profile and a healthier cardiovascular system.

- **The Capacity to Confide:** James W. Pennebaker, Ph.D., a psychologist at Southern Methodist University in Dallas, Texas, has demonstrated that individuals who confide their secrets, traumas, and feelings to themselves and others have livelier immune responses, healthier psychological profiles, and far fewer incidences of illness.

- **Hardiness—Commitment, Control, and Challenge:** Suzanne Ouellette, Ph.D., a psychologist at the City University of New York, originated the concept of personality *hardiness*. Hardiness includes the "three Cs": a sense of *control* over one's quality of life, health, and social conditions; a strong *commitment* to one's work, creative activities, or relationships; and a view of stress as a *challenge* rather than a threat. People who exhibit the three Cs suffer far fewer chronic illnesses and symptoms than those who don't. Other investigators have found that hardy individuals have stronger immune systems.

- **Assertiveness:** George F. Solomon, M.D., an early pioneer of psychoneuroimmunology, conducted the earliest studies on personality and immunity. He has shown that people who assert their needs and feelings have stronger, more balanced immune responses. They more readily resist and overcome a range of diseases associated with dysfunctional immunity—from rheumatoid arthritis to AIDS. Solomon has found Immune Power connections to other traits as well, including the ability to find meaning in stressful life circumstances.

- **Affiliative Trust:** A world-renowed motivational psychologist, David McClelland, Ph.D., of Boston University, has discovered that individuals who are strongly motivated to form relationships with others based on unconditional love and trust—rather than frustrated power—have more vigorous immune systems and reduced incidence of illness.

- **Healthy Helping—The Trait of Altruism:** While heading the Institute for the Advancement of Health, investigator Allan Luks conducted a large survey showing that people committed to helping others get a "helper's high" that is not only mental and spiritual but physical as well. These individuals, displaying the personality trait of altruism, suffer fewer illnesses than others who are not similarly motivated or engaged. Luks has become a one-man clearinghouse for the research of scientists and psychologists who have verified findings from his own survey.

- **Self-Complexity—The Healthy Hydra:** Patricia Linville, a psychologist at Duke University, has demonstrated that people who explore many facets of their personalities—called "self-aspects"—can better withstand stressful life circumstances. In her research, people with many "self-aspects" were less prone to stress, depression, physical symptoms, and bouts of flu and other illnesses in the wake of stressful life events. They also had higher self-esteem. Linville found that individuals high in "self-complexity" have strengths to fall back on when one part of themselves is lost or wounded.

I have interviewed these investigators, studied their data, and spoken with many of their patients. In each case, a story emerged with important ramifications for our health and well-being. They are stories of scientists on a path of discovery who overcame the biases of both traditional and alternative medical communities. They are also stories of new and penetrating visions of human functioning and advances in the mind-body field that will change the face of medicine.

Other scientists have investigated health-promoting personality traits, but these seven have emerged with the most sophisticated theories, substantial research findings, and practical approaches for self-development. With one exception, they are psychologists or psychiatrists who have conducted original studies published in leading scientific journals. (Please consult References for their published papers, and related scientific findings.) The only exception is Allan Luks, a nonscientist whose vision propelled him to conduct a large survey on the role of helping and altruism in health. (Luks has collected hard data from other scientists confirming conclusions of his survey—that people motivated by altruism experience better health.) Despite the fact that their findings have challenged the conventional wisdom of established medicine, the rigor of their scientific methods has been recognized. Indeed, many are viewed as pioneers in their respective fields. And, interestingly, the researchers themselves exhibited Immune Power traits, often the very ones they studied. They had to be assertive to survive professionally in an academic community that is skeptical about psychological factors in health. Their sense of commitment, control, and challenge in confronting academic and scientific roadblocks was unerring. They designed and advocated methods that empower people to benefit from their discoveries.

THE STRESS MODEL—AND BEYOND

Why isn't stress reduction enough? Why do Immune Power traits represent a leap forward in mind-body medicine? The current—but increasingly outdated—model of mind and body teaches us that stress is bad, plain and simple. The public continues to be fed this old dogma in trivialized form: "Avoid stress in your life, stay positive, and you'll remain healthy." At times, it seems as if prescriptions for mind-body health can be reduced to Bobby McFerrin's famous lyric: "Don't worry, be happy!"

The mind-body researchers whose work forms the heart of this book have abandoned this overly simple model. From both a scientific and a practical perspective, they have concluded that mere stress reduction and having a "positive attitude" are insufficient guides to mind-body wellness. One of these scientists, Suzanne Ouellette, who originated of the concept of hardiness, scoured the literature on stress and turned up this finding: If you were to predict illness from a knowledge of stressful life events, you would be right less than 15 percent of the time. Her work, and the work of the other scientists, demonstrates that how we *respond* to stress—emotionally, cognitively, and behaviorally—is critical in determining whether stress will make us sick.

For instance, during hard economic times, it's unrealistic to think that we can remain hermetically sealed off from the uncertainties, the job insecurity, or the financial difficulties that have become part of our lives. Moreover, we weren't built to avoid stress. Could our prehistoric ancestors, whose survival depended on dangerous hunting forays into the wilderness, have stayed cloistered in their caves in the name of stress management? Certainly not. In the modern era we cannot sidestep the stress that accompanies our pursuit of financial stability and creative enrichment in our work; our quest for more gratifying relationships; and our search for meaning as we confront everyday problems and inevitable losses. Consider the Chinese symbol for "crisis," which combined two words: danger and opportunity. When confronted with personal upheaval, we face the danger of regression or collapse, but we also are presented with opportunities for growth. Immune Power trait research is defining forms of personal growth that promote mind-body health.

IMMUNE POWER TRAITS IN THE AGE OF AIDS

Of course, any discussion of immunity raises the issue of AIDS, acquired immune deficiency syndrome. During the early years of the AIDS epidemic, people diagnosed with the disease were not expected to live long. The media relentlessly hammered home the message that AIDS was an automatic, swift, and harsh death sentence. Only the lucky, we were told, would live as long as one year. Given the immense suffering wrought by AIDS, some patients were considered fortunate *not* to live that long. I recall a conversation with a physician who thought AIDS patients were better off without illusions about extended survival. Borrowing a line from poet Dylan Thomas, he suggested that such patients need not "rage against the dying of the light."

I shared these early 1980s assumptions. But they were shattered in late 1984, when I met Michael Callen. He was twenty-nine years old and had been living with AIDS for three years. Callen was the first person I encountered with the disease. He was not emaciated or covered with lesions, the way AIDS patients usually appeared in the media. Free of any visible signs of illness, Callen was an anomaly—a man who, for the time being, had beaten the odds against the virulent plague of our times.

By the late 1980s, it became clear that many people infected with HIV, the AIDS virus, would remain fit and functional for years. (Basketball star Magic Johnson is a perfect example.) However, when Callen was first diagnosed, he was not simply infected with HIV. He had full-blown AIDS, replete with the opportunistic infections that were supposed to herald a quick demise. Yet here he was in 1984—robust, energetic, and upbeat.

I met Callen at a New York conference on the role of psychological factors in AIDS. His brief talk was the weekend's most moving moment. He spoke of his struggle to reject the media's insistence that AIDS patients would invariably die quickly and painfully, which he called a "propaganda of hopelessness." With regard to his own long survival, he claimed he was not alone. Many others were outliving medicine's dire predictions. (Studies later proved him right.) Callen also chronicled his political battles against the established medical community, which cast a blind eye toward AIDS prevention and research. He was fighting for causes he believed in, and he was fighting for his own life.

Later I had several opportunities to speak with Callen, who confided his personal struggles with AIDS. How had he coped with such a devastating diagnosis? He found a doctor whom he trusted, and together they developed a healing partnership. He did not deny the seriousness of his condition, but he was resolute in rejecting a death sentence. He was motivated by love and a search for meaning in his life's work and relationships. A revitalized singing career buoyed his spirits. I was struck by Callen's intelligence, compassion, and grit. As in Dylan Thomas's poem, he *did* rage against the dying of the light, and his light kept burning.

I couldn't help but wonder if his personality had contributed to his unexpected survival. The passage of time would only reinforce my suspicion that it had. Michael Callen lived for twelve years after his original diagnosis. In 1993, he may have been the longest AIDS survivor on record. During those years, he lived his life with passion and intensity. When he died at the end of 1993, he left a legacy of hope to countless other people with AIDS.

On a personal level, I found Michael Callen's courage inspiring. But I also was encouraged by his example to further investigate the role of personality in recovery from illness. Callen's story begged the question: Could an individual's personality traits enable him to resist a disease with the pathological power of AIDS? As I will detail further, in recent years, mind-body scientists have in fact turned up scientific evidence that Immune Power traits can help people infected with the HIV virus to resist collapse into full-blown AIDS for extended periods of time.

The significance of these discoveries go far beyond AIDS, however. Immune Power traits have been associated with resistance and recovery from many diseases associated with dysfunctional immune systems—including cancer, arthritis, lupus, asthma, allergies, chronic fatigue, herpes, and other viral infections.

For over twenty years, the popular press has informed us that various vitamins, herbs, dietary regimens, and holistic practices balance or boost the immune system. Many of these factors can be effective, but we've too long neglected the healing potential of our own hidden characterological strengths.

DEVELOPING AN IMMUNE POWER PERSONALITY

In each chapter, I present experiments, data, and case histories showing that Immune Power traits *demonstrably, materially improve physical health.* I also will provide therapeutic suggestions and specific exercises you can apply to cultivate Immune Power traits and better health for yourself. These strategies include:

- Therapies and mind-body approaches for cultivating Immune Power traits, implemented by the scientist whose research is the focus of the chapter.
- Strategies for cultivation of Immune Power traits developed by other mind-body practitioners.
- Specific practices and exercises you can follow on a regular basis. These clinician-tested mind-body practices—including medita-

tions and guided imagery exercises—are specifically tailored to evoke that Immune Power trait.

I have been asked one question most frequently about Immune Power traits: Can people really change aspects of their personalities?

The researchers represented in this book have shown, with varying degrees of specificity, that Immune Power traits *can* be cultivated. They are *not* fixed parts of character that some of us have been fortunate enough to inherit. They are healthy capacities we all have from birth, that each of us experiences and manifests differently. At the same time, Immune Power traits are not rigid molds into which we must twist ourselves to achieve some idealized mind-body state. They are healthy potentialities each of us can maximize and express in our own unique way. As I will show, Immune Power traits can be reawakened in adulthood through short-term therapy or specifically tailored mind-body methods.

Since each Immune Power trait has demonstrable links to health, the person who develops all seven traits will optimize his or her potential for mind-body wellness. That is why the transformative program I present involves a stepwise approach to cultivating each trait, one at a time. Mind-body pioneer George Solomon has observed that exceptionally healthy individuals, and those who overcome disease, manifest a unique combination of Immune Power traits.

Chapter 1, "Deeper into the Mind-Body Connection," traces the scientific developments that led to the discovery of Immune Power traits. Beginning with chapter 2, each chapter is devoted to the work of one investigator, the story of his or her research, a description of the Immune Power trait, and the strategies you can apply in your own life in order to cultivate that characteristic. Taken together, these strategies amount to an overall program of Immune Power Personality development. The available evidence strongly suggests that all of us can develop the seven Immune Power traits, as long as we apply the strategies in ways that meet our singular needs and express our individuality.

I have established an order for developing an Immune Power

Personality based on the distinct but overlapping qualities of these traits. The strategies for developing each trait touch upon many different levels of mind-body awareness but tend to focus more on one particular level. The program starts with an Immune Power trait rooted in an awareness of the body (the ACE Factor), then moves forward with traits that emphasize emotions, thoughts, the need for meaning, interpersonal relationships, and spirituality. Thus, in developing Immune Power traits, you start with a simple mindfulness of your physical state of being and progress to more complex levels of feeling, thought, and relations to others and the world.

I recommend that you read each chapter in order and follow the program's progression. However, as you move through each chapter, it may become clear that you already possess certain Immune Power traits, to a greater or lesser degree. Feel free to skip over program strategies or traits you already possess and move on to areas where you feel you require more development. Trust your intuition.

The last chapter, on "self-complexity," brings together elements from all previous chapters, in suggesting that we optimize our state of mind-body health when we accept and nurture *all* facets of ourselves. Psychologist Patricia Linville has proposed a model of psychophysical well-being, in which our personalities are like broad rivers with many tributaries. Following those tributaries leads us to new terrain—previously unexplored aspects of ourselves that include valuable, untapped resources. When we self-discover these facets, we find alternatives to old, habitual patterns; new ways of coping with stress; and new sources of pleasure and meaning in our lives.

In the Appendix, I briefly recount my own experience in following the program set forth herein. Because I was able to obtain a complete workup of my immune system before and after, I found out whether developing the seven traits actually bolstered my immunity.

In a conversation I had with him eight years ago, Lawrence LeShan, a psychotherapist who treats cancer patients and an early pioneer in the mind-body field, summed up the approach underlying the Immune Power Personality. Each one of us, he said, must develop "a fierce and tender concern for all parts of ourselves so that no part of our being is standing outside the door, whimpering, 'Is there nothing for me?' " That "fierce and tender concern" is essential to the development of an Immune Power Personality.

Before detailing the seven Immune Power traits, the next chapter presents an overview of developments in the mind-body field and a primer on the immune system itself. Breakthroughs in mind-body research have led inevitably to the work I describe throughout, work that has shown how basic human characteristics—not just transitory emotions or "techniques"—are keys to vibrant good health.

DEEPER INTO THE MIND-BODY CONNECTION

BEFORE LONG, MEDICAL RESEARCHERS MAY DISCOVER THAT THE HUMAN BRAIN HAS A NATURAL DRIVE TO SUSTAIN THE LIFE PROCESS AND TO POTENTIATE THE ENTIRE BODY IN THE FIGHT AGAINST PAIN AND DISEASE. WHEN THAT KNOWLEDGE IS DEVELOPED, THE ART AND PRACTICE OF MEDICINE WILL ASCEND TO A NEW AND HIGHER PLATEAU.

—NORMAN COUSINS

Most of us harbor wisdom about the inseparability of mind and body. We may have had grandparents or parents who taught us that we get sick when we overwork or when our family lives are in turmoil. As adults we remember these lessons and come to accept that our thoughts, moods, and feelings are powerful influences on our health. Or we eventually learn these lessons through personal experience.

We rarely get colds when our lives are going well, but the sniffles begin, as if on cue, when a problem at work or home overwhelms our capacity to cope.

Our blood pressure reading is high when external pressures are high—whether from our bosses, our families, or an accumulation of taxing demands.

We develop a serious infection or disease when we feel fatigued, fearful, or downright depressed.

We may even be subject to symptoms that "express" what we cannot.

In the vicelike grip of an impossible expectation on the job, we get constant headaches.

After a death in the family, we take on more responsibilities than we can bear. With the "weight of the world" on our shoulders, we suffer debilitating back pain.

We hold back our tears after the breakup of a long-term relationship and suffer one respiratory infection after another.

Experiences such as these help us to recognize that our state of mind is a critical factor in our physical health and well-being. Yet many of our doctors and medical scientists cast doubt upon this native wisdom. A mere quarter century ago, mainstream medicine spurned ideas about the mind-body connection that were embraced by a large sector of the public. Medical scientists do not accept concepts that cannot be empirically demonstrated, and research on psychological factors in illness did not meet their standards.

Until the 1970s, those who studied the mind-body connection lacked the sophisticated research tools to ground their theories in biological fact. In order to buttress popular beliefs with scientific proof, mind-body researchers had one overriding task. They had to show that the mind could influence our primary biological system responsible for preventing and healing disease—the immune system.

Our immune system stands guard against the intrusion of noxious invaders—bacteria, viruses, cancer cells, or any organism that threatens harm to our tissues. An interactive network of cells and substances, the immune system is our body's monitor, its police force, its protector. It has the necessary "intelligence" to distinguish between elements that belong to the "self" and those that are foreign, or "nonself." It is a multiarmed tool for fine-tuning our biological responses, thus maintaining balance between our internal and external environments. It resolves the crisis of an invasion by fighting the interlopers, repairing the damage, and cleaning up the remnants of battle. The immune system is the healer within.

In the absence of hard evidence, the reigning medical experts refused to believe that the immune system could be regulated by any other biological system. It was viewed as a stand-alone entity—a network that operated independently to eliminate disease agents and heal insults and injuries to the body. For medical scientists to accept the mind's powers over disease and healing, they required proof that the immune system did not stand alone—that it somehow relied on signals from the brain. But before the late 1970s the idea of brain-immune connections was considered as preposterous as the notion that the Atlantic and Pacific oceans are joined by previously uncharted waterways.

Today, the idea that the brain and the immune system are interconnected is no longer considered preposterous. It is an incontrovertible fact.

Research from a burgeoning field known as *psychoneuroimmunology* (PNI, for short) has taught us that the brain and nervous system are intimately involved in the activities of the immune system. So, too, is the endocrine system, our network of glands and the hormones they secrete. PNI research is building a scientific base for a viewpoint long held by advocates of "holistic" medicine: that all our biological systems, including those governing "mind" and "body," are integrated into a seamless whole. Our healing network—the immune system—is an integral part of a larger entity, the "bodymind." We can no longer carve up our biological systems into separate work forces based on a false division of labor.

In a language consisting of cell products, our nervous, endocrine, and immune systems "talk" to each other. But their dialogue is more than occasional chatter. It is nonstop communication along a superhighway of cellular information. These continuous exchanges enable our systems to act in concert to eliminate outside invaders and maintain the integrity of the body.

To the astonishment of many immunologists, it turns out

that our thoughts and feelings are mediated by brain chemicals that also regulate our body's defenses. These chemicals, called *neurotransmitters,* are not restricted to the brain. They circulate throughout the body, carrying messages to other systems and cells—including our immune system. In other words, the chemical "carriers" of our human emotions directly influence our physical health.

As PNI scientist Candace Pert has said, "In the beginning of my work, I matter-of-factly presumed that emotions were in the head or the brain. Now I would say they are really in the body as well. They are expressed in the body and are part of the body. I can no longer make a strong distinction between the brain and the body."

So our native wisdom about mind and body, whether garnered from our grandparents or from personal experience, is grounded in scientific reality. Many of the so-called mind-body myths were not myths at all. They were truths.

Soon I will describe the recent breakthroughs in PNI research, which are heralding a sea change in the way we practice medicine in this country. Farsighted doctors are beginning to apply mind-body techniques for the healing and prevention of disease. These are methods for calming the mind, relaxing the body, expressing emotions, changing negative thoughts, and controlling physical functions. Commonly referred to as "mind-body medicine," such techniques have proven benefits for people suffering with chronic pain and illness.

The methods of mind-body medicine include meditation, biofeedback, guided imagery, hypnosis, group therapy, behavior therapy, cognitive "restructuring," and individual psychotherapy. These treatments are being applied to an encyclopedic list of disorders, from AIDS, cancer, and heart disease, to arthritis, allergies, back pain, and headaches.

But mind-body science is still young. Investigators are mapping mind-body interactions on the molecular level, yet gaps remain in our understanding of how our thoughts and emotions "trickle down" to influence cells, tissues, and organ systems. Mind-body techniques have proven their value, but mysteries linger regarding why they work, how they work, and which treatments are most effective for specific disorders.

We do know that the mind can either sap or strengthen our bodies' defenses, contributing to illness or nourishing states of health. Still, the title of Bill Moyers's recent PBS television series, "Healing and the Mind," prompts the critical question: "Exactly *what* aspect of the mind is healing?"

In an effort to simplify research into the mind-body connection, the media have emphasized such concepts as "relaxation," "reduced stress," and "positive emotions." The scientists whose work is the subject of this book are not satisfied with these maxims, based as they are on a dated model of stress and illness. Although "relaxation," "reduced stress," and "positive emotions" *can* be healing, the mysteries of mind and body are deeper still, and more complex.

Yes, we must reduce certain unnecessary stressful influences. But a strategy of avoiding stress makes little sense, because our creativity is stretched, our intellect challenged, and our emotions engaged when we confront and actively cope with hardship. We benefit most—in mind and in body—by adapting to change and loss. What determines our capacities for coping and adaptation? To a great extent, our personalities.

A large body of research over the past several decades has investigated "harmful" personality traits that contribute to ill health. However, in recent years a coterie of scientists has moved to understand the nature of health and has discovered positive personality traits—ways of coping and being that nourish our physical health. Though some will disagree, I believe that research on the health-promoting personality is a radical turn in the history of medical science. For decades, legions of biologists, pathologists, psychiatrists, and psychologists have trained their scientific sights exclusively on the causes of sickness.

This problem has been partly societal. Our media culture emphasizes pathology on every front: disorganized economies, disordered cities, dysfunctional families, and diseases of the individual, from addictions to physical afflictions. Our obsession with pathology has had an especially powerful impact on medical research, which has produced far too little data on factors that promote health.

Abraham Maslow claimed that his fellow psychologists knew a great deal about mental illness and almost nothing about mental health. But of course, the psychologists' limitations are but a reflection of our own. We know too little about our own potential for healthy development. As William James has written: "Compared to what we ought to be, we are only half awake. Our fires are dampened, our drafts are checked, we are making use of only a small part of our mental and physical resources."

As James suggested, we awaken to our potential by drawing upon heretofore untapped inner resources. What is our potential? The establishment of a meaningful and successful life in all spheres, including work, creativity, relationships, and health. Indeed, personal growth in work, creativity, and relationships is inseparably linked to our physical well-being. To extend James's metaphor, when we relight our fires, our biological systems are invigorated and our defenses are fortified.

This book is about relighting our fires by recovering parts of ourselves that are capable of creating joy, meaning, *and* physical health. Before proceeding, I provide you with essential background on the scientific developments that led to research on the Immune Power Personality.

THE GERM, THE TERRAIN, AND THE HISTORY OF MIND-BODY SCIENCE

The roots of the mind-body medicine can be traced back to 400 B.C., when Hippocrates wrote, "Natural forces within us are the true healers of disease." The Greek physician, whose imprint on medicine has lasted through the millennia, taught his students to consider, as a regular part of medical practice, their patients' life circumstances and emotions. Aristotle was arguably the first forceful advocate of a philosophy of holism. The Greek philosopher and biologist believed that the soul was inseparable from the body and that our bodily systems functioned cooperatively to serve the whole organism.

For centuries, the holistic concepts of Hippocrates, Aristotle, and the Greek physician Galen held some sway over medical practice. A historical turning point occurred in the mid-seventeenth century, when René Descartes, the influential French philosopher, set forth the doctrine that mind and body were entirely separate entities. Known as Cartesian dualism, this absolute split between mind and body became the philosophic basis for Western medicine. For 350 years, medical scientists have largely based their research, and doctors have largely based their practice, on the notion that the body is a mere biological version of a machine. Cartesian dualism held that this machine was unregulated and untouched by the "ephemeral" entities of mind and spirit.

Renewed stirrings of the ancient philosophy of mind-body interactions could be detected in the writings of certain renowned nineteenth-century physicians and scientists. Sir William Osler, a Canadian physician who practiced in Britain and was considered the preeminent clinician of his time, is famous for having said "It is much more important to know what sort of patient has the disease than what sort of disease the patient has." His remark represented an early glimmer of recognition by traditional medicine that personality could play a part in health.

In the nineteenth century the Western world had come to embrace the notion that every disease had one cause and one cure. The researches of the German physician Robert Koch and French physician Louis Pasteur led to *the theory of specific etiology*—the idea that diseases were caused by a single microorganism and could be eradicated by a single strategy for destroying the invader.

Koch solved the mystery of anthrax, a bacterial disease of sheep and cattle and occasionally of humans. And in 1905, he won the Nobel Prize for identifying the germ that caused tuberculosis, a signal achievement in medical science. Pasteur made his indelible mark on medicine by translating Koch's bacteriologic breakthroughs into cures. He developed a vaccine that used weakened versions of a virulent organism to inoculate animals against anthrax. Later he used similar methods to vaccinate humans against rabies. Koch and Pasteur set the stage for the development, in the early twentieth century, of antibiotics and other "magic bullets" designed to rid the body of the specific pathogens that cause disease.

Enter Claude Bernard, the mid-nineteenth-century French physiologist who established his reputation by discovering that blood sugar was stored in the liver and released to meet the body's energy needs and that the nervous system helps to regulate blood flow. Bernard was also a great philosopher of medicine, with an overarching view of human biology. Long before the word "stress" entered the lexicon, he spoke of the need to prevent our organisms from being overwhelmed by environmental demands. He also spoke of the need for balance within our organisms, which he called the *milieu interior*—the interior environment. Our cells, bodily chemicals, and organs would function efficiently, he claimed, when there was harmony in our systems.

In Bernard's view, harmony implied a balanced biochemistry—a vigorous yet finely tuned biological apparatus. Health was predicated on balance, and disease was a by-product of imbalance in the interior environment. Bernard did not view germs as omnipotent invaders that caused disease whenever they managed to gain access to our insides. "Diseases float in the air," he said. "Their seeds are blown by the wind but they only take root when the terrain is right." Thus, Bernard's metaphor was one of "the germ and the terrain." The germ could cause disease only when it found a hospitable home in a weakened terrain. Otherwise, it would be overcome by our natural resistances.

Bernard's emphasis on the germ and the terrain called into question the widely accepted theory of specific etiology. Pasteur may himself have recognized that germs were not the only consideration in disease. An apocryphal story is told about Pasteur's last words, which were reported to have been "Bernard was right. The germ is little—the terrain all."

Bernard's emphasis on the terrain, largely ignored in his time, laid the groundwork for twentieth-century forays into the mind-body relationship. In the 1930s and '40s, Harvard physiologist Walter B. Cannon concluded that humans have built-in mechanisms that help us to sustain a vital balance ("homeostasis") within the body. Cannon theorized that we are self-regulating creatures. Under ideal circumstances, we maintain our own health by making constant biological adjustments in response to inner and outer stimuli. Our central nervous system—the brain—is the master regulator of homeostasis, including such processes as blood pressure, body temperature, heart rate, and blood sugar levels. Cannon also showed how life experiences (namely "stress," although the word had yet to be popularized) alter a whole gamut of bodily functions via the nervous system. When faced with threatening situations, the sympathetic branch of our nervous system goes into overdrive. Cannon called this the *fight-or-flight* response, because the brain's message and body's reply readies us for a confrontation or a quick exit.

Cannon brought rigor to the nascent field of mind-body science, but his sights were set on physiological rather than psychological processes. Little was known or even proposed about the specific mind-states that either sapped or strengthened our defense against disease. However, a few years earlier Sigmund Freud had made an appearance on the mind-body stage, though from a completely different side of the scientific and cultural theater.

Freud believed that people who repressed unbearably painful emotions in the wake of a trauma would "convert" those feelings into bodily symptoms, such as temporary paralysis, nervous conditions, and chronic pain. Called *conversion disorders,* these otherwise unexplained symptoms could be relieved when the person expressed and resolved the feelings he or she had blocked. With this theory, Freud opened the door to the study of illness as unconscious metaphor for a person's suffering.

Freud's notion of conversion disorders was elaborated in the 1940s, when one of his students, Chicago psychiatrist Franz Alexander, developed a form of medicine based on principles of psychoanalysis. He believed that "many chronic disturbances are not caused by external, mechanical, chemical factors or by microorganisms, but by the continuous functional stress arising during the everyday life of the organism in its struggle for existence." His ideas led to the formal development of the mind-body field called *psychosomatic medicine.*

Alexander believed that emotional turmoil and conflict were especially powerful factors in specific diseases, later dubbed the "psychosomatic seven." They were: hypertension, hyperthyroidism, rheumatoid arthritis, neurodermatitis, asthma, ulcerative colitis, and peptic ulcers. Psychosomatic medicine peaked in the 1950s and lost some favor by the 1960s and '70s, due in part to the failure of research to prove that mind-states were *overriding* causes of the "psychosomatic seven." Also, psychosomatic researchers could not link emotions to immunity, because they lacked the tools and the knowledge base to demonstrate interconnections between the nervous, endocrine, and immune systems.

A crucial step toward mapping these interconnections was taken in the 1950s by Hans Selye, the celebrated biochemist, while he was conducting animal research at McGill University in Montreal. The leading proponent of the concept of stress, defined as "the nonspecific response of the body to any demand made on it," Selye charted a winding psychophysiological pathway through which external events and pressures influenced health. Simply put, during stress the brain triggers a veritable "cascade" of hormonal secretions that act as messengers to the rest of the body. To use a corporate analogy: As soon as the brain registers danger or difficulty, a stress message is "written" and passed along by various couriers from one neural or hormonal office to another, each time stimulating a different functional responsibility.

The process begins in the hypothalamus, a walnut-size piece of tissue located deep within the brain, which sends a hormonal signal to the pituitary gland at the base of the brain. In turn, the pituitary is activated to secrete ACTH, a messenger that stimulates the adrenal glands, which sit like triangular hats upon each of the kidneys. The adrenals produce two classes of vital hormones, the corticosteroids (which include cortisol) and the catecholamines (which include adrenaline), that have potent effects on our nervous and musculoskeletal systems. The "stress" message, translated by these neural and hormonal messengers, is the alarm that readies us for fight or flight. Our hearts beat faster, our breaths deepen, sugar stored in the liver is released, and blood flows away from the skin and in toward the brain and skeletal muscles.

The stress response was obviously an innate survival mecha-nism—our body's preparation for action in the face of imminent danger. But Selye also understood that excessive stress, or a habit-ual pattern of responding to nonthreatening circumstances as if they were threatening, would overwork our sympathetic nervous systems, overtax our endocrine systems, and harm our cardiovascu-lar systems. Coronary-prone Type A personalities, who react to ev-eryday hassles as if they were threats to their integrity, have been found to have higher blood levels of stress hormones. These very hormones also have been shown to damage coronary arteries—the precursor of full-fledged heart disease.

The missing link in the work of biologically oriented scien-tists such as Selye and Cannon and psychologically oriented phy-sicians such as Freud and Alexander was the immune system. No one sufficiently understood the mechanisms of immunity to dem-onstrate how stress, fight or flight, or repressed emotions had any-thing to do with our cellular defense against disease.

If the physical seat of consciousness—the brain—could be shown to regulate immune reactions, the mind-body field would gain instant credibility. But how could the brain possibly control white cells floating around the bloodstream in search-and-destroy missions for foreign invaders? How could the brain influence the glands that harbored those white cells, when there was no appar-ent anatomical connection? How could the brain send messages to the countless different types of cells and cell products involved in the killing and cleanup process known as an immune response?

It would take decades before any serious scientist had the in-struments, the imagination, or the daring to ask and answer these questions, which were central to the mind-body mystery.

THE PNI BREAKTHROUGH

The first American to navigate the previously uncharted waters of the mind's complex relationship to the immune system was psychi-atrist George F. Solomon, M.D. At Stanford University in the 1960s, Solomon was treating patients with rheumatoid arthritis, an autoimmune disorder in which immune cells attack tissues in the joints, causing painful and sometimes crippling inflammation. Observing that his patients' symptoms flared up during difficult times in their lives, he reasoned that the immune system—which reacts inappropriately in rheumatoid arthritis—must be affected by the presence of stress.

Based on these observations, he theorized that our immune systems were highly sensitive to stress and emotions. While that may not seem like a breathtaking insight, at the time it was quite startling in its implications, and Solomon realized it. For the immune system to be responsive to stress and emotions, the brain *had* to be involved in immune regulation. If proven, brain-immune connections would topple medicine's long-standing credo that our immune network functioned independently of any other bodily system.

To test his theory that the brain regulated immunity, Solomon sought the help of a farsighted immunologist, Alfred Amkraut, for an elegant series of animal studies. First, Solomon and Amkraut stressed rats by placing them in crowded cages and administering electric shocks. Compared to the control group of animals that were not subjected to shocks, tumors implanted in these rats grew at a rapid rate. Clearly, this type of stress suppressed the rats' immune defenses responsible for clearing cancer from the body.

This study implied but did not prove that electric shocks influenced the immune system via the brain. But Solomon had come across an obscure Soviet study that suggested that the hypothalamus was the brain's "headquarters" of immune regulation. He and Amkraut devised an experiment in which they used electric probes to burn out the hypothalamus in a group of rats. What they found confirmed their hypothesis: The rats suffered a marked decline in their immune reactions.

As a psychiatrist and immunologist working together, Solomon and Amkraut demolished traditional barriers separating medical specialties of "mind" and "body." It is not surprising, then, that their unprecedented collaboration produced one of the first significant pieces of hard evidence that the brain was involved in immune regulation. However, Solomon's 1960s research was so far ahead of its time that few specialists could make sense of his endeavors. With no scientific precedent for his data, his findings were assumed to be mistaken. Solomon's funding sources dried up, and he took a prolonged leave of absence from a field that now appeared to be stuck in its infancy.

It would take a stroke of genius to find an airtight way of proving linkage between mind and immunity. That stroke of genius was supplied by an experimental psychologist, who wondered if classical concepts of conditioning—the basis for learning—could be applied to the immune system. The psychologist was Robert Ader, Ph.D., who in 1974 proceeded with his conditioning experiments at the University of Rochester. Just as Pavlov's dogs had been conditioned to salivate at the sound of a bell, Ader and his colleague, Nicholas Cohen, attempted to condition rats to suppress their immune systems at the taste of saccharin-sweetened water. Ader did so by repeatedly feeding rats the sweet water, while simultaneously administering an immune-suppressing drug. Long after the drug was withdrawn, the sweet water *alone* caused the rats' immune cell reactions to plummet. Like Pavlov's dogs, Ader's rats no longer required the stimulus—an immune-suppressing drug—to elicit the response.

In his next experiment, Ader went even further. He studied a group of rats with lupus erythematosus, an autoimmune disease in which immune cells attacked the rats' own cells, causing crippling symptoms. (Humans with lupus suffer from a variety of disabling symptoms, all resulting from overactivity in the immune system, which destroys the body's tissues.) Using methods similar to his earlier study, Ader conditioned the rats to tone down their immune reactions. The results represented an astonishing clinical success: The rats' symptoms of lupus were markedly relieved.

Ameliorating lupus in rats hinted at the long-range prospects for a medicine based on conscious mental or behavioral control over the immune system. One day, perhaps, human beings suffering with autoimmune disease could use their minds to dampen their own immune systems and reduce their symptoms. Or, perhaps, they could mentally *boost* their immune responses to fight infections or slow the growth of cancer. But the immediate revelation from Ader's work was the recognition—now irrefutable—that the brain and immune system "talked" to each other.

Recognizing the ramifications of his discovery, Ader christened a new field of research. George Solomon had once called the nascent field psychoimmunology. Ader used the tongue-twisting name psychoneuroimmunology, known more simply as PNI. By demonstrating material connections among the mind (*psycho*), the nervous system (*neuro*), and the immune system (*immunology*), this young field took over where psychosomatic medicine left off. George Solomon's visionary work of the 1960s had been vindicated, and he returned to the field.

Ader's work opened the floodgates for other scientists who began to investigate brain-immune connections. The late 1970s and '80s saw a veritable explosion of interest in PNI, with new studies helping to piece together the inordinately complex mind-body puzzle. High-tech advances in neurology and immunology enabled PNI researchers to decipher mind-body communication on the level of cells and molecules.

The nitty-gritty of early PNI endeavors was research depicting the brain as the orchestrator of our immune responses. One of the most innovative demonstrations came from Swiss researcher Hugo Besedovsky. He measured the electrical activity in the hypothalamus of rats' brains before and after injecting them with foreign substances called *antigens*. Within a short time, the rats generated a full-fledged immune response to the antigens, with cells increasing in number and activity to combat the invaders. When this occurred, Besedovsky also detected a 100 percent increase in electrical activity in the hypothalamus of these animals. The brain had apparently received messages from the immune system that the body was under attack. In turn, the hypothalamus began buzzing with activity as it orchestrated the immune system's symphonic dance of cells and substances, all for the purpose of upholding the organism's integrity.

Even more direct anatomical connections were uncovered between the brain and immune system. University of San Diego neuroscientist Karen Bulloch investigated the thymus gland, located in humans behind the breastbone. Our T-cells, which lead an entire branch of the immune system, are produced and "schooled" in the thymus, where they "learn" how to become mature cells that act in the interests of the body. Bulloch discovered that rats' thymuses were laced with fibers of the vagus nerve, which descends down directly from the brain. This same pattern of nerves in the thymus is present in other animals and humans as well.

The thymus is not only hard-wired to the brain, it depends on nerve fibers to function at all. Without these hookups, the thymus was weakened or even crippled in its ability to produce T-cells that protect the organism from infections and cancer. University of Rochester scientist David Felten expanded on Bulloch's work when he used fluorescent dyes to trace the pathways of these same nerves. He not only observed connections to the thymus, but also to the spleen, lymph nodes, and bone marrow—all the major organs that produce and house the various cells of the immune system. (I describe the many types of immune cells later.) Nerve networks even extended to areas near blood vessels, through which immune cells passed, suggesting that nerve impulses could directly influence the behavior of these cells.

But anatomical connections between the brain and immune system did not fully explain how immune cells swimming throughout our blood and lymphatic systems could be influenced by the central nervous system. Nerve networks could not possibly extend to every fluid corner of the bloodstream. There had to be another line of communication.

That mysterious line of communication was the focus of PNI's other major breakthrough, which occurred in the early 1980s. It was made by neuroscientist Candace Pert, Ph.D., then chief of the brain biochemistry branch of the National Institute of Mental Health. Pert discovered that certain brain chemicals—usually called *neuropeptides*—acted as messengers between the mind and the immune system. How was this possible? Along with Michael Ruff, Ph.D., Pert showed that a class of immune cells (the monocytes) were studded with molecules on their surface—called *receptors*—that were perfect fits for neuropeptides. Each receptor had a biochemical shape, like the interior grooves of a door lock, that was designed to receive a specific neuropeptide "key."

These receptors, or "locks," were the signs that our immune cells interacted with chemical "keys" made by the brain. Molecular biology has taught us that the presence of a receptor means that the substance it's designed to receive can adjust the growth patterns or activities of that particular cell. Put differently, the existence of a lock proves that a door can be opened. In the world of cells, an open door implies a message received, and a message received means that a new course of action will be taken.

Thus, Pert's discovery meant that brain chemicals present in the bloodstream could alter the behavior of immune cells. These receptors were proof that the brain helped to orchestrate the immune system. Other researchers demonstrated that neuropeptide receptors were present on not just one but *every* major type of immune cell. Apparently, the brain's reach extended to every nook and cranny of the body, sending messages to immune cells that patrol the bloodstream and lymph system for evidence of injury or invasion. That's why Candace Pert once referred to white blood cells as "bits of brain floating throughout the body."

Neuropeptide "keys" are chemical carriers of emotions: Their synthesis in the body changes when our thoughts, moods, and feelings change. Endorphins, those natural painkillers and mood modifiers produced in the brain, are but one of many classes of neuropeptides that hook onto immune cells. In light of Pert's findings, little doubt remained that our shifting emotions are accompanied by biochemicals that *also* modify our immune system.

The impact of moods and emotions on immunity was no longer conjecture, it was biochemical fact. Moreover, recent studies reveal that the messages exchanged by the brain and immune system travel a two-way street. The brain does not simply deliver edicts to the immune system; it must know what is happening in the field of the body in order to orchestrate defensive maneuvers. Thus, the immune system also "talks" to the brain by producing its own messengers—ones with chemical structures that are stunningly similar to the neuropeptides made by the brain.

Thus, the language of mind and body is a language of messenger molecules that can be decoded by both the nervous and the immune systems. This mind-immune dialogue is a nonstop, two-way conversation in which massive amounts of information are transmitted with great specificity and subtlety. Without such dialogue, our bodies could never coordinate the immensely complex immune responses that keep us healthy.

MINDING THE MIND'S ROLE IN HEALTH

With PNI's remarkable work on brain regulation of immunity, the field gained its foothold in the world of modern biological research. A parallel track of research was followed by scientists investigating the specific psychological states and traits that influence immune functions.

A series of animal studies, carried out by groups of investigators working independently, showed that rats who are helpless to reduce a stressor, such as shocks delivered to their tails, suffer damage to their immune systems. Other rats who got the same number of shocks, but were able to control their delivery by pushing a lever, did not suffer the same losses to immunity. The culprit in immunosuppression was not stress per se. It was helplessness.

Helplessness in animals is considered roughly comparable to hopelessness in human beings. People who feel chronically hopeless appear to be at risk for a variety of illnesses, including cancer. In the 1950s, Lawrence LeShan observed that cancer patients often suffered a loss shortly before their diagnosis. But LeShan was not as impressed by the fact that a loss occurred as he was by the strikingly similar reactions these patients had to their loss: They felt utterly hopeless. Whether they had lost a job, a dream, or a loved one, they believed there was no escape from despair. In his research on 152 cancer patients, LeShan detected this pattern in 72 percent of the participants, compared with 12 percent of a control group.

Such studies provided the first inkling that stress was harmful to the immune system *when the organism's capacity to cope was overwhelmed.* Sir William Osler's statement that it was "more important to know what kind of patient had a disease than what kind of disease the patient had" required amendation. It was more important to know *what kind of coping abilities a person had* than what kind of stress the person had.

All of us have experienced the pressure-cooker conditions of examination time in high school or college. To find out whether these conditions affected immunity, psychologist Janice Kiecolt-Glaser and immunologist Ronald Glaser of Ohio State University studied a group of first-year medical students undergoing exams. Kiecolt-Glaser and Glaser discovered that the students suffered a drop in the activity of their natural killer (NK) cells—a group of immune cells that ward off infections and cancer. But the students who experienced the most precipitous loss of NK-cell activity were *not only stressed but also lonely.* Loneliness had compounded the normal effects of stress and further weakened the students' immune defenses.

The Glasers' findings confirmed another trend in mind-body research: People with strong networks of social support are more able to handle stress. In a landmark paper published in 1988, University of Michigan epidemiologist James House, Ph.D., reviewed a series of studies of a total of more than 22,000 men and women. House determined that people without many friends and supportive relationships were two to four times more likely to die early than those with rich, substantial networks of support.

But a strong support network depends on more than the luck of having good friends and loving family members. Those of us who maintain close, supportive relationships are also adept at coping. We know to seek out friends and family when we are overwhelmed, fatigued, or depressed. We know how to nurture those relationships through communication and commitment. Those of us who handle hard times by seeking support can prevent stress from disabling our immune defenses.

Effective copers not only seek support, they generally express emotions, assert themselves, and develop action plans to handle complex problems. When people lack coping skills, or the strategies they rely on stop working, they become susceptible to depression. Scientists at Mount Sinai Hospital in New York showed that clinically depressed individuals had weakened immune functions. Dr. Steven Locke examined a group of Harvard undergraduates for levels of life stress, coping skills, and immunity. He discovered that "poor copers"—those who reported high levels of depression and anxiety in response to stress—had significantly weaker natural killer cells.

The more researchers explored the widely accepted notion that stress alone weakens immunity and causes disease, the more trouble they had with the concept. In both animals and humans, stress definitely altered the immune system. However, in some studies, immunity was weakened by stress, while in others, immunity was actually *enhanced* by stress. The type of stress experienced by the research subjects—whether chronic or acute, escapable or inescapable—had some bearing on the outcome. But no crystal-clear pattern emerged.

The earliest and most serious effort to challenge conventional wisdom about stress came from Suzanne Ouellette, Ph.D. (then Suzanne Kobasa), whose studies at the University of Chicago are detailed in chapter 4. Ouellette began by questioning the statistical strength of the stress-illness link being trumpeted by the media. Her careful review of the literature revealed this finding: If you were to predict illness on the basis of stressful life events, you would be right only 15 percent of the time. One reason why stress was a poor predictor of illness was the presence of many individuals who stayed well *despite* high levels of stress.

Ouellette was intrigued by these anomalous people, whose lives were filled with disruption at work or at home but who remained free of significant health problems. She theorized that these individuals had "resistance resources"—aspects of their lives and/or personalities that enabled them to defuse the dangers of stress. Her research on a large group of telephone company executives showed that people who stay healthy under stress possess the trait of hardiness, which consists of commitment, control, and challenge.

With Ouellette's research, human potential finally entered the stress-illness equation. The old view of stress presented us with a classic double bind: Seek new challenges and you risk being stressed to death; avoid challenges and you risk being bored to death. Her findings (and others') liberated us. We can draw upon the strengths in our own character to take on challenges and weather losses over which we have no control. Those of us who engage in the life of our times—with its inescapable pressures of career, finances, creativity, and redefined family relationships—don't have to see ourselves as victims of stress.

The message that stress was not the crux of the mind-body issue, but that how we cope with stress was, gradually took hold in the research community. *Behavioral medicine* became the academic term for the study of psychological and social factors in illness and the mind-body treatments that ameliorate disease. Leaders of behavioral medicine, known more simply as *mind-body medicine,* designed therapies that moved away from stress avoidance and emphasized the individual's own resources.

With this new vantage point, other traditional mind-body approaches were retailored. Relaxation techniques—including meditation, yoga, self-hypnosis, and deep breathing—were no longer applied as twenty-minute escape valves from everyday tensions. Instead, they became part of a grander scheme for *actively* and *effectively* handling the myriad problems of work, relationships, and family.

The recognition that coping was paramount began to shape mind-body medicine. But, as so often happens, the lag time between scientific advances and media coverage has been interminable. To this day, the understanding that our psychological resources are more important than the number and intensity of our stressful life events has yet to be "popularized." Our culture persists in selling simplistic "stress-busting" approaches, based on fear that our health is ruined by the roller-coaster ride of everyday existence. Leading-edge clinicians have gotten the message about coping, but many others, riding the wave of a new trend, have yet to deepen their mind-body practice.

During the 1980s, PNI researchers became even more sophisticated in their understanding of the mind-body problem. They depicted us humans as organisms who use our highly developed brains to maintain equilibrium in the face of pressure, instability, and loss. When, for whatever reason, we lose our equilibrium, we experience increasing levels of inner *distress*—the real culprit when our immune systems break down.

The vital distinction is that *distress is not stress.* Stress is the objective event or ongoing problem. Distress is the inner reaction when one is psychologically overwhelmed by stress.

What do we experience when we feel distress? Helplessness. Hopelessness. Depression. Anxiety. Panic. Isolation. Pent-up rage. Fatigue. Demoralization.

These are the states most powerfully linked to immune dysfunction. The research findings were clear: Helpless rats had helpless immune systems. Hopeless cancer patients had worse outcomes. Depressed spouses had more illness. Anxious individuals had more skin disorders. Panicky people had more heart disease. Isolated individuals had shorter lifespans. Bottled-up arthritis sufferers had more flare-ups. Fatigued breast cancer patients had fewer fighting cells. Demoralized workers had weaker defenses. The problem is not stress, but distress. *And distress is not an emotion to be avoided, it is a signal that our coping methods are not working.*

As PNI scientists began to target distress as the disabler of immunity, clinicians took these laboratory lessons seriously. Therapists who treated medical patients in the hopes of boosting their immune systems could no longer rely on simple stress reduction. They recognized the need to reduce their patients' feelings of hopelessness, despair, anxiety, isolation, and depression.

By their behavior, cells were teaching immunologists the same lesson that human beings were teaching psychologists. What we need, they were both saying, is not an escape but a way of coping that keeps us from breaking down. Defender cells cannot function when the larger organism is out of balance and the brain is sending them the wrong messages. And human beings cannot function when their lives are out of balance and their brains are sending them the wrong messages about how to solve their emotional, financial, or spiritual problems.

The lessons being learned about cells and the ones learned about human beings were also intertwined. Why? When our coping strategies falter, and we're flooded with feelings of distress, our immune systems are *also* flooded—with too much, too little, or the wrong kinds of messenger molecules. Once the immune system receives inappropriate messages, it malfunctions, setting the stage for disease. When our minds cannot effectively defend us from the ravages of stress, our immune systems cannot effectively defend us from the onslaught of microbial invaders.

With a deeper understanding of the links among stress, coping, and immunity, mind-body practitioners began to design treatments that helped people to cope more effectively with their travails—including illness itself.

With new knowledge and a sound footing, mind-body medicine faced its next set of questions. How can people combat depression, hopelessness, pent-up rage, anxiety, panic, and isolation? What coping strategies reduce these feelings? How can people handle stress in a balanced, healthy way? The focus returned to the persistent inquiry: *What aspect of the mind is healing?*

BACK TO BASICS: PERSONALITY AND HEALTH

"We know what mind-states are bad for our health," said David McClelland, Ph.D., a renowned researcher of human motivation and health. "Yet we pay little attention to psychological factors that *promote* health."

McClelland was right—our culture pays little attention to mind-states that promote health. But that is changing. We have had impressive data on mind-states that are bad for our health, but now we're learning what mind-states prevent distress and keep us healthy.

I have emphasized that the key to mind-body health is how we respond to stress. Do we respond with hopelessness or hope? Helplessness or a sense of control? Despair or fighting spirit? Depression or grief that is felt and resolved? Bottled-up rage or healthy anger? Anxiety or tranquility? Panic or rationality? Demoralization or commitment?

Note that the healthy counterparts to each of these unhealthy states are either normal, healthy emotions or proactive ways of coping. Mind-body researchers are honing in on these two aspects of the healing mind. The first aspect is emotional, and the second is behavioral.

Let's start with the healing emotions, which are not necessarily positive. Research has shown that our health is protected when we express the *full range* of emotions, including the so-called negative ones. When we find constructive ways to express anger, grief, and fear, we *prevent* lapses into hopelessness, depression, and passivity. Bottling up these feelings makes it more likely that we will get stuck in chronic states of distress. The reason? Unless we explore and express these primary human emotions, we cannot receive the information they carry. In the next chapter, on the ACE Factor, I explore the informational aspect of emotions, explaining why attending to negative feelings is good for our immune systems.

On the other side of the coin, positive emotions are clearly beneficial to health and well-being. Yet some of us are blocked in our expression of joy, pleasure, and hope. Lydia Temoshok, Ph.D., who studied psychological factors in cancer for over a decade, showed that disease-prone individuals often have difficulty expressing negative *and* positive emotions. In one study, patients with melanoma (an aggressive form of skin cancer) who expressed emotions had more cancer-killing immune cells and slower-growing tumors. Temoshok's research, and other scientists' data, showed that we promote our health by gaining access to the full palette of human emotions.

The behavioral aspect of the healing mind involves proactive coping. How we feel is not all that's important; what we do about our feelings is also. We must take actions that redress imbalances in our environment that cause us to experience negative emotions in the first place. For instance, if we suspect that someone is stalking us, we must attend to the "fear" message and then take action by calling the police.

Thus, the healing mind processes emotions and conceives real-world actions in an appropriate and effective manner. But there is an even deeper issue. What part of our being generates emotions? Can we simply manipulate our own psyche to produce desired emotions and actions? Does wishing or willing positive mental states make them materialize?

On the behavioral side, what part of our being generates plans of action to cope with stress? What causes us to act against our own interests, or not to act at all?

The answers to all these questions involve our personalities. Our tendency to respond to circumstances with certain emotions and our behavior patterns in the face of stress are expressions of our character. We are all born with traits that are shaped and transformed throughout our life cycle. Genetic inheritance is part of our personality blueprint. Experiences in infancy and childhood also lay down powerful personality imprints. Each of us possesses a prismatic configuration of these traits. Personality psychologists believe that this configuration helps to shape our emotional and behavioral tendencies over the course of a lifetime. Free will and choice enable us to undergo remarkable transformations. But we are dealt certain cards, by nature and by nurture, and we must work with them.

For instance, if passivity is an ingrained trait, then we will let our abusive boss ride roughshod over us. If assertiveness is ingrained, we will stand up for our rights. If resignation is an in-grained trait, then we will become hopeless after the breakup of a romantic relationship. If optimism is ingrained, we will grieve but get on with our lives.

The template for what we feel, and how we express those feelings, is anchored in our personalities. So is the template for how we behave when stressed.

Psychotherapy is one arena where we can explore our personality templates. Patients who make these explorations discover active traits that stand in their way, preventing them from expressing emotions and taking effective action in their own behalf. They recognize that they are stubborn, or repressed, or hostile, or timid, or rigid, or narrow in their thinking.

But psychotherapy patients also discover healthy traits—parts of themselves they have "lost," whether as infants, young children, or young adults. These traits, involving healthy ways of handling emotions and real-world problems, did not disappear. They simply became inactive after years of negative conditioning. Such healthy traits can often be coaxed out of their lair within the psyche.

We are all born with the capacity to feel the full spectrum of emotions. And most of us are born with the potential to develop active, intelligent, and socially adaptive ways of handling our problems. Genes may determine vast differences in *how* we express emotions or handle problems, but they cannot disable us from feeling or coping. Only early conditioning by parents and/or society can do that. Such conditioning lays down new imprints that cover the healthy impressions we were born with. These imprints are so powerful that they fool us (and others) into thinking that our dysfunctional traits are the sum and substance of our personalities.

I do not mean to suggest that our true selves are defined by purely healthy traits, and our "false" selves—the masks we wear that reflect our conditioning—are defined by purely unhealthy traits. At bottom, we all have a mixture of traits, some of which are "desirable" and "adaptive," some of which are not. The purpose of Immune Power Personality development is not to extinguish our dark sides, but to reopen channels to parts of ourselves we have split off from consciousness.

Many people remain unconvinced that we can develop healthy traits. Our personalities are fixed in stone, they contend. But psychotherapists have documented successful transformations for decades. As William James wrote sixty years ago,

The potentialities of development in human souls are unfathomable. So many who seemed irretrievably hardened have in point of fact been softened, converted, regenerated, in ways that amazed the subjects even more than they surprised the spectators. . . . We have no right to speak of human crocodiles and boa-constrictors as of fixedly incurable things. We know not the complexities of Personality, the smouldering emotional fires, the other facets of character, the resources of the subliminal region.

What aspect of the mind is healing? The researchers covered in this book looked to our personality templates, below the layers of conditioning and habitual behaviors, to discover the health-promoting traits we share. They are traits that enable us to experience and express emotions. They empower us to use our intelligence, energy, and hope in the service of problem-solving. They allow us to establish healthy relationships with others. They uplift our spirits and our spirituality. Ultimately, they are traits that encompass and express the best in us.

Moreover, they are traits that keep us healthy. As I document in the chapters ahead, each scientist showed statistical correlations between a particular trait and a stronger immune system and/or better health. The aspects of the mind that are healing are Immune Power traits.

The seven Immune Power Personality researchers have taken pains not to oversimplify the mind-body link. The model they embrace accepts that personality and emotions are only one set of contributors to disease and health. Moreover, it is difficult to specify precisely the degree to which Immune Power traits contribute to overall disease resistance. And wide variations in their contribution are due largely to individual differences. For some, genetic makeup is the overriding factor; personality has less to do with health outcomes. For others, Immune Power traits appear to be major role-players. The notion that personality is the *only* factor in health is not only unscientific, it can lead people to blame themselves for diseases, including cancer and AIDS.

I must add that research indicates that the various Immune Power traits are linked to somewhat different immune enhancements and resistance to different illnesses. Each Immune Power trait has its own track record, but, taken together, these traits cover an extraordinarily wide spectrum of health benefits, including resistance to: viral infections from influenza to HIV; autoimmune diseases from arthritis to lupus; many types of cancer; chronic fatigue; chronic pain associated with inflammations; asthma and allergies. Certain Immune Power traits also are linked to reduced risk of heart disease. Although the mechanisms of this benefit do not centrally involve the immune system, I have included discussions of heart disease* in certain chapters because the purpose of Immune Power Personality development is, ultimately, the health of every bodily system.

The Immune Power Personality is founded on a realistic, scientific basis for mind-body empowerment, not omnipotence. Our brains do not grant us total conscious mastery of our immune systems. And we are *not* 100 percent responsible for any disease, or even for recovery, because there are many factors in illness that we realistically cannot control. But we can change our behavior, thoughts, and feelings, and doing so can change our physiology— including our immune responses. We don't create our biological reality, but we can affect it. For people struggling with disease, this measure of control yields significant returns in their quality of life and health.

THE IMMUNE SYSTEM: A PRIMER

The immune system is a fluid network designed to protect us from agents of disease and to heal wounds delivered by injury or invasion. One immunologist called it a "roving bag of cells" that patrols our bodies on missions of resistance and restoration. In order to do its job properly, our immune system must be exquisitely sensitive in detecting the surface features of other cells and substances. It must distinguish the "fingerprints" of intruders from those of family members—our own cells and molecules. That is why scientist Ted Melnechuk once remarked that "The immune system is a sensory organ for molecular touch." But our defense network is called upon to be as aggressive as it must be sensitive. Its task is to identify and then eliminate foreign agents—whether they are bacteria, viruses, fungi, toxic chemicals, or cancer cells— with precision and dispatch.

Except for the nervous system, the immune system is the most

---

* Recent studies suggest that the immune system *is* involved in the generation of coronary artery disease, via inflammatory responses that cause or worsen atherosclerosis, but research has yet to be conducted on a mind-immune linkage with heart disease.

complex biological system we have. It consists of master glands, principally the thymus; various sites that harbor immune cells; and different classes of "soldier" cells, which carry out specialized functions—including cells that prompt, cells that alert, cells that facilitate, cells that activate, cells that surround, cells that kill, even cells that clean up. Many immune cells also synthesize and secrete special molecules that act as messengers, regulators, or helpers in the process of defending against invaders.

ANTIGENS: THE SIGNALERS

Antigens are the fingerprints of immunity. They are identifying molecules that reside on the surface of cells and are unique to the cells that bear them. All of our body cells have antigens that signal "self-self-self"—a message that they are part of us and therefore not to be attacked.

Microorganisms, viruses, or any agent that invades our bodies also have identifying antigens on their surfaces, which signal "foreign-foreign-foreign" to the immune system, readying it for immediate attack. That's why organ transplants are difficult; the antigens on newly introduced cells sound the "foreign" alarm. To prevent the rejection of transplanted tissues, a patient is given drugs that suppress the immune system.

If the immune system overreacts to an outside antigen, the result is an allergy. Hayfever, for example, is a hyperresponse to grass, pollen, or ragweed antigens. When our immune system reacts inappropriately to the antigens on our own cells, the result is an *autoimmune* disorder. Lupus erythematosus and rheumatoid arthritis are examples of autoimmune diseases, in which our own tissues are attacked from within by our immune defenses.

If our immune systems fail to react properly to an outside agent—say a virus or bacterium—the result is an infection. Finally, if our immune systems fail to identify and destroy our own cells after they become malignant, the result is cancer-cell development and, possibly, the growth of tumors. How can the immune system react to our own cancer cells if the antigens on our cells are supposed to signal "self" to ward off attack? The answer reveals the special mechanism by which our bodies may prevent cancer.

Once a cell turns malignant, certain antigens on its surface also change. These altered molecules—known as *cancer-specific antigens*—signal "foreign" to the immune system. Cancer antigens are the giveaway—the slight change in fingerprints that can enable our defenses to detect a dangerous "inside job." Fortunately, our immune cells are not only guards, police officers, and soldiers; they're detectives as well. They have to be, because the outlaw cancer cell often cloaks its identity as a traitor to the community of cells. (These antigens have been found in some cancer types but not all. Immunologists continue to search for them, because cancer-specific antigens can be used in vaccines or other immunological approaches to preventing and treating cancer.)

ANTIBODIES: THE KEYS

Antibodies are the body's complement to antigens. Think of each antigen as a unique lock, and the protein molecules called antibodies (or immunoglobulins) as custom-made keys for every variation of lock. Antibodies are marvels of immunity that can fit into the "keyhole" of any one of millions of different antigens. Each one has a unique molecular configuration, and we can produce antibodies that latch perfectly into every conceivable antigen.

Antibodies are carried throughout the body by white blood cells called *lymphocytes,* the prime movers of the immune system. Lymphocytes are divided into two main classes—T-lymphocytes and B-lymphocytes (T-cells and B-cells, for short). It is the B-cells that manufacture, display, and secrete antibodies.

Imagine the immune system as a tree with two monumental branches—the *cell-mediated* arm, led by T-cells, and the *humoral* arm, led by B-cells and the antibodies they produce. The T- and B-cell branches themselves have offshoots: subpopulations of cells, cell products, and messengers that enable each branch to carry out its broad goal—effective destruction of foreign substances. The cell-mediated and humoral branches also communicate with each other for the purposes of a coordinated attack.

B-cells circulate throughout the body with antibody molecules on their surfaces. When they pick up the signal of a particular antigen, they multiply and transform into plasma cells, which are essentially minifactories with one purpose: to churn out the precise antibodies that hook onto the antigens of the interloper. Antibodies not only neutralize foreign substances or microbes, they signal other immune sentries into battle. An antigen-antibody bond is a call to arms, and a cascade of immune reactions follow the initial "connection." This cascade—the sum total of activity by both branches of the immune system—is called an *immune response.*

Certain B-cells also remember their encounters with foreign agents. As a result, antibodies are produced swiftly when the same invader attacks again. Immunologic memory is the basis for vaccines, which introduce small amounts of antigen to prime our bodies for subsequent attacks.

T-CELLS: THE PRIME PLAYERS

T-cells are the stars of cell-mediated immunity, the branch consisting of subgroups of interacting cells. T-cells are so named because they "grow up" in the thymus, the walnut-size gland located under the breastbone. Although all immune cells are "born" in the bone marrow, different types follow different developmental pathways. T-cells migrate to the thymus. There, with the aid of various thymic hormones, immature T-cells grow, learn to recognize and attack antigens, and develop a range of specialized activities. The thymus is the master gland of cell-mediated immunity, a veritable training school for different classes of T-cells. Mature T-cells are harbored in the spleen and lymph nodes, waiting there for the sound of an alarm signaling an intruder. As with B-cells, the T-cell line also generates memory cells that prime the body for repeat attacks by a familiar invader.

There are three main subcategories of T-cells: T-helper cells, killer T-cells, and suppressor T-cells.

T-helper cells. These cells orchestrate the actions of other immune cells. They are essential to the performance of their fellow

B-cells of the humoral branch; certain antibody reactions depend on help from the helper Ts. T-helpers, which are also referred to as *CD4 cells* (so named for one of their cell-surface receptors), are the primary targets of HIV, the virus that causes AIDS. HIV's destruction of T-helpers, which are crucial conductors of immunity, is the reason why people with AIDS eventually lose their capacity to fight off infections and cancer cells.

Killer T-cells. These cells, also known as *cytotoxic T-cells*, are able to liquidate invading microbes, viruses, or cancer cells. Once alerted by other immune cells and activated by messenger molecules, the killer Ts go into action. They have nimble receptors on their surface that reconfigure their structure to fit snugly into their adversaries' antigens. Once attached, the T-cell injects a load of toxic chemicals into the invader, puncturing its surface membrane and causing its insides to gush out into the fluid environment.

Suppressor T-cells. These cells are vital to maintaining properly balanced immune responses. Sometimes called *CD8 cells*, they are able to suppress or dampen the actions of other immune cells. Without the activity of suppressor Ts, immunity could easily get out of hand, resulting in allergic or autoimmune reactions. But CD8 cells are multifaceted—they also can destroy virus-infected cells. That's why their strength and numbers are considered crucial to individuals infected by HIV.

BIG EATERS AND NONSPECIFIC FIGHTERS

A third class of immune cells are the multitalented scavenger cells. Also called *phagocytes*, they engulf microbes or other unwanted products in the bloodstream. The most ubiquitous scavengers, comprising two-thirds of all white cells, are the granulocytes, so named because they have large granules in their structures, visible under a microscope. Granulocytes represent a first line of defense against bacteria, viruses, and cancer cells.

Another critical type of phagocyte is the macrophage, which literally means "big eater," based on its ability to gobble up foreign substances. Macrophages, which begin their cellular lives as monocytes, are the garbagemen of the immune system. They clean up waste products in the aftermath of an immune cell attack. But macrophages are also critically involved in the earliest phases of our immune responses. They kick off the immunologic cascade by processing and presenting antigens to lymphocytes, which then initiate full-fledged cellular and humoral reactions. Macrophages also release messenger molecules, such as interleukin-1, that stimulate and inform lymphocytes during the course of an attack. Another product of macrophages, tumor necrosis factor (TNF), is like the body's own chemotherapy—it has the noteworthy ability to liquidate cancer cells.

Immune responses require breathtakingly complex interactions throughout the entire immune network. T-helper cells need antigens presented to them by macrophages, and they depend on numerous signals from other cells and messenger molecules. B-cells depend on T-helpers to do their job, so both branches—cell-mediated and humoral—ultimately depend on macrophages.

Unlike T- and B-cells, macrophages are "nonspecific": They don't latch onto invaders in a perfectly targeted lock-and-key fashion. But they do swallow up and present invaders to specific T-cells and clean up the messy aftermath. Another group of nonspecific immune cells, from neither B- or T-cell lineages, forms the natural killer cells, or NK cells.

NK cells have the capacity to recognize viruses and cancer cells without having encountered them before, without having antigens served up to them by other cells, and without a specific lock-in-key receptor. Through mechanisms not fully understood, NK cells execute "quick strikes" against virus-infected and cancer cells, killing them with stunning efficiency. In animal studies, NK cells have been shown responsible for stopping the spread of cancer cells throughout the body. Immunologists suspect that NKs serve the same life-saving function in humans as well.

A vital mind-body connection has been uncovered with NK cells. A multitude of methodologically sound studies have demonstrated relationships between how we cope with stress and the vitality of our NK cells. These cells represent a bridge between psychological factors and our resistance to viral and malignant diseases.

CELL PRODUCTS AND MESSENGER MOLECULES

Our immune cells manufacture a vast number of biological products. These are molecules whose functions vary as widely as the scientific names given them: biological response modifiers, cytokines, cell products, growth factors, messenger molecules, and just plain biologicals. Regardless of their titles, these substances carry information and instructions from one group of immune cells to another, changing behavior and coordinating immune responses. These molecules are couriers, communicators, helpers, growth inducers, and suppressors.

Among the most well-known immune-cell products are the *interferons,* which have antiviral and anticancer properties, and the *interleukins,* many of which fight cancers as well. There are many subtypes of interferon and interleukin, each of which performs distinct functions—but all are critical links in the immunologic chain reaction. Scores of other products, each with its own name and properties, regulate the activities of our immune cells.

As mentioned, one of PNI's most surprising discoveries is that brain chemicals—the neuropeptides and neurotransmitters—also carry messages to immune cells. (Receptors for these brain chemicals have been found on lymphocytes, macrophages, and natural killer cells.) Moreover, recent research has shown that the immune system itself produces neuropeptidelike molecules, and brain cells appear to make immune chemicals, such as interleukin-1. We are just beginning to understand the true reciprocity of the brain-immune dialogue. Brain and body make and receive the same kinds of chemicals in order to communicate effectively. They "speak" the same language—the language of messenger molecules.

DEVELOPING IMMUNE POWER TRAITS

George Solomon has noted intriguing analogies between our immune systems and our psychological systems. For example:

- Our brains and immune systems both have the capacity for memory.
- Our minds and immune systems are both designed for adaptation. Psychologically, we adapt to environmental stressors. Immunologically, we adapt to environmental invasions.
- Our minds and immune systems both serve functions of defense. Psychologically, we defend against intolerable pain and overloads of information. Immunologically, we defend against attacking organisms and agents.
- In both systems, inadequate defenses result in vulnerability.
- In each system, inappropriate defenses lead to disease—to allergies in the immune system and neurosis in the psychological system. For instance, ragweed pollen is not truly dangerous to the allergy sufferer. Nor are garter snakes to the person with a phobia.
- In both systems, prior exposure to a noxious agent can lead to either tolerance or extreme sensitivity. When we repeatedly encounter low doses of an antigen, we develop either resistance or allergy. When we experience early emotional traumas, such as the loss of a parent, we respond to later losses either with the strength that comes from hard experience or by succumbing to episodes of depression.

These analogies add depth to the notion that mind and body are inextricably intertwined. The researchers in this book did not rely on analogy, having shown statistical associations between specific traits and stronger immunity. But similarly intriguing, nonmeasurable analogies exist between the seven Immune Power traits and immune system functions. The healing personality and the healthy immune system both demonstrate qualities of keen attention, expressive communication, hardiness (being committed, in control, and seeking challenge), assertiveness, trust (immune cells must recognize and "trust" the vast majority of "self" cells they encounter, or else they will lash out with self-destructive consequences), helping (an entire population of immune cells are devoted to helping), and self-complexity (the immune system is incredibly multifaceted).

These analogies don't necessarily explain *why* Immune Power traits are linked to immune functions. But the congruence between our psychological and immunological systems suggests that both are devoted to the same overriding goals for our organisms: balance and harmony, communication and connectedness, and maintaining our bodymind integrity.

One recurrent theme of the Immune Power Personality is that the power of mind-body techniques may lie in their ability to elicit Immune Power traits. Hypnosis and meditation fine-tune our attention and connection to bodymind states. Relaxation, biofeedback, and guided imagery enhance our sense of control. Cognitive therapies increase hardiness by changing a relentlessly negative perspective into a more positive one. Group and individual therapy nourish our capacity to confide and to assert ourselves. Psychotherapy and even meditation can help us recognize our desire for healthy relationships; cognitive-behavioral treatments teach us skills to pursue them responsibly. Support groups foster helping behaviors, and combinations of mind-body therapy bring out our multifaceted potential.

Arguably the most astonishing findings in the past decade of mind-body medicine have been the effect of multifaceted group therapies on people with life-threatening illnesses. In brief:

- Stanford University psychiatrist David Spiegel, M.D., studied metastatic breast cancer patients who participated in a group therapy program that emphasized social support, emotional expression, assertiveness, and self-hypnosis for relaxation. Women who participated in these groups lived twice as long as members of a control group who did not participate.
- University of Miami psychologist Michael Antoni, Ph.D., has shown that group therapy for stressed HIV patients—including relaxation, emotional expression, cognitive restructuring, and social support—helped prevent decline of their CD4 cells. Patients who stayed with the program after its completion were less likely to develop AIDS two years later.
- UCLA psychiatrist Fawzy I. Fawzy, M.D., provided group therapy to melanoma (skin cancer) patients and followed their progress

for six years. The treatment included relaxation, cognitive therapy to develop active coping, and psychological support. Compared with nonparticipants with the same disease, the group members had *one-third* the rate of recurrence and death.

- Univeristy of California cardiologist Dean Ornish, M.D., led a landmark study in which heart disease patients participated in a group lifestyle change program, including dietary modification, exercise, relaxation, yoga, visualization, and group therapy that emphasized the sharing of emotions, "opening your heart," and spirituality. Participants experienced marked reversal of heart disease, proven with scans that showed the opening of previously blocked arteries.

Based on my own readings and discussions with these investigators, it became clear that all these programs stimulated development of Immune Power traits. Indeed, these groups may have facilitated healing by evoking patients' resiliency characteristics. Being in a group with others undergoing the same fear and anguish creates an atmosphere in which people's strengths—their self-care, compassion, and fighting spirit—can flourish. The goal of the Immune Power Personality program is to tap these same powers, in formal group contexts or not, for the promotion of optimal health and healing.

All of us can cultivate Immune Power traits. We each have a unique way of communicating love, confiding in others, becoming hardy, asserting ourselves, attending to our needs, finding our purpose, and expressing our many-sidedness. The differences among us are based on variations in culture, upbringing, and genetic makeup. We must therefore find our own path to each of these health-promoting traits. They are not blueprints for who we should become, they are conduits to realization of our authentic selves. According to seven visionary scientists, realizing our authentic selves is among the most powerful health prescriptions we can adopt.

THE ACE FACTOR: ATTEND, CONNECT, EXPRESS

IN THE GREATEST CONFUSION THERE IS STILL AN OPEN CHAN-
NEL TO THE SOUL. IT MAY BE DIFFICULT TO FIND.... BUT THE
CHANNEL IS ALWAYS THERE, AND IT IS OUR BUSINESS TO KEEP
IT OPEN, TO HAVE ACCESS TO THE DEEPEST PART OF OUR-
SELVES—TO THAT PART OF US WHICH IS CONSCIOUS OF A HIGHER
CONSCIOUSNESS.

—SAUL BELLOW

The year 1973 was not an easy one for Gary Schwartz, Ph.D.,
a young psychology instructor at Harvard University. He was teaching his first course, an introduction to mind-body relationships
that was among the first such offerings at a major university. Excitement and registration ran high. But the mind-body field was in its
infancy—no textbooks existed. Schwartz would have to create his
own curriculum and live up to the soaring expectations of his students. For two hours every Wednesday morning, he was a nervous
wreck.

He'd prepare his lectures on Tuesday. By Wednesday morning, he had a burning stomachache.

"I was really sick," Schwartz recalled. "It was obviously linked to the stress of teaching the course. And the stomachache augmented my anxiety. I began to get really furious at my stomach. I was at the point where I wished I could rip it out and replace it with another one."

Having no such option, Schwartz relied upon a string of over-the-counter medicines. But Pepto-Bismol, Alka-Seltzer, Maalox, and Rolaids provided only temporary relief.

A vicious cycle had begun. The more antacids Schwartz took, the more ineffective they became. The more ineffective they became, the more tense and frustrated he grew—which only worsened his stomachaches. Yet this brilliant young professor, teaching a class on the mind-body connection, still didn't get the message his body was sending him.

The absurdity of his predicament finally hit home when Schwartz saw it mirrored on TV. He began noticing a series of commercials for Alka-Seltzer, one of which depicted a huge man in a pie-eating contest. Fruit filling smeared on his face, the man found himself with a horrendous stomachache. But the sure-fire cure was readily at hand: "Plop, plop, fizz, fizz, oh what a relief it is!"

Schwartz characterized the commercial:

The message was: "Eat all you want. If you get a stomachache, don't change your behavior and listen to your body. Instead, take Alka-Seltzer." The commercial captured our culture's approach to symptoms: Neglect them for as long as possible, then suppress them with drugs. What happens when Alka-Seltzer stops working? We get a prescription for something stronger. What if that doesn't work, and we get an ulcer? We go to a surgeon. What's really happening is that the stomach is telling the brain that it can't work under those circumstances. And we're being taught to say, "Darn you stomach, don't you interfere with my behavior."

He realized that he was behaving like the man in the pie-eating contest. The pie-eater ignored his stomach's signal that he'd had enough. Schwartz ignored his stomach's signal that he needed a better way to handle his stress. In both instances, the tablets, liquids, and bromides only stifled the signal. When he finally paid attention to his stomach, Schwartz took more time to relax before classes. He prepared materials earlier. Most important, he stopped hating his stomach and began heeding its messages. Schwartz's self-directed anger, and the medicines he used as silencers, had fueled the vicious cycle of pain. When he transformed his approach, the cycle was broken.

Gary Schwartz's reaction to his stomachaches reflected his evolving concept of mind-body interactions. He believed that the human organism functions well when "information" is effectively transmitted and received between biological and psychological systems. And his bellyaches were just that—a form of body-mind information. The discomfort was "feedback" to his conscious brain, carrying the message that Schwartz needed to handle his stress more effectively. Cutting off this feedback with over-the-counter remedies was merely a stop-gap measure.

When we repeatedly reach for symptomatic relief—whether it's aspirin for headaches, bromides for bellyaches, or any other palliative drug—we buy ourselves time. Eventually, however, the pills and potions can lose their efficacy, because we continue to neglect the underlying causes. Schwartz began to view all symptoms and sensations—including pain—as forms of feedback that we must attend. As his theory and research broadened, Schwartz recognized that emotions were also forms of feedback. Grief, anger, and fear carry information that is vital to our well-being. When we *attend* to these feelings, *connect* them to consciousness, and *express* them appropriately, we restore balance to our body-mind systems.

What did this "systems" approach tell Schwartz about personality and health? Some of us *characteristically* attend to feedback signals, whether they are symptoms, sensations, or emotions. We connect them to consciousness and discover their meaning. Let's say our headaches reflect tension at work. Or heart palpitations indicate that we're exhausted from taking on too many responsibilities. Or chronic anger over minor problems is a sign of major conflicts in our marriage. Once the "message" is received, we can take expressive action to reestablish harmony in our inner and outer environments. When we block out the message, disharmony reigns. According to Schwartz, such disharmony affects mind and body—including our cardiovascular and immune systems.

Those of us who characteristically *dis*attend (ignore) symptoms, *dis*connect (cut off) sensations and feelings, and repress (bottle up) emotions will suffer ongoing imbalances in our bodymind systems. The result is a chronic state of *dis*order that eventually leads to *dis*ease—which literally means "lack of ease."

Gary Schwartz has discovered that our capacity to Attend, Connect, and Express—or the *ACE Factor*—is a trait that upholds our health and well-being. Currently a professor of psychology at the University of Arizona, Schwartz has spent two decades researching the importance of the ACE Factor in human health. Through a series of experiments, he demonstrated that the ACE Factor is associated with a strong heart and a strong immune system.

Schwartz's research on the healing power of ACE reached fruition in the late 1970s and the 1980s when he was a professor of psychology at Yale University. He began by studying the opposite of ACE, known as *repressive coping*. Repression is a psychological defense mechanism in which people push away painful thoughts, feelings, fantasies, or memories, and store them in their unconscious mind. For all intents and purposes, they no longer know that these mind-states even exist. Repressive copers use this defense as a way of handling stress. They generally do *not* attend to sensations and symptoms; do *not* connect feelings to consciousness; and do *not* express emotions or take actions to rectify bodymind imbalances. As a result, they are prone to physiologic *dis*order and *dis*ease. As Schwartz studied the health-damaging effects of repression, he also discovered its counterpart: our natural capacity to attend, connect, and express.

From the start, Schwartz's goal was to define ACE and measure its effects on immunity and health. His odyssey began with observations of patients in his own laboratory and climaxed with experiments that revealed mechanisms of the healing brain.

"SUPERNORMALS" AND THE ILLUSION OF HEALTH

Charles Darwin observed that human beings express emotions on the face in patterns that are predictable, no matter their nationality. For instance, people from widely varying cultures—from British high society to Australian aborigine—display anger with retracted lips and clenched teeth. Since then, researchers have confirmed that a wide range of emotions—including disgust, embarrassment, pleasure, and sadness—involve specific configurations of facial muscles. The same configurations for particular emotions have been noted in people with backgrounds as divergent as those found in the American West and the African coast.

By the 1970s, sophisticated equipment enabled scientists to confirm Darwin's observations. Using the electromyelograph (EMG), which can measure the activity of facial muscles, investigators have identified configurations of facial muscles that are activated when we experience specific emotions, from happiness to hostility. For instance, we tense the corrugator muscles, located above the eyebrows, when we feel sad or depressed. The corrugators are now simply known as the "grief muscles."

In 1973, the discovery of grief muscles piqued the interest of a pharmacologist at the Food and Drug Administration (FDA). He'd been searching for an objective way to test whether clinically depressed patients benefited from antidepressant medication. He hypothesized that a drug that genuinely alleviated a person's suffering would also cause his or her grief muscles to relax. The pharmacologist decided to use EMG technology to measure the grief muscles of patients taking antidepressants. The FDA supported his proposal, and the pharmacologist brought in Gary Schwartz, an emerging expert on the physiology of mind-body interactions.

Schwartz evaluated fifty psychiatric patients and thirty controls from the Massachusetts hospital system. Before investigating the effects of antidepressants, Schwartz had to confirm that depressed patients had more active grief muscles to begin with. He administered psychological tests among both the patients and controls, and he studied the facial muscles of both groups using EMG technology.

Schwartz was perplexed by his findings. The depressed patients did have more active grief muscles. But the overall statistical relationship between depression and grief muscle activity was weak. He also found weak correlations between anxiety and the activity of the "fear" muscles.

"Needless to say," Schwartz comments now, "the findings made me quite anxious and depressed."

Schwartz carefully combed his data. When he did, an intriguing subgroup of individuals emerged. These were people who claimed to be free of depression. But their grief muscles were as active as psychiatric patients mired in clinical depression! Another group reported little anxiety, but their "fear" muscles were as active as those who were highly anxious.

Because these individuals *reported* no anxiety or depression, Schwartz dubbed them the "supernormals."

"The supernormals were people who claimed that their lives were perfect," said Schwartz. "Superficially, you'd think they were the healthiest population."

But there was a marked discrepancy between their reports of anxiety or depression and the EMG data that revealed their facial muscles. The "supernormals" had completely skewed the study's statistical findings. Schwartz wondered: "Why this gap between the story told by their words and the story told by their facial muscles?"

To Schwartz, there was but one logical answer: There had to be a "disconnect" in their bodymind systems. While the "supernormals" said they weren't sad, depressed, or anxious, the deeper truths were registered on their countenances. Schwartz did not believe that the "supernormals" were liars. Rather, they had come to believe their own illusory story, developed over years of denial. The "supernormals" had learned to say "I'm fine" no matter what pains or problems had plagued them. Eventually, they'd come to *believe* they were fine, even when sadness or fear was etched in their faces.

Soon thereafter, Schwartz was approached by a group of students who practiced Transcendental Meditation (TM). As much a movement as a practice, TM was led by the Maharishi Mahesh Yogi, who many remember as the short-lived personal guru to the Beatles. During the early 1970s, TM was the most visible attempt to popularize ancient Eastern practices of meditation. The students tried to convince Schwartz that TM brought them inner peace, and he should be studying them.

Schwartz did not doubt the sincerity of the TM followers. But certain aspects of their behavior made him doubt the veracity of their view of themselves. They all wore the same suits and mouthed the same platitudes. Despite their claims of inner peace, they appeared to be quite nervous.

"There was a discrepancy between what they were saying and the emotions they were subtly expressing," said Schwartz. "The discrepancy frankly disturbed me. I wanted to understand it. I was beginning to see that under certain circumstances, people can use relaxation, meditation, and biofeedback as a way to disconnect rather than connect them to aspects of their lives."

Schwartz saw more evidence of this problem in his own lab. He'd been conducting research on biofeedback, a form of therapy in which people are hooked up to electronic instruments that convey information about bodily functions. This information—whether it is heart rate, blood pressure, brain wave activity (electroencephalograms), muscle tension (electromyograms), or skin resistance—is translated into beep tones, video images, or readings on a dial. Once patients become aware of their own physiological processes, they learn to alter them through psychological shifts. Biofeedback trainers often teach patients the mental means—such as hypnosis, visualization, deep breathing, or simple concentration—to change their physiology. (Patients know their technique is working when beeps slow down, video images change, or dials move in the proper direction.) This "biological feedback" guides people as they seek to calm both mind and body.

In his biofeedback research, Schwartz came across medical patients who began by saying they felt calm. But their vital signs reflected high levels of anger, anxiety, and tension. Like the "supernormals" and the TM followers, the story told by their words diverged sharply from the story told by their bodies. And many of these patients had a strange reaction to biofeedback: It made them feel worse instead of better.

"These people came to the clinic looking for a nonpharmacologic pill for their symptoms," he remarked. "They just wanted their illness cured by biofeedback, without having to make any other changes in their lives. They didn't want to make emotional connections."

When these patients underwent biofeedback, they often became upset. The feedback from their bodies carried distressing news that contradicted their claims of inner peace. When the same individuals were taught relaxation techniques, they became more tense than tranquil. Schwartz had discovered a phenomenon later confirmed by other scientists: Disconnected people feel temporarily worse when they calm down enough to get in touch with their bodies. Distress signals they'd ignored or repressed suddenly rise to the surface of consciousness. A few of Schwartz's patients fled therapy, afraid of the very feedback that could guide them toward balance and well-being.

Schwartz was gathering evidence for his theory: People who disconnect from bodymind feedback experience disharmony; while people who attend to feedback maintain harmony and physical health.

Viewing the bodymind as a "system," Schwartz evolved a lucid model of the dynamics of health and illness. He likens the bodymind system to the common household thermostat. When the house temperature falls below the set point, the thermostat signals the furnace to turn on. The heat rises through the pipes, and the temperature gradually rises to the set point. After it exceeds the set point, the thermostat signals the furnace to shut off. The temperature gradually lowers, and over time a rhythmic ebb and flow occurs.

What if the wires between the thermostat and furnace are disconnected? The system loses its capacity to self-regulate.

This same principle holds for human systems. Metaphorically speaking, if the "wires" are cut between body and mind, we don't get the feedback we need to establish order, ease, and self-regulation in our own systems. Eventually, the result is bodymind disorder and disease. Our states of anxiety, rage, or depression become chronic when we disregard them. However, when we heed our own distress signals, we reconnect with our bodies. We take control of our current life circumstances. And we take action to re-establish balance and health.

VICTOR'S HEADACHES AND THE BODYMIND THERMOSTAT

Victor, a thirty-five-year-old corporate lawyer, had reached a pinnacle of financial and professional success when migraine headaches threatened his ability to function. His frequent attacks started with strange sensations and ended with blindingly intense pain. He'd been to doctors, neurologists, and headache specialists, but none of their medicines offered him substantial relief. With few options left, Victor turned to the Yale Behavioral Medicine Clinic and its director, Gary Schwartz.

"Victor appeared to be a very uptight, angry young man when I first saw him," recalled Schwartz. "But he said his life was going fine, with no major problems. His work was great, he was happily married. I wondered why he seemed so tense."

Like many migraine patients, Victor's hands were cold. Mind-body therapists have shown that when migraine sufferers use relaxation and biofeedback to warm their hands, their headaches often disappear. Apparently, if you can dilate constricted blood vessels in your hands, the same thing occurs in your head. Then you can ameliorate one source of migraine headaches—vasoconstriction.

Schwartz used this approach, but in a unique way. He resisted applying biofeedback and relaxation just to rid people of their symptoms. From Schwartz's perspective, using mind-body techniques as if they were pills to vanquish symptoms could be counter-productive. The whole point of mind-body medicine, he believed, was to *tend* to symptoms in order to learn their deeper causes and cures.

Rather than handing Victor a set of relaxation tapes or hooking him up to biofeedback equipment, Schwartz asked him to first "collect some data" on his daily experiences. What was he doing or feeling when his hands were cold? What was he doing or feeling when his headaches began? One purpose of the exercise was for Schwartz to learn what was going on in Victor's life. But the larger purpose was for *Victor* to learn what was going on in Victor's life—particularly when his headaches exerted their vicelike grip.

Victor followed Schwartz's instructions and returned for his weekly sessions with information about his daily life and symptoms. However, within a few weeks, he wanted to stop therapy. The procedure had become "too distressing." Schwartz suspected that the exercise was forcing Victor to pay attention to the realities of his life and the disturbing emotions he'd kept at bay. His belief that "everything was okay" was wobbling under the scrutiny required by Schwartz's procedure. An unnameable anxiety began to rise in Victor, an anxiety he wanted to go away.

Schwartz decided to take another therapeutic tack. He asked Victor what in his life brought him *joy*.

"My baby Frances," he said.

"What else?" queried Schwartz.

"My work. I love my work. I really enjoy being a lawyer."

Schwartz didn't doubt that Victor believed what he was saying. But he detected another level of experience of which Victor seemed unaware.

"Were you aware of what your face was doing while you answered my questions?" asked Schwartz.

Victor shook his head. "What do you mean?"

"Of course you were not aware. Most of us typically are not conscious of our facial expressions and what they reveal. What was your first response to my question of what brings you joy?"

"My baby Frances. I really love her." Victor paused, then remarked, "I'm smiling, aren't I?"

"Yes, you're actually beaming."

Victor began to elaborate, telling sweet stories about Frances. He showed his pleasure with her every new movement, sound, expression. He described his giddy anticipation when coming home from work, knowing he would be spending the better part of his evening playing with his baby daughter.

Schwartz didn't need scientific instruments to detect the vibrant quality of his joy. "Okay, what was the next thing you told me?"

"How I enjoy my work, how I love being a lawyer."

"Are you smiling now?"

"I guess I'm not."

"You weren't smiling the first time I asked either. But you weren't aware of it then. You are now."

"Yes, I am."

"Let's explore this. Why do you think you aren't smiling, even though you say you love your work?"

As Victor began to open up about his law practice, it soon became apparent that success had come at a steep price. His firm was a veritable viper's pit of competitive maneuvering, and Victor strove especially hard to maintain his position. Higher-ups in the firm, fearful of Victor's further ascension, gave him no secretarial support. The stress on him was psychological and physical, as he was riddled with anxiety about his position and drained by ridiculously long hours. In the midst of all this, Victor maintained a rigid positive focus on his achievements and current standing. He was so caught up in the struggle at work that he was blind to the effect of these pressures on his bodymind. Victor was a classic *repressive coper,* who blocked out thoughts and emotions that rocked his psychological status quo.

As Victor spoke, both he and Schwartz had the impression that a Pandora's box had been opened. He and his wife had problems Victor never previously revealed. They'd recently purchased an ostentatious house way beyond their financial means. The pressure to maintain his standing at the firm and continue his rise was intensified by the financial stress of high monthly mortgage payments. Ongoing conflicts with his in-laws exacerbated the tensions between him and his wife. And the headaches themselves had become one more source of stress.

The emotional upset that almost drove Victor from therapy

had fully surfaced. Now, instead of being frightened by his feelings, he was relieved to be facing and expressing them.

Over fifteen weeks of therapy Victor unraveled a Gordian knot of problems. After raising Victor's awareness of his objective difficulties and emotional responses, Schwartz proceeded to use biofeedback as a tool. Electronic instruments "fed back" information to Victor—via graphs and digital beeps—about the temperature of his hands and the muscular tension in his face and head. The instruments guided Victor as he attempted to raise his hand temperature and relax his head and neck.

But Schwartz also used biofeedback to continue teaching Victor about the gap between his conscious thoughts and deeper feelings. Thus, "external" feedback in the form of electronic instruments were used to reconnect him with his own "internal" feedback. He would discuss his problems with Schwartz, and the instruments would inform Victor whether his body was in sync with his beliefs. Victor learned that disconnecting only worsened his problems and his health. The buried issues and feelings continually resurfaced in the form of splitting headaches. (The term "splitting" seems apt, since disconnection is the root problem.) By finally confronting these issues and feelings—*attending* and *connecting*—Victor became temporarily more upset. But his ability to "tolerate" his upset, in increasingly larger "doses," enabled him to undergo a healing transformation.

Victor's development of ACE was gradual. But his work with Schwartz quickly reduced the frequency and severity of his headaches. Expressing rather than stifling his feelings lessened his physical tension. Over time, Victor learned that confronting his problems set the stage for effective solutions. To prevent the backstabbing of his colleagues, he became more assertive at work. He insisted on the secretarial help he so badly needed. He worked to improve communication with his wife, so they could deal with their financial problems—and her parents—with calm and creativity. They refinanced their mortgage and revitalized their marriage. These expressive actions represented the "E" in Victor's healing sequence.

By educating Victor to attend, connect, and express, Schwartz enabled him to overcome his migraines. But Schwartz's therapy was not like a "pill," because symptomatic relief was not the only goal. Alleviating his distress—the underlying cause of his migraines—was the overriding goal. Victor's distress would never have been relieved through more denial and disconnection. Only acceptance and action would prove to be healing.

THE RIDDLE OF REPRESSION

Patients like Victor presented Gary Schwartz with clinical evidence that repressive coping can cause bodymind imbalance and *dis*ease. And his early therapeutic work demonstrated that people like Victor *can change.* They can develop the ACE Factor, generate harmony in their bodymind systems, and heal many of their medical disorders. But neither Schwartz nor any other scientist had been able to fully explain the health-promoting power of ACE. To do that, Schwartz would have to develop an objective measurement of the ACE Factor and its opposite, repression. He'd also have to demonstrate that ACE influences our biology, including our immune systems. In the mid-1970s, Schwartz began to pursue these ambitious scientific goals.

During that period, Schwartz was approached by a bright, far-sighted psychology student, Daniel Weinberger. "Dan was convinced that Freud was right, that there really was this phenomenon called repression," recalls Schwartz. "He wanted to prove that repression existed, by showing that 'repressed' people have a particular set of physiological responses. He heard about me through the grapevine and thought that I might be able to help him."

"The essence of repression," Freud wrote in 1915, "lies simply in turning something away, and keeping it a distance from the conscious." Freud saw repression as a psychological defense that people used to banish painful emotions—and socially unacceptable impulses—from their conscious minds. In Schwartz's view, certain repressors relied too heavily on this defense to cope with life's travails. By blocking so many thoughts, memories, and feelings, they lost their capacity to attend, connect, and express. With so few

ACE abilities, rigid repressors can no longer regulate their bodymind systems: The wires to their "thermostat" have been virtually cut.

But how could this be scientifically proven? Schwartz and Weinberger—currently professor of psychology at Case Western Reserve in Cleveland—first had to measure repression, which amounts to a form of mental sleight-of-hand. The problem was this: How can you ask a person if she represses thoughts and feelings? By definition, the repressor is *unaware* of her reliance on repression, not to mention the feelings she's repressed. There had to be a psychological instrument that bypassed the conscious mind.

An oft-used psychological test—known as the Manifest Anxiety Scale (MAS)—asks a subject whether he experiences high or low levels of anxiety. But Schwartz realized that repressive copers would not be aware of their anxiety. By contrast, people with ACE abilities would be aware of anxiety when it arose, but most of the time they'd be calm. Why? Because their ongoing attention to feedback enabled them to maintain a relaxed "set point." If anxiety arose, they'd tend to it, connect it to consciousness, and take effective action that restored tranquility. People high in ACE were *authentically* calm, while repressive copers only *believed* they were calm.

Thus, despite their differences, repressors and ACE personalities would *both* claim to be calm. Schwartz wondered how he could scientifically distinguish between these two groups, who seemed similar on the surface but could not have been less alike on the deeper level of personality.

A solution presented itself when Schwartz and Weinberger used another psychological test, called the Marlowe-Crowne Social Desirability Scale, or M-C, for short. The M-C test revealed whether people characteristically put the best face on their life circumstances and emotions, no matter how distressing. High M-C individuals firmly agree with statements such as:

• I never resent being asked to return a favor.
• I almost never feel the urge to tell someone off.
• I am always courteous, even to people who are disagreeable.

• I don't like to gossip at all.
• I don't find it particularly difficult to get along with loudmouths.

High M-C scorers deceive themselves ("I never want to tell someone off"), whereas low M-C scorers tell themselves and others the truth, even when it isn't socially "desirable." ("I *often* want to tell people off.") Schwartz and Weinberger would use the M-C to double-check the validity of people's claims of tranquility. Could a person who reported low anxiety be trusted? The answer would distinguish repressors from people high in ACE.

Schwartz and Weinberger administered these two tests—the MAS anxiety test and the M-C. The following list depicts how people were categorized, depending on whether they scored low or high in self-deception and self-reported anxiety. Thus, each individual could be placed in one of four coping categories:

1. *True Low Anxious* (low in anxiety, low in self-deception). True low anxious people tell the truth to themselves and others, and thus their claim of tranquility can be believed. They are high in the ACE Factor, because their self-awareness enables them to maintain an authentic state of bodymind balance.

2. *Repressive Coper* (low in anxiety, high in self-deception). Repressive copers deceive others, not because they are liars but because they deceive *themselves* so thoroughly that they're unaware of negative or "unacceptable" feelings. Thus, they cannot be believed when they claim to be free of anxiety. Their lack of self-awareness and bodymind connection makes them low in the ACE Factor.

3. *True High Anxious* (high in anxiety, low in self-deception). True high anxious people tell the truth to themselves and others, and thus their report of anxiety can be believed. They have ACE abilities, because they are aware of their real feelings. But they do not necessarily complete ACE sequences that resolve their anxiety and return them to a set point of genuine tranquility.

4. *Defensive High Anxious* (high in anxiety, high in self-deception). Defensive high anxious people score high in self-deception *and* anxiety. They try to block out negative feedback (unpleasant

sensations or feelings) but are unable to do so. They rely on psychological defenses (such as repression) to keep up a good front, but these defenses are faltering. Anxiety begins to "leak through" into consciousness, leaving them in a state of confusion or helplessness. Defensive high anxious people are caught midway between repression and ACE.

With these categories, Schwartz and Weinberger had solved one riddle of how to study repression and the ACE Factor. But they needed scientific proof that repressors were out of touch with bodily feedback and that their defenses bred disorder and disease. They also needed proof that ACE personalities were connected with bodily feedback, generating order and ease in their systems.

In a watershed 1979 study, Schwartz and Weinberger gave the MAS and the M-C to a group of subjects, all of whom fell into one of the four coping categories. The participants were then hooked up to equipment measuring physiologic signs of inner stress: heart rate, skin resistance, and muscular tension. Each person was asked to perform a moderately stressful task: completing sentences with overtly aggressive and sexual content. Here are the results:

1. The true low-anxious individuals showed little physiological evidence of internal stress.
2. The true high-anxious individuals showed high physiological evidence of internal stress.
3. The repressive copers (who claimed low anxiety) showed physiological evidence of *skyrocketing* internal stress—in many cases, even higher than the true high anxious.
4. The defensive high-anxious individuals showed physiological evidence of internal stress at a level midway between the true low and high anxious individuals.

These findings fit Schwartz and Weinberger's thesis perfectly. ACE personalities (the true low anxious) maintained stability in heart rate and muscular tension when stressed. People with ACE potential (the true high anxious) did exhibit increases, but they were seldom as severe as repressors who denied feeling anxiety!

The repressors experienced the most severe increases in heart rate, muscular tension, and other physical signs of overstimulation.

Among repressors, the gap between conscious thoughts and biological reality could not have been more dramatic. Simply put, repressors did not know what forces gripped their unconscious minds and agitated their bodies. By contrast, ACE personalities were not overstimulated by stressful tasks, because they didn't have to engage in so much physiological "work" to repress threatening emotions.

These findings led Gary Schwartz to believe that repressive copers were at greater risk for heart disease, because they fooled themselves into believing everything was okay while their vital signs ran amok. Following that lead for fifteen years, he's produced a compelling body of evidence linking repression and heart disease.

In one study, he compared repressive coping among healthy people and those with high blood pressure. While a mere 11 percent of a healthy population were repressors, a whopping 45 percent of hypertensives kept a lid on their feelings—a *fourfold* increase. In another experiment, Schwartz asked patients a series of reflective questions, and measured their heart rate and respiration for fifteen seconds. He concluded that "beat-by-beat homeostatic control of heart rate during the mental task was disrupted in repressive subjects more than in true low anxious subjects. In other words, the repressor's cardiovascular systems . . . responded in a more disordered fashion."

Out of sync with their bodies, people who lack ACE are at risk for heart disease. Their fight-or-flight mechanism is easily triggered, but without their knowledge. Their sympathetic nervous systems stimulate a continuous cascade of stress hormones that not only spike their heart rate and blood pressure, but contribute to arterial blockages that cause heart attacks. When people are unaware that fight-or-flight is constantly in motion, they become unwitting victims of the physiological havoc it wreaks on their cardiovascular systems. We also know that stress hormones (such as adrenaline) associated with fight-or-flight *can suppress the immune system*. Repressors' overactive nervous systems may be as bad for their immune defenses as it is for their hearts.

We all have an image of the stressed-out executive who relentlessly pushes himself, throwing himself into a cauldron of high anxiety on a daily basis. He rides roughshod over his body's messages, toiling for such long hours that the clock seems to fade into oblivion. He never gets enough sleep, forgets when to eat, and spends too little "quality time" with his family. We also have another stereotypical image of this executive: At a tragically early age, he suffers a massive heart attack. This stereotype has not arisen out of thin air: Many studies confirm that such individuals run the risk of heart disease.

Gary Schwartz's research adds a new dimension to the link between behavior and heart disease. Chronic states of hostility and anxiety damage the heart, *but so does the tendency to ignore bodily sensations and feelings.* If the high-strung executive paid attention to his body, he'd recognize his jazzed-up emotions, his fatigue, his overwork, his ceaseless struggling, and his physical discomfort. Then he might do something about these bodymind states and the conditions that cause them. When such individuals cultivate ACE, they slow down, turn inward, and transform their behavior and environment. Developing ACE breeds order and ease in their cardiovascular systems.

What about the role of ACE in other diseases? Does ACE help us prevent or overcome colds, viral infections, or even cancer? Does the ACE Factor balance not only our cardiovascular systems, but our immune systems as well? Gary Schwartz began searching for answers in the 1980s.

THE ACE FACTOR, IMMUNITY, AND HEALTH

During the 1980s, the Yale Behavioral Medicine Clinic (YBMC) established a reputation as a unique mind-body treatment center. Patients were referred to the clinic with a wide variety of illnesses, ranging from back pain to asthma to cancer, that had not responded to conventional medical treatment.

The YBMC patients would undergo a medical evaluation like no other. Based on an approach developed by psychiatrist Hoyle

Leigh, M.D., and Gary Schwartz, the clinic's directors, every person who walked through the clinic's doors would get a complete physical exam *and* a complete psychological evaluation. Patients would report their mood state, personality, early experiences, and family relationships. The doctor in charge would also gather information about their diet, environment, work status, medical history—even past experiences with doctors and hospitals. The result was a genuinely holistic examination, which was necessary to design treatments for the whole person. All this occurred in a setting replete with X-ray machines, brain wave instruments, electrocardiograph (EKG) devices—all the high-tech provisions of mainstream medicine.

When Gary Schwartz began studying personality and health, he used personality tests (including the MAS and M-C) in his initial evaluation of the clinic's patients. This enabled him to place each patient into one of the four coping categories. Schwartz knew he had a unique opportunity: He could study whether his patients' immune systems were influenced by their personalities—a revolutionary concept then and now.

THE ACE FACTOR AND IMMUNE CELLS

Schwartz joined with Larry Jamner, Ph.D., to investigate whether repression—and the ACE Factor—had a demonstrable effect on immunity. They studied 312 of the YBMC patients who'd come for treatment during the previous five years. Blood was drawn from each patient and a series of immune and endocrine tests were performed. Schwartz and Jamner were interested in whether personality influenced the number of circulating monocytes—cells that are critically involved in defending against infectious diseases and cancer.

Their findings are depicted in Panel A of Figure 2.1. It shows:

- Both repressive copers and defensive high-anxious individuals had a reduced number of monocytes in their bloodstream. Thus, *individuals who lacked ACE abilities had weaker immune function.*
- Both true high-anxious and true low-anxious individuals had a

higher relative number of monocytes in their bloodstream. Thus, *individuals who demonstrated greater ACE abilities had stronger immune function.*

• The true low-anxious individuals, considered to have the strongest ACE abilities, had the greatest number of circulating monocytes—a sign of *Immune Power.*

These findings shattered the simplistic myth that "negative emotions" cause immune dysfunction. If the myth had been fact, then the true high-anxious people—who reported feeling great distress—would have had the weakest immune function. But the true high-anxious individuals had greater Immune Power than repressors, who said they felt fine! The pivotal issue is not the presence of negative emotions, but whether the person represses or expresses them.

The defensive high-anxious subjects had the fewest monocytes. Schwartz speculated why their immune function was even weaker than the repressive copers: They were individuals whose psychological defenses were faltering. Although repressors rely upon a psychological defense that weakens their immune system, at least their defense is "working." (Repression can prevent a complete psychological collapse.) But defensive high-anxious people are often flooded with feelings of anxiety, confusion, or depression. Because they lack ACE, they cannot express and resolve these difficult emotions. Overwhelmed by negative feedback, their immune system suffers along with their spirit.

ACE personalities also had fewer signs of *over*sensitive immune systems. They had fewer eosinophiles, white blood cells that are activated during allergic reactions, and fewer allergies to medications. (See Panel B of Figure 2.1.) By contrast, repressive copers had the most eosinophiles and the most allergies to medications. The powerful immune system is the balanced immune system: one that does not overreact to foreign substances—as in allergies—or underact—as in infections and cancer. Schwartz and Jamner had uncovered evidence that ACE personalities have not only stronger but more finely tuned immune systems.

One mystery continued to surround these findings: In the

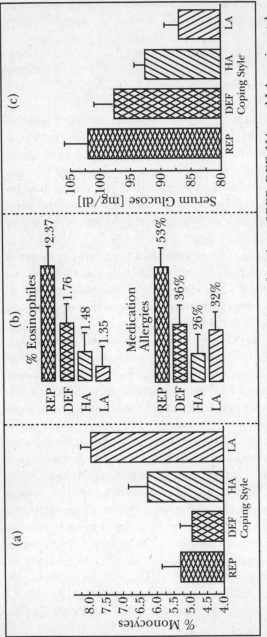

Fig. 2.1. (a) Mean monocyte count (per 100 leukocytes) as a function of REP, DEF, HA, and LA coping styles. (b) Mean eosinophile count (per 100 leukocytes) and group percent of patients reporting allergies to medication as a function of coping style. (c) Mean serum glucose levels (mg/dl) for REP, DEF, HA, and LA groups.

Key: REP: Repressive copers
DEF: Defensive high anxious individuals
HA: High anxious individuals
LA: Low anxious individuals

68

body, how does the ACE Factor translate into stronger immune defenses? How does repression weaken immune defenses? Gary Schwartz had a hunch, and it was confirmed by a revealing panel of data from his study.

THE ACE FACTOR, BLOOD SUGAR, AND ENDORPHINS

ACE personalities had normal serum glucose levels, a measure of blood sugar. But repressors who lacked ACE had *elevated* serum glucose. (See Panel C of Figure 2.1.) What was the significance of these blood sugar findings? The answer requires a bit of biochemical background.

Schwartz suspected that repressors had high levels of endorphins, brain chemicals that serve a natural painkilling function in our bodies. In order to block out "negative" bodymind feedback—pain, anxiety, anger, sadness, and tension—the repressors synthesized a continuous stream of these chemicals, which dulled their experience of discomfort.

In an earlier study, Schwartz and Jamner had administered mild shocks to subjects who'd been psychologically tested for repression. The intensity of the shocks was gradually increased, while the subjects were asked how much pain they could tolerate. The repressors accepted twice as much electric current as nonrepressors before saying they'd reached their tolerance level. The findings were so strong that Schwartz was persuaded: Repressors must produce extremely high levels of painkilling endorphins in their brains and bodies.

Schwartz began to patch together a psychophysical portrait of repressors. He combined his observations of repressed patients at his clinic, who he'd come to know and understand, with his biochemical findings, which suggested that they churned out excess endorphins. The repressor can be likened to an injured racehorse that gets injected with painkillers so it can compete in a big-money derby. The horse won't get any pain feedback, and once the drug wears off, its injury may be dangerously aggravated. Likewise, the repressor often struggles in stressful jobs, relationships, or family situations without making changes, because he's inured to the pain. He may sustain "injuries"—fatigue, loss, or failure—that require dispensation of more internal painkillers, the endorphins. The brain complies. The cycle intensifies as the psychic wounds accumulate. Only a major alteration in the repressor's life will interrupt the circuit of pain and repression. Often it takes a psychological collapse, physical illness, or personal revelation before the individual changes his pattern.

Gary Schwartz knew, however, that endorphins (and other "opioid peptides") serve a vital function in our minds and bodies. Normal levels of these neuropeptides lift our mood, calm our anxieties, reduce our experience of severe pain, and boost our immune systems. Endorphins have gotten great press over the years, especially since we've learned that joggers experience a health-promoting "high." This fed popular opinion that the more endorphins we make, the better we'll feel. But Gary Schwartz, whose watchword of health is balance, saw evidence that we are harmed by too much *or* too few endorphins.

The subtle role of endorphins in health had been revealed by UCLA psychologist Yehuda Shavit, Ph.D. In 1985, he conducted an ingenious experiment in which shocks were administered to mice who were helpless to turn them off. The helpless mice demonstrated increases in endorphins that were linked to sudden drops in NK cells—a key litmus of Immune Power. Their NK deficits hindered the animals' ability to reject implanted tumors. In another study, Shavit injected mice with morphine (a chemical cousin of endorphins), and their resistance to tumors was substantially weakened. Clearly, endorphin overload dampened the immune system's strength and sensitivity.

Schwartz believed that human repressors rely so heavily on pain-numbing defenses that their immune systems become hampered by excess endorphins. For complex biochemical reasons, a lack of endorphins appears to have the same dampening effect. But research strongly suggests that *appropriate* levels of endorphins *bolster* the immune system.*

---

* Research also suggests that various types and structures of endorphins may enhance or suppress immune cells, and that different individuals respond differently to endorphin surges. However, the issue of endorphin *balance* appears to be critical.

Which returns us to the finding that repressors had high blood sugar compared to ACE personalities. Schwartz had unearthed studies proving that endorphins elevate blood sugar. One researcher injected endorphins directly into the brain, which caused an immediate rise in blood sugar. Therefore, the repressors' high blood sugar probably reflected higher levels of endorphins. By contrast, the ACE personalities' *normal* blood sugar reflected *normal* levels of endorphins.

The blood sugar discovery confirmed Schwartz's hunch: The ACE personality—who is sensitive to pain but not oversensitive; aware of feelings but not overwhelmed by them—*makes endorphins in proper amounts.* His or her immune cells receive *appropriate* signals from these messenger molecules: They signal "attack" when the body is invaded and "desist" when no threat is imminent.

As in battle, the most effective responses to attack are both powerful and proportional. Schwartz reasoned that the ACE personality demonstrated such balance in both psychological reactions to negative events and immunological reactions to foreign invaders. The ACE personality displays the right amount of sensitivity to distress signals; the right amount of endorphins; and the right amount of immunological firepower against outside attack.*

Repressors who lack ACE evidence other biochemical imbalances. Schwartz's earlier studies showed that the sympathetic nervous systems of repressors react powerfully to stress—even when they say they feel fine. Their heart rate, blood pressure, and muscle tension increase—evidence that stress hormones are being released into their bloodstream. We know that chronically high levels of corticosteroids and catecholamines—the primary stress hormones—can weaken our immune cells. Here was yet another mechanism by which repression could diminish our Immune Power.

---

* A 1993 study by Brian Esterling and his colleagues at the University of Miami confirms the immune-protecting role of ACE. Using Schwartz's measures, the researchers found that people highest in ACE had better immune control over a latent virus (EBV) than repressors and defensive high anxious people.

DOES THE ACE FACTOR PREVENT DISEASE?

One question raised by Schwartz and Jamner's study: Is the ACE personality, who has more monocytes, really less vulnerable to infections or cancer? Although more research is needed, immunologists have documented the importance of monocytes in fighting microbes and malignant cells. One research team used monocyte counts to accurately predict whether medical patients would contract infections.

Schwartz's discovery also must be perceived in the context of many other studies linking repression to disease and the ACE Factor to health. Schwartz cited the following findings, some of which came from his own laboratory.

Asthma. Research in the 1970s by A. A. Mathe and P. H. Knapp uncovered a link between repression and asthma. People lacking ACE had imbalanced immune systems that were more vulnerable to asthma and allergies. With William Polonski, Ph.D., Gary Schwartz had asthma patients use mental imagery to shift their attention from an external focus to an internal one—concerned with sensations and feelings. These patients demonstrated improvements in their immune functions consistent with the healing of asthma.

Rheumatoid Arthritis. George Solomon, M.D., showed that patients with rheumatoid arthritis, an autoimmune disease, had a marked tendency toward repressive coping: They blocked awareness and expression of so-called negative emotions. Solomon observed repressive coping in patients with lupus, allergies, asthma, cancer, and infectious diseases.

Diabetes. Lauren Abramson, Ph.D., of Johns Hopkins University and David McClelland, Ph.D., of Boston University found that diabetics were more likely than controls to suffer from *alexithymia,* a condition of people who "do not have conscious or verbal access to their own emotions." (The condition is in many respects comparable to repression.) Diabetics with the least access to their emotions had the *poorest control over blood sugar levels.*

In diabetes, the person's control of blood sugar is already

impaired. A fascinating possibility is raised by Schwartz and Jamner's previous discoveries: Repressors may be vulnerable to diabetes because they churn out excess endorphins, which in turn raise blood sugar. Could diabetics reverse their condition by cultivating the ACE Factor? More study is needed, but Richard Surwit, Ph.D., of Duke University has already proven that relaxation and biofeedback—which foster attention to bodymind signals—lower blood sugar and reduce symptoms in many diabetes patients.

Cancer. Steven Greer, M.D., of Britain, and Lydia Temoshok, Ph.D., while at the University of California, San Francisco, have both shown powerful associations between repressive coping and the development of cancer. Temoshok demonstrated that cancer patients who *expressed* emotions had more cancer-fighting lymphocytes at the base of their melanoma tumors. Translation: ACE personalities had greater Immune Power in response to cancer cell invasion.

In collaboration with Gary Schwartz, Mogens R. Jensen, Ph.D., followed a group of breast cancer patients for two years. Women who suffered more rapid spread of cancer shared certain personality traits: repressive coping, nonexpression of emotions, feelings of helplessness, and comforting daydreaming. They *avoided* attending, connecting, and expressing the difficult emotions associated with their illness. By contrast, women who displayed the ACE Factor (nonrepressors) had a rate of remission that was 46 percent less than women who repressed emotions.

Schwartz believes that the ACE Factor is important for people wishing to prevent or recover from cancer. People who lack ACE may be prone to biological imbalances, such as endorphin overload. Their immune systems are hampered and they become vulnerable to cancer cell growth. But it's never too late for cancer patients to transform their response to illness. Patients who recognize their symptoms, get an early diagnosis, seek the best available treatment, procure emotional support from friends and family, and express their sadness and anger are *developing the ACE Factor.* They attend (symptoms), connect (levels of information), and express (needs and emotions). Some of these ACE activities, such as early diagnosis, lead to better medical care. Others, such as expressing emotions, strengthen immune functions within the body. Whether ACE engages external (medical) or internal (immune) defenses, such patients may enhance their prospects for recovery.

In the landmark 1990 study, Stanford University psychiatrist David Spiegel followed a group of eighty-six women with metastatic breast cancer, all of whom received the same medical treatment, but only half of whom participated in group therapy. Spiegel's treatment, called Supportive/Expressive Therapy, encouraged patients to:

- Relax and tune into their bodymind through self-hypnosis.
- Become aware of their needs and feelings, then share them with group members.
- Procure social support from group members and loved ones outside the group.
- Become more expressive and assertive with doctors and family members.

Each of these features touches upon the development of attention, connection, and expression. The group participants, whose ACE abilities increased over time, lived twice as long as the breast cancer patients who did not participate. David Spiegel's astonishing discovery suggests that people can cultivate ACE and better their odds against cancer. And Gary Schwartz's data offers a likely explanation: The ACE Factor is an Immune Power trait that strengthens their internal defense against malignant cells.

David Spiegel is now studying the specific effects of Supportive/Expressive Therapy on the immune systems of cancer patients. In recent years, however, scientists have already shown that certain ACE-positive treatments bolster immunity. At Ohio State University, psychologist Janice Kiecolt-Glazer taught "progressive muscle relaxation" to a group of geriatric patients. During this exercise, the person mentally travels through the body, attending and relaxing each part. *Blood tests revealed a marked increase in the vitality of natural killer cells among patients who practiced this form of bodymind attention.* Natural killer cells are vital to our defense against infections and cancer.

When we develop the ACE Factor, we generate balance, order, and power in our immune systems. As a result, our efforts to prevent or heal *any* illnesses caused by immune dysfunction—from arthritis to cancer to AIDS—are strengthened. Jungian philosopher Thomas Moore writes eloquently about care of the soul. ACE is an expression of care of the bodymind, the human repository of soul.

DEVELOPING THE ACE FACTOR

In her book *The Alchemy of Illness,* Kat Duff writes poetically of her struggle with chronic fatigue syndrome. Listening to her body's messages was a central part of her healing journey:

> My body has taught me many things, all of them filled with soul: how to dance and make love, mourn and make music; now it is teaching me how to heal. I am learning to heed the shifting currents of my body—the subtle changes in temperature, muscle tension, thought, and mood—the way a sailor rides the wind by reading the ripples on the water. Sometimes I am surprised by the feedback my body gives me; after being a vegetarian for twelve years I was astonished—and mortified—to discover that my body thrives on an occasional serving of organic red meat, at least for now. Apparently, ideology has no place in the delicate rhythms of healing.

Kat Duff's approach mirrors Gary Schwartz's own therapeutic philosophy. Over fifteen years, Schwartz has treated patients suffering from an extraordinary range of medical disorders, including chronic fatigue, chronic pain, asthma, allergies, diabetes, temporomandibular joint syndrome (TMJ), viral infections, migraines, ulcers, hypertension, and cancer. He designed a treatment program in which each person was encouraged to develop the ACE Factor. Like Kat Duff's sailor, patients would learn to ride winds of stress by reading ripples on the water—the fluctuations of their own bodies.

In evolving his treatment program, Schwartz discovered that traditional mind-body therapies—including biofeedback, meditation, and guided imagery—did not always enhance the ACE Factor. The key to effective mind-body treatment, he found, lies in how these treatments are applied. Relaxation techniques can be used to cut off bodymind feedback, or they can be used to reconnect bodymind feedback. They can be applied in a one-size-fits-all fashion, or with respect for individual differences. They can be prescribed as the sole focus of mind-body healing, or they can be integrated into a holistic program that fosters ACE on every level of being.

Gary Schwartz found that the healing potential of meditation—or biofeedback, or guided imagery—is realized when such methods are custom-tailored to enhance the ACE Factor. Consider the case of a man suffering with asthma. He does not recognize that his condition is exacerbated by stress on the job—in particular, a corrosive relationship with his boss. The boss mistreats him, and the man sees no escape from his daily trap of humiliation. He knows he is stressed, but does not connect his worsening asthma to his painful dilemma at work. If this man goes to a stress reduction clinic, where he imagines himself lying on the warming sands of a beautiful beach, his symptoms may improve temporarily. But the asthma will not abate, because he does not connect this symptom to his relationship with his boss. He never attends to the underlying problem.

If, however, he uses relaxation to tune into his own bodymind experience—rather than a prefabricated "tranquil" experience—he'll discover *just how distressed he really is.* While this realization is unpleasant, a mind-body therapist can help him make sense of his distress by relating it to his job and helping him recognize that his distress is normal, justified, and completely human. The final stage is to find empowering solutions: ways for him to become more assertive, or alternative job options if his boss continues to abuse him. Throughout this process, the man continues using relaxation to tune into his bodymind. As his external situation improves, his relaxation practice becomes more truly relaxing. His asthma may heal on a deeper level, because he's confronted the stressor that has contributed to his immunological *dis*ease.

As in this case, Gary Schwartz uses mind-body techniques to elicit the patients' own truths, but he never pushes them to feel more distress than they can handle. His respect and care for his patients is built into his therapeutic approach.

REPRESSION AS CURSE, REPRESSION AS GIFT

In seeking to cultivate ACE, Schwartz has confronted one particular challenge. The patients who most need to develop ACE are repressors. By encouraging them to change, was Schwartz indicting them for a bad psychological defense that caused them to become sick? Would this implication make them feel worse about themselves, instead of better? He confronted this problem by going deeper into the origins of repression and sharing his insights with his patients. Surprisingly, one of the most powerfully healing aspects of Gary Schwartz's therapy is his ability to communicate that repression is not a sickness but a talent.

Repression begins in childhood, and it helps children maintain emotional stability in painful circumstances. Children subjected to sexual, verbal, or emotional abuse often must repress their anger, sadness, and fear. Expressing these feelings can expose them to disapproval, humiliation, punishment, or the withdrawal of parental love. The children squelch their own negative emotions until, eventually, they completely lose touch with them. Banishing these threatening feelings from consciousness, the children feel safer. The feelings no longer threaten their psychological integrity or their appointed role within the family.

Said Schwartz:

Of all the coping strategies a child can develop to deal with terrible stress, one could argue that repression is ultimately the healthiest and even the kindest. Consider the child who grows up in a household where there is tremendous strife between the parents, or there is emotional or physical abuse, and the child has little support from other loved ones. What are the child's options? One of them is to get severely depressed and become unable to function, which happens to many. They may resort to drugs to take away the pain. They may run away or act out.

But they may also repress their pain and anger. This enables them to stay in the household, to provide some support for others within the home, and to function. These are exceptionally good, often shy children, perhaps too well behaved. They tend to do well in school. These children survive the experience and eventually leave the home intact. If repression becomes a chronic way of dealing with emotional difficulties, it will catch up with them later. In the short term, however, repression is profoundly adaptive.

Schwartz recognized a therapeutic paradox: He could help his patients undo rigid repression by showing them how it saved their lives. Here is his explanation from a recent paper:

> The patients I saw were veritable masters of repression. My approach in therapy was to help them discover this "talent" (rather than "sickness") and to help them relabel their repressiveness as a highly mastered tool of the mind they should be proud of rather than ashamed of. . . .
>
> However, they were helped to discover that what was once a necessary and adaptive coping strategy was no longer necessary and adaptive. They were helped to discover that it was now safe for them no longer to rely primarily on this overlearned mental tool and learn new, more flexible coping tools.
>
> The process of coming to trust the therapist and unlearn some of the automatic repression is, of course, easier said than done. However, with time, this strategy helped these patients become more hopeful, more realistic, and more openminded, to see therapy as a positive challenge that in a safe context could help free them.

An adult who cannot shed his repressive defense is like some-one who continues to wear a heavy fur coat in spring and summer. No one would suggest that the coat is useless, just inappropriate under changed weather conditions. The repressor should not dis-card his protective psychic coat. Instead, he can "hang up" this coat, grateful for the cover it provided in harsh weather and secure in the knowledge that he can don it once more if necessary.

We can develop ACE only when we experience our bodymind in trust and self-care. When we blame ourselves for past repression and disconnection, we impede this growth process. When we ac-cept our past patterns with compassion and insight, we accelerate the growth process. The groundwork for development of the ACE Factor is laid with kindness.

The following sections break down Gary Schwartz's therapy into components that foster attention, connection, and expression, respectively. Included are specific guidelines you can follow, pro-vided by Schwartz and other practitioners who have honed the art of cultivating ACE.

ATTENTION: BALANCE AND LOVING-KINDNESS

Gary Schwartz's ACE-enhancing therapy begins with instruction on the gentle art of self-attention. The goal is to monitor symptoms, sensations, and emotions carefully but not obsessively. When we pay keen attention to each of these realms of our being, we move effortlessly to the next stage of connection. When we listen to mes-sages hidden in our headaches, ulcers, or tumors, we learn what our bodymind has lacked and what it needs now. When we tune into sensations of fatigue, hunger, yearning, discomfort, or arousal, we uncover sources of dissatisfaction—or pleasure—in our daily lives. When we explore inner qualities of anger, sadness, or fear, we tap a motherlode of information about our relationships, creativity, and spirituality.

But these connections cannot be forged until we cultivate that fine-tuned quality of attention.

Many techniques engender attention. Meditation, biofeedback, and guided imagery can be used to heighten awareness of symptoms, sensations, and emotions. Each of these methods requires that we take time out of our day. A daily practice of meditation and/or guided imagery requires a commitment to paying attention. Making this commitment is a first step toward healthy attention. But it is not the only step. We can allow the quality of attention cultivated in twenty-minute blocks of time to spread into all corners of our lives.

For those of us who tend toward repressive coping, increasing attention can be a difficult task. Our body-sense and awareness of emotions may be attenuated after years of "pressing down." According to Gary Schwartz, a first step toward change is keen attention to physical symptoms.

You can start by keeping a record of your symptoms. It should indicate when they arise and precisely what you are thinking, feeling, and doing at those times. By keeping track in this manner, you foster attention to the area of greatest concern and conflict. Often you have ignored or medicated the symptoms just to function. You may have developed a fierce hatred for your symptoms. Now you focus a gentle awareness on the symptoms and listen to their messages. At the end of this chapter, you will find an imagery exercise that enables you to deeply attend to your symptoms.

The purpose of record keeping, in which you note events and feelings on other levels of your being, is to enhance the quality of your attention and set the stage for connection. On page 95 I have provided a record-keeping template for your convenience that will enable you to view temporal relationships among your symptoms, emotions, thoughts, and life events.

Record whatever symptoms arise, whether they are headaches, muscle pains, a flare-up of allergies, a worsening cold, or the progression of a particular disease. Your symptoms also may be psychological—depression, anxiety, panic, compulsive behavior, difficulty concentrating, and so on. If so, record those symptoms and the corresponding feelings, sensations, and circumstances.

Take note of the situations, times of day, and emotional contexts in which your symptoms worsen or abate. Then you will be better able to notice the changes *when they happen*. Your attention will become tuned to the frequency of the present moment.

The Buddhist practice of *mindfulness* involves moment-to-moment awareness. Mindfulness is both a way of being and a specific meditation. In life or in meditation, mindfulness is a non-judgmental acceptance of inner and outer realities. The essence of mindfulness is a simple attention to the moment, without either rejecting or clinging to any one mental state. Many of us dwell ceaselessly in the past, holding fast to old hopes and regrets; or in the future, postponing pleasures to some faraway time. The revelation of mindfulness is that experience exists in one realm only: the present.

A key to mindfulness: What we think or feel in any one moment is not the totality of who we are. Sadness, anger, terror, joy, excitement, anxiety, pleasure, and pain move in and out of consciousness, coexist in clusters, appear and subside. In mindfulness meditation, the goal is not to push feelings in or out the door of awareness. The goal is to "entertain" them, until their time for a graceful exit naturally arises.

Jon Kabat-Zinn, Ph.D., is director of the Stress Reduction Clinic at the University of Massachusetts Medical Center. He has designed and led this unique program for twenty years, teaching six thousand patients suffering from a wide range of disorders how to cope and live with their illnesses. The basis of his rigorous eight-week program is training in mindfulness. In his book *Full Catastrophe Living*, Kabat-Zinn discusses mindfulness as a form of healthy attention: "The way of mindfulness is to accept ourselves right now, as we are, symptoms or no symptoms, pain or no pain, fear or no fear. Instead of rejecting our experience as undesirable, we ask, 'What is this symptom saying, what is it telling me about my body and my mind right now?' "

Kabat-Zinn also emphasizes balance when bringing to bear what he calls "wise attention" to our bodymind signals. "When we fail to honor these messages, either through denial or by an inflated and self-involved preoccupation with symptoms, we can sometimes create serious dilemmas for ourselves."

Gary Schwartz makes a similar point: Obsessive attention is as unhealthy as lack of attention. The purpose of attending symptoms is not to become frightened by every ache, pain, and twinge. And the purpose of attending emotions is not to become self-conscious about every melancholy moment or angry impulse. When we properly practice attention, we achieve a balanced state of awareness characterized by relaxed acceptance of whatever arises in the moment. We do not hold tight to symptoms and sensations. We fully investigate their qualities and move on.

Today, many people are compulsively concerned about every morsel of food they consume. Others beat themselves emotionally for one breach of a strenuous exercise regimen. Still others view all health problems as solvable with one alternative medical solution—acupuncture, homeopathy, herbs, crystals, or psychic healing. Referring to the obsessiveness of some health "fanatics," Schwartz remarked, "That's not a flexible way to bring order into your life."

Schwartz's concept of "flexible order" has radical ramifications for health. He sees order in the universe and order in our bodymind systems. Our job is not to impose that order with one narrow health-promoting technique or another. Our job is to let that order unfold naturally.

The health fanatic, exercise freak, and person committed to expressing every one of his innermost feelings will ultimately answer to the law of diminishing returns. On the other hand, the person who stays in the middle of the road—never daring to risk radical steps toward change—also can become hamstrung in her quest for health. Schwartz sums up his approach when he calls for "moderation in all things, including moderation."

How does one go about sharpening attention to bodily sensations, emotions, and thoughts? One structured way is psychotherapy with a professional who helps us to explore repressed emotions and their connection to difficult issues in our present. However, with or without psychotherapy, another way to accomplish this end is a meditation practice known as "sweeping the body." See the "ACE Exercises" on page 91 of this chapter for instructions on this practice.

CONNECTION: THE "AHA" EXPERIENCE

Making connections is an intrinsic aspect of psychotherapy; it is also essential for bodymind healing. Reconnecting feedback loops that have been severed through years of inattention and repression is the pivotal step in developing the ACE Factor.

The record-keeping template I have provided offers you the opportunity to connect your symptoms with corresponding levels of being: emotions, moods, memories, physical sensations, and life circumstances, including work and relationships. You also can connect these levels to each other. After one week of record keeping, search for these patterns:

- Do particular symptoms worsen when certain emotions are activated?
- Do particular symptoms worsen when certain events take place?
- Are particular emotions associated with other physical sensations?
- Are certain sensations associated with particular moods?
- Are certain relationships linked to especially troubling emotions?
- Do certain memories arise when you participate in specific activities?
- Do your worst symptoms occur at work? During interactions with particular individuals?

These are questions Gary Schwartz asks his patients in ACE-enhancing therapy. You can ask yourself these same questions, and forge the connections that facilitate bodymind healing. Gary Schwartz described this endeavor.

What I do in therapy is help people make connections between their past and present; thoughts and feelings; how they're feeling and how someone else is feeling; and between symptoms and what's going on in the present. The purpose is to increase self-awareness. To accomplish this, I ask Socratic questions that encourage self-discovery. I give people feedback they themselves have lost touch with. I facilitate people's ability to jump from one level of awareness to another, seeing connections between levels and discovering how they are more than a collection of disparate parts. I encourage patients to consider alternative ways of looking at things. Ultimately, I try to help people accept their past and accept who they are—with all their gifts and limitations.

Schwartz has observed a common reaction to meaningful connections: We say to ourselves "aha." Whether the connection occurs in therapy or in life, "aha" experiences spark immediate insight. They represent a unique interface between intellectual recognition and visceral understanding: What we have always known on some level finally hits home. Perhaps long-repressed memories emerge. Or connections between illnesses and unmet emotional or spiritual needs become crystal clear. Or relationship difficulties are suddenly seen to reflect an earlier conflict with a parent. Or sadness and anger about present-day career troubles rise to awareness.

For individuals who've relied on repressive coping, "aha" experiences repair the bodymind split. According to Gary Schwartz, this repair is more than metaphorical. *It may be actual repair of a neurophysiological split in the brain.*

For twenty years, Gary Schwartz has studied disconnection within the brain. He has found that repressed people have a functional disconnection between their left and right hemispheres. ("Functional" means that the disconnection is not the result of an organic disease or injury. This implies it can be reversed.) Neural information from the right hemisphere, where "negative" emotions originate, is not adequately transferred to the left hemisphere, where analytic and verbal functions originate. This theory explained how so many people—the "supernormals," TM followers, and others—seemed to operate on two different levels of consciousness.

Gary Schwartz has used PET (positron emission tomography) scans, brain wave studies, and other high-tech strategies to produce strong evidence that repressors have a verifiable disconnect between the two hemispheres. Years of reliance on this mental defense impeded the flow of information between the right and left sides of their brains. The repressors' cerebral disconnection is reflected in psychological splits: between positive and negative emotions, negative emotions and consciousness, intellect and feeling. Schwartz is convinced that when ACE-enhancing therapies heal psychological splits, they help to heal the split within the brain. "You know the saying that healthy people 'have their heads together'?" said Schwartz. "That is more than a turn of phrase. Their left and right hemispheres freely communicate. Much of what I do with repressed individuals is to facilitate such connections."

One of Jon Kabat-Zinn's patients, Nancy Horniak, was able to make such powerful connections. She came to Kabat-Zinn's Stress Reduction Clinic with a host of conditions, including migraine headaches, rheumatoid arthritis, Raynaud's disease, and a rare autoimmune disorder called Sjogren's syndrome. The most aggravating to her was the Sjogren's syndrome, in which the body's immune cells mistakenly attack the salivary glands and tear ducts, causing horrendous dryness of the mouth and eyes. Digestion becomes difficult, and crying produces no tears.

By the time Nancy came to the clinic, she had not cried for five years. In her work with Kabat-Zinn, she learned to practice mindfulness and a "body scan" meditation. One day, shortly after her fourth group session, she experienced one of her splitting migraines. This time, instead of fighting her pain, she attended to her physical sensations. She breathed deeply and imagined her breath traveling down into her toes and out of the top of her head. Nancy completely let go of her tension, then found herself wiping tears from her face.

"All of a sudden it dawned on me," Nancy recalled. "I'm crying!"

Nancy's migraine disappeared as her tears flowed freely. And there was more to come. By sharpening her attention, Nancy had allowed deep-seated emotions to break through into consciousness. Her tears were mixed with feelings of joy and relief at her discovery that she could produce tears. She understood the joy and relief. What was the sadness about?

Weeks later, Nancy attended an all-day session at the University of Massachusetts Medical Center Stress Reduction meeting room. This time, her neck, back, and head were throbbing with pain. But hours of "sitting meditation," a rigorous exercise in self-attention, allowed Nancy to become deeply aware of her inner and outer environment. Suddenly she felt the presence of her father, who had died suddenly seven years earlier of a heart attack at the age of fifty-two. For Nancy, then thirty-two, the loss had been heartbreaking. She described her father as a devoted family man to whom she'd felt very close.

Her eyes popped open. She focused on the rug beneath her, which caught her by-now sharp attention. The color, burnt orange, vibrated with familiarity. Memories began to pour forth: of her fifteen-year-old self, and her father, a construction worker who a quarter century earlier had helped build the University of Massachusetts Medical Center. She could actually remember watching as the burnt-orange rugs were brought into the just-completed building.

I looked up from the rug and out the window. All of a sudden I could see the center being built, the medical school undergoing construction. And I recalled sitting on the truck with my father, waiting for those rugs to come in. I was just being a kid with my dad. It happened to have been one of our happiest days together. We sat together and had a wonderful conversation. I hadn't cried from missing him. Now I thought, my God, he's here with me today. It was like I had gone back in time. The tears started to flow again.

Nancy said she cried tears of grief and joy. Grief because she realized how profoundly she missed him; joy because the memory was happy and renewed her sense of connection with her father. She left feeling "terrific," cherishing the memory and the opportunity to release her sadness, relieved of her physical pain and at peace with herself.

For Nancy, a rigorous practice of attention led to powerful healing connections. The burnt-orange rug was a striking coincidence, but had her mind and heart not been open, the memory would never have reached to her consciousness. "I had been in that room before, for many yoga and meditation sessions," said Nancy. "But during that all-day session, I was ready for what happened."

EXPRESSIVE ACTION: CONSCIOUS CHOICE, CLEAR COMMUNICATION

Diane was a middle-aged university professor, also married to a professor, who suffered from high blood pressure. The person who referred her to Gary Schwartz gave her the impression that she'd learn simple relaxation techniques to lower her blood pressure.

When Diane showed up for her appointment with Schwartz at the Yale Behavioral Medicine Clinic, she was surprised by what transpired. Instead of instruction in relaxation, Schwartz gave Diane a home blood pressure monitor. He told her to keep a record of when her blood pressure rose, and what she was thinking, doing, and feeling at the time. She was game, if only because she was worried about her hypertension.

Following Schwartz's instructions, Diane discovered that her blood pressure would skyrocket after certain social gatherings—even though she thought she was relaxed during them. But her blood pressure wouldn't rise after every social gathering. Schwartz encouraged her to continue keeping records, to search harder for a pattern.

As it happened, there was a pattern. Diane's blood pressure skyrocketed after large social gatherings—primarily parties attended by her husband's professional associates. By contrast, her blood pressure went *down* after small social gatherings and dinner parties with close friends. Why did the large gatherings produce so much stress? And why was she unaware of this connection until she began monitoring her blood pressure?

Diane's attention to her bodymind signal set the stage for connection. She realized that she felt intense social pressure at the large gatherings because her husband felt that his academic stand-

ing depended on their joint appearances. She resented the obligation and disliked the role of academic wife. She also disliked many
of the people for whom she was expected to perform. The gatherings triggered anger, anxiety, and strain—sure-fire contributors to
high blood pressure. But Diane had barely been aware of these
feelings until she made a conscious effort to attend.

Diane's "aha" experience begged the question: What expressive actions would protect her integrity and her health?

Gary Schwartz emphasizes that expressive action is not about
venting unbridled emotions. The key is a clear understanding of
your objectives. Then you can choose how to express needs and
feelings so that your objectives are met. For Diane, the answer was
not to tell her husband to go to hell, or to scold the snobbish and
obnoxious partygoers. Nor was the answer to avoid these gatherings altogether. Diane empathized with her husband's desire to
have his spouse appear with him.

Then what could she do to protect herself from internal stress
and high blood pressure? Together, Schwartz and Diane created
a strategy for expressive action, which included a list of options
she would employ flexibly—how and when she deemed them most
appropriate. These options were as follows:

1. Become aware of the people who most irritate you. Acknowledge your aggravation. Decide that you are not obliged to engage in repartee with them. If you do, and they exhibit rude
   behavior, politely excuse yourself. If they are overtly insulting,
   plainly state your objection and excuse yourself.
2. Become aware of those people you feel comfortable with, and
   spend most of your time with them. Don't be afraid to be selective. Remember your discovery that small, nurturing social gatherings actually lowered your blood pressure. To the extent that
   you can, transform the large unpleasant events into small pleasant ones by creating your own social space.
3. Tune into your body during the course of your conversations. If
   you are aware of tension, allow yourself to conduct a private
   body-scan relaxation technique. Be particularly aware of your

hands and face, which hold much of your tension, and let the muscles go slack.

4. Find the humor in the situation! Observe people's behavior (and your own) and recognize the amusing predictability or absurdity of it all.

5. Consider taking antihypertensive medication before such events, as a preventive measure. You would not have to take medication all the time—only in anticipation of such events. Knowing that your blood pressure can be controlled during such events might relax you sufficiently to reduce additional stress. Eventually, the other options may prove so effective that you would no longer require preventive medication.

6. Continue to monitor your blood pressure to learn how well your strategies succeed in reducing your stress and blood pressure. This is a form of biofeedback, in which you discover behaviors that meet your needs and reduce your symptoms. Don't feel that you always have to come home from social gatherings with normal blood pressure! Don't turn ACE development into another form of health fanaticism.

Diane used all of these approaches, in varying degrees and combinations. Over time, she not only controlled her blood pressure, she learned creative ways of coping. She discovered sides of herself she'd neglected—including her body-sense and her sense of humor. And she stopped feeling subterranean resentment toward her husband.

Diane's options for expressive action are a good guide for developing the "E" in ACE. Since there is no end to the variety of circumstances in which you might need to take expressive action, there can be no simple blueprint. But Diane's list demonstrates several fundamental principles:

1. In interpersonal, familial, and work circumstances that call for expressive action, recognize your range of choices. Don't take on obligations simply to please; discover your own reasons for accepting or rejecting them.

2. When a problem in a relationship or at work calls for change or

confrontation, you can employ communication skills to assert your needs, express your anger, or share your distress.

3. Uncover your needs and develop creative solutions to meet them.

4. Alter your attitudes toward unavoidable stressful circumstances by experimenting with other points of view—including a humorous outlook.

5. Find ways to protect your psychological well-being and prevent aggravation of symptoms—through relaxation, prophylactic medication, or any other health-promoting behaviors.

Every emotion carries a message. As in Diane's case, we should choose expressive actions based on an accurate reading of that message. With regard to anger, the best outlet is not the most explosive one. The best outlet is one that most effectively redresses the unfairness, insult, or injustice that you perceive. This calls upon your communication skills—a key to effective action. You will find a guide to assertive communication in chapter 5, "Assertiveness: The Hub of the Wheel."

The ACE Factor is an intrinsic capability that all of us share. When we tap this capacity, we access the wisdom of the bodymind. The quality of *attention* has been the focus of twenty-five hundred years of meditative practices in the East. The ability to *connect* sensations and emotions to consciousness has been a goal of Western psychology since Freud. Taking *expressive* action is a central feature of contemporary cognitive and dynamic psychologies.

When we attend, connect, and express, we make the best use of our internal compass—the bodymind. Relying on the guidance of our own feedback, we learn what paths to take in terms of diet, exercise, stress, creativity, family relationships, and spiritual concerns. We can discover how much work is too much; how much support we need; how much sleep we require; what kind of vacation we should take; how much time we need to grieve a loss; how actively we must fight for our interests at work. Then we can take expressive action to correct the present imbalances that weaken *all* of our systems.

ACE personalities are less likely to get sick, because they respond efficiently to stress. When the ACE personality attends, connects, and expresses, her bodymind systems return to homeostasis, that graceful state of balance described by physiologist Walter B. Cannon. When she does develop symptoms, her ACE abilities reduce the risks of full-blown disease. When she does develop disease, her ACE abilities may enhance her prospects for recovery.

Immune Power Personality development begins with the ACE Factor, because this trait encompasses an elemental awareness of our thoughts and feelings. A basic "mindfulness"—or moment-to-moment awareness—should be the starting point for bodymind healing. Why? Because we can work with sensations and emotions only when we can access them and properly interpret their meanings. Cultivating the ACE Factor starts with a simple awareness of the body, that fount of information vital to the healing endeavor.

ACE EXERCISES

EXERCISE 1: "SWEEPING THE BODY" MEDITATION

This first exercise is for enhanced attention. Stephen Levine uses a version of sweeping the body founded in Buddhist traditions.*

Levine suggests that you begin by lying down on a bed or mat in a comfortable position, breathing deeply and easily. Focus your attention on each discrete area of your body, starting with the very top of your head. Often it is useful to imagine your breath flowing into that region as you inhale and your breath flowing out of that region as you exhale.

As you linger on each area of the body, allow yourself fully to receive the sensations and feelings present in that moment. Try to accept those feelings—whether they are painful, pleasurable, frightening, unsettling, or delightful—with as little judgment as possible. Cultivate an attitude of loving acceptance toward your

---

* For tapes of Stephen Levine's guided meditations, write to Warm Rock Tapes, P.O. Box 108, Chamisal, NM 87521.

body and the sensations that arise from each region. Kindness toward yourself is the healing perspective.

The most difficult aspect of this practice is being able to tolerate the psychological or physical distress that may surface. Accepting those feelings without judgment—indeed, with loving kindness—is an intrinsic aspect of bodymind healing. Healthy attention to "negative" feelings does not mean holding fast to them, dwelling on them, or drowning in them. It means allowing them to flicker in and out of consciousness.

EXERCISE 2: LISTENING TO YOUR SYMPTOMS

The purpose of the second exercise, one of guided imagery, is furtherance of attention and connection. Gary Schwartz uses imagery because it involves mental processes closely linked to the brain's emotional centers and physiologic activators. In her book *Imagery and Healing*, Jeanne Achterberg argues that nonverbal images are a specialty of the right brain, where negative (emotional) feedback is centered. She adds that "the specific functions attributed to the right hemisphere, and the connections between it and other brain and body components, support the premise that images can and do carry information from the conscious fore to the far reaches of the cells."

Martin L. Rossman, M.D., is a leader in the use of guided imagery for the purposes of attention, connection, expression, and healing. He developed the following imagery exercise, excerpted here from his book *Healing Yourself,* in which your physical and/or psychological symptoms are the launch pads for inner exploration. This exercise will be most effective when practiced after "sweeping the body."

To begin, find a comfortable position in a quiet room. You can either read the script to yourself, have someone else read it, or make a recording of it on audiotape, to use as your own guide through the process.

Script:

Take a couple of deep, slow breaths, and let the out breath be a real "letting go" kind of breath. . . . Imagine that any unnecessary tension or discomfort begins to flow out of your body with each exhalation. . . . Then let your breathing take its own natural rate and rhythm, allowing yourself to sink a little deeper and become more comfortable with each gentle breath. . . .

When you are ready, direct your attention to the symptom or problem that has been bothering you. . . . Your symptom may be a pain, weakness, or dysfunction in some part of your body or a mood or emotions that are uncomfortable for you. . . . As you focus on the sensations involved, allow an image to appear that represents this symptom. . . . Simply allow the image to appear spontaneously, and welcome whatever image comes—it may or may not make immediate sense to you . . . just accept whatever comes for now. . . .

Take some time just to observe whatever image appears as carefully as you can. . . . If you would like it to be clearer, imagine you have a set of controls like you do for your TV set, and you can dial the image brighter or more vivid. . . . Notice details about the image. . . . What is its shape? . . . Color? . . . Texture? . . . Density? . . . How big is it? . . . How big is it in relation to you? . . . Just observe it carefully without trying to change it in any way. . . . How close or far away does it seem? . . . What is it doing? . . .

Just give it your undivided attention. . . . As you do this, notice any feelings that come up, and allow them to be there. . . . Look deeper. . . . Are there any other feelings present as you observe this image? . . . When you are sure of your feelings, tell the image how you feel about it—speak directly and honestly to it. (You may choose to talk out loud or express yourself silently.) . . .

Then, in your imagination, give the image a voice, and allow it to answer you. . . . Listen carefully to what it says. . . .

Ask the image what it wants from you, and listen to its answer. . . . Ask it why it wants that—what does it really need? . . . And let it respond. . . . Ask it also what it has to offer you, if you should meet its needs. . . . Again allow the image to respond. . . .

Observe the image carefully again. . . . Is there anything about it you hadn't noticed before? . . . Does it look the same or is it different in any way? . . .

Now, in your imagination, allow yourself to become the image. . . . What is it like to be the image? . . . Notice how you feel. . . . Notice what thoughts you have as the image. . . . What would your life be like if you were this image? . . . Just sense what it's like to be this image. . . .

Through the eyes of the image, look back at yourself. . . . What do you see? . . . Take a few minutes really to look at yourself from this new perspective. . . . As the image, how do you feel about this person you are looking at? . . . What do you think of this person? . . . What do you need from this person? . . . Speaking as the image, ask yourself for what you need. . . .

Now slowly become yourself again. . . . The image has just told you what it needs from you. . . . What, if anything, keeps you from meeting that need? . . . What issues or concerns seem to get in the way? . . . What might you do to change the situation and take a step toward meeting the image's needs? . . .

Now choose one way that you can begin to meet your symptom's needs—some small but tangible way you can fill part of its unmet needs. . . .

When you have thought of a way to begin meeting its needs, recall again the image that represents your symptom. . . . Ask it if it would be willing and able to give you tangible relief of symptoms if you take the steps you have thought of. . . . If so, let the exchange begin. . . . If not, ask it to tell you what you could do in exchange for perceptible relief. . . . Continue to dialogue until you have made a bargain or need to take a break from negotiating. . . .

Consider the image once more. . . . Is there anything you have learned from it or about it? . . . Is there anything that you appreciate about it? . . . If there is, take the time to express your appreciation to it. . . . Express anything else that seems important . . . and slowly come back to your waking state and take some time to write about your experience.

	SUN. 8 A.M.-5 P.M./ 5 P.M.-11 P.M.	MON. 8 A.M.-5 P.M./ 5 P.M.-11 P.M.	TUES. 8 A.M.-5 P.M./ 5 P.M.-11 P.M.	WED. 8 A.M.-5 P.M./ 5 P.M.-11 P.M.	THURS. 8 A.M.-5 P.M./ 5 P.M.-11 P.M.	FRI. 8 A.M.-5 P.M./ 5 P.M.-11 P.M.	SAT. 8 A.M.-5 P.M./ 5 P.M.-11 P.M.
Symptoms							
Activities							
Events							
Thoughts							
Emotions							
Body Sensations							

THE CAPACITY
TO CONFIDE

THEN, WHEN THE OTHERS HAD GONE, EACH MAN ABOUT HIS
BUSINESS, ROBIN TURNED ONCE MORE TO THE YOUTH. "NOW,
LAD," SAID HE, "TELL US THY TROUBLES, AND SPEAK FREELY. A
FLOW OF WORDS DOTH EVER EASE THE HEART OF SORROWS; IT IS
LIKE OPENING THE WASTE WEIR WHEN THE MILL DAM IS OVER-
FULL. COME, SIT THOU HERE BESIDE ME, AND SPEAK AT THINE
EASE."
—HOWARD PYLE, *THE MERRY ADVENTURES OF ROBIN HOOD*

Fifteen years ago, James Pennebaker, Ph.D., a psychology professor
at Southern Methodist University (SMU) in Dallas, was building a
theory about the healing mind. One aspect of his theory wasn't
new: that people who confide their deepest thoughts and feelings
about traumatic events will benefit psychologically. Pennebaker's
thesis was rooted in a venerable tradition that began with Freud,
one that lives on today in the offices of countless psychotherapists. But the other aspect of his theory was nothing short of radical: those who confide their deepest thoughts and feelings about

96

traumas will experience dramatic improvements in their *physical* health. Their cardiovascular systems will become more resilient. Their immune systems will respond with greater balance and vigor. And those who confide will resist and perhaps defeat diseases that would otherwise have overtaken them.

While a handful of mind-body scientists agreed with him, none had methodically tested whether people bolstered their health by confiding painful memories and feelings. The ramifications of this theory were monumental, but so was the scientific challenge to providing proof, hard evidence about the healing power of confession.

It all began in the 1970s, when Pennebaker's curiosity was piqued by a dramatic representation of the healing power of confession. He was asked by the FBI to deliver a series of talks to polygraph instructors, individuals trained to administer lie detector tests to crime suspects. Pennebaker spent time with these experts and was stunned when they all reported the same unusual finding. When suspects are initially hooked up to physiologic monitors—whether they are guilty or not—their nervous systems are racing. If the polygraph expert is able to induce a confession (something they are well trained to do), the suspect is booked and readied to go to jail. In most instances, the person is still required to take a further, confirming polygraph. That is when the peculiarity occurs.

"The person has already confessed, and now he's hooked up again to the monitors," explained Pennebaker. "He's about to go to jail, his personal life is ruined, his financial life—everything. His world is about to collapse. But it turns out he is physiologically very relaxed. His heart rate is low, his skin conductance is low, his blood pressure is low. Just before the handcuffs are put on and he's carted off, every polygraph instructor I've talked to says that the suspect will get up, warmly shake his hand, and thank him."

That's when Pennebaker realized that confession had potentially powerful effects on mind and body. He also surmised that the opposite of opening up—*inhibition*—was as stressful as confession was relieving. This led Pennebaker to two logical questions: If inhibiting thoughts and emotions is associated with internal stress, is it also a cause of ill health? And if confession is associated with relaxation, does it herald good health and well-being?

Shortly thereafter, Pennebaker recognized several opportunities to test whether inhibition is linked to physical illness. He was researching the causes of the eating disorder bulimia, in which people binge and then purge their food repeatedly. He decided to include this question on his survey of over 700 female undergraduates: "Did you have a traumatic sexual experience prior to age seventeen?" At a time when the prevalence of sexual abuse was not well understood, the fact that 10 percent of the college women answered "yes" took him aback. But no link turned up between early sexual trauma and bulimia. However, the students who reported sexual traumas did tend to suffer more illnesses in general.

The very same day he was pondering these results, Pennebaker got a call from an editor of *Psychology Today* magazine. "She asked if I had any ideas for questions for her general health survey to be completed by readers of *Psychology Today*. Funny she should ask."

Over 24,000 people completed and returned the survey, which included Pennebaker's question about early sexual trauma. Twenty-two percent of the women and 10 percent of the men said that they had experienced such a trauma before the age of seventeen. These respondents were more likely, later in life, to have developed ulcers, infections, heart problems, and illnesses in virtually every other health category. While Pennebaker was cautious in interpreting these results (it was not a truly random survey), he still thought they were "riveting." And Pennebaker was particularly intrigued by one fact revealed in the *Psychology Today* survey: *The vast majority of people who'd experienced early sexual trauma had not discussed the event with anyone.*

Pennebaker strongly suspected that the sexual traumas caused later illness primarily when people inhibited their painful thoughts and feelings about these experiences. Evidence was accumulating that supported his belief: In terms of physical health, how we handle trauma may be more significant than the trauma itself. By confiding our pains and fears, we reverse the harm to our bodymind caused by inhibition.

THE HEALING POWER OF CONFESSION

What damage is wrought by inhibition, and how does confession prevent disease? Pennebaker theorized that when we inhibit thoughts and feelings—particularly those tied to traumas—we engage in intense physiological "work." Inhibition is associated with high blood pressure, faster heart rate and breathing rate, and high skin conductance readings—all of which indicate that our autonomic nervous systems are working overtime. When we can never acknowledge or share our thoughts and feelings, this inner work intensifies until our nervous systems are chronically overtaxed. Confession can relieve that stress and enable our nervous systems to relax—often for the first time in years.

To test this theory, Pennebaker and his colleague, Sandra Beall, rounded up forty-six male and female students attending Southern Methodist University, and gave the following instructions to one group:

Write continuously about the most upsetting or traumatic experience of your life. Write about anything you want. Ideally about something you have not talked about with others in detail. Don't worry about grammar, spelling, or sentence structure. In your writing, I want you do discuss your deepest thoughts and feelings. Try to let yourself go and touch those deepest emotions and thoughts that you have. In other words, write about what happened and how you felt about it, and how you feel about it now.

Each student was then left alone in a room to write continuously for twenty minutes, a procedure that was repeated on the four following days.

After the study was completed, Pennebaker asked the participants to report their psychological reactions to the weeklong experience. The typical student said that the first day was disturbing. Anger and grief associated with his most private and painful memories had surfaced—feelings he hadn't quite realized were still simmering inside him. He grappled with these emotions for another day or two. By the fourth day of writing about this trauma, he began to feel better. By the fifth, he experienced a sense of calm and resolution. When it was all over, he realized that the exercise had had a healing effect on his mind and spirit. Whether it also had a healing effect on his body remained to be seen.

"The immediate impact of the study was far more powerful than we had ever imagined," said Pennebaker. "Several of the students cried while writing about traumas. Many reported dreaming or continually thinking about their traumas. Most telling, however, were the writing samples themselves. Essay after essay revealed people's deepest feelings and most intimate sides."

Pennebaker and Beall instructed a second group of students to write about the most traumatic event they could remember, but only the facts involved—not the feelings. A third group was told to write about their worst trauma, but only the feelings it aroused—no facts. A fourth group was asked to write each day about trivial events, such as the layout of their dorm room. They were the experimental control subjects.

The students completed the exercise and were followed for six months. They were asked about their general health, the number of days they had to restrict their activities or school attendance, and the appearance of specific symptoms—including colds, flu, ulcers, high blood pressure, skin disorders, gastric difficulties, and heart problems. Finally, records at the student health center were checked for the number of visits they made for illness. The study began in early November, and an increase in colds and flu was expected during the winter months.

When Pennebaker and Beall tallied their final results, they found that students who wrote about the facts and feelings involved in past traumas experienced significant health benefits for the six months following the weeklong writing experience. They had the fewest visits to the health center for illness and had to restrict their activities for the least number of days.

Students who wrote only about their feelings reported fewer symptoms of illness, but the overall health benefits to the facts-and-feelings group was far greater. From before the study to six months afterward, the control group—who wrote about trivial events—only got sicker. They reported more illnesses and logged many more visits to the health center.

Interestingly, students in the facts-and-feelings group were sicker before the experiment began, having visited the doctor more frequently during the prior two and a half months. After the procedure, however, their health improved while the number of illnesses among all other students jumped dramatically. The winter months took their toll on everyone—*except those who wrote about facts and feelings*. This finding would be Pennebaker's first strong clue that confiding was an Immune Power trait.

Pennebaker believed that confession was healing when people expressed their emotions *and* organized their thoughts about an upsetting event. Catharsis—the venting of emotion—would not be enough. And a dry representation of the facts would certainly bypass the person's emotional experience. Doing both offered people the prospect of catharsis *and* insight, which appeared to represent a powerful form of bodymind integration.

The final results would strike many people as bizarre. Skeptical observers found it hard to accept that students who sat and wrote about past traumas for twenty minutes on four consecutive days remained healthier for six months afterward. Even Pennebaker knew that these findings were so remarkable that they could not be fully trusted. So he continued his investigations.

Over the next five years, Pennebaker ushered a variety of populations—university staff members, unemployed white-collar workers, Holocaust survivors, and more students—through this same exercise. Over and over he demonstrated the astonishing benefits that come from writing about traumatic events. He's shown that the participants in his studies not only feel better emotionally, their physical health improves markedly. Compared to control groups, people who wrote about traumas made significantly fewer visits to the doctor and reported fewer symptoms of illness for months afterward.

Why was writing Pennebaker's preferred mode of confession? One reason was his own powerful experience of writing through a period of depression eight years earlier. Another was that writing bypassed the scientific muddle involved in having people confide to others. If research subjects unleashed their traumas to a confessor, their experience could be altered by the confessor's responses, no matter how subtle or seemingly dispassionate. Writing offered a unique opportunity for people to work through their pains with the fewest perceived expectations.

Nevertheless, Pennebaker wanted to find out if talking about traumas had similar healing effects. Avoiding the confessor problem, he had groups of students speak their confessions into a microphone, while control groups spoke of trivial matters. Those who spoke about their traumas experienced the same health benefits as those who'd committed them to writing. They not only suffered fewer bouts of illness, but they had a sense of emotional well-being that lasted months.

"Just putting upsetting experiences into words," Pennebaker explained, "has profound psychological and physical benefits for our participants."

One of the revelations of Pennebaker's work is that the capacity to confide appears to be stunted in a remarkably high percentage of people, whatever their age, class, or ethnic background. The students in Pennebaker's early research were all eighteen-year-olds with high grade-point averages who were attending an upper-middle-class college. "These are people portrayed as growing up in the bubble of financial security and suburban tranquility," said Pennebaker.

The irony is that story after story revealed deceit, tragedy, and misery. . . .

Our first study and every study since has completely shocked me in terms of the stories people tell. Someone in every study has experienced parents' divorce, sexual abuse, incest, rape, family suicide, drug and alcohol problems, public humiliation, or family violence. Occasionally, they've suffered from the death of a parent, a sibling, or a pet. The more common difficulties included coming to college, moving to a new town, the death of a grandparent.

Most of Pennebaker's studies, including his first, demonstrated that healing confessions had certain qualities. People invariably felt worse during the first few days, but if they allowed free rein to their thoughts and feelings, the rage or grief would lift and they'd start coming to terms with the painful events of their past. This unique letting-go experience was directly tied to health.

Consider the experience of Martha, one of Pennebaker's subjects. She was nine years old when she was molested by a teenager. When she first began writing about the abuse, Martha emphasized her feelings of embarrassment and guilt. By the third day, she expressed anger at the boy who'd victimized her. By the last day, she began to put the whole experience into perspective. Six weeks after the experiment, she reported, "Before, when I thought about it, I'd lie to myself. . . . Now I don't feel like I even have to think about it because I got it off my chest. I finally admitted that it happened. . . . I really know the truth and won't have to lie to myself anymore."

Martha's story exemplifies the healing sequence experienced by so many other writers in Pennebaker's studies. After several days of anger or grief, they develop new insights—connections between old feelings and current problems—and a broader perspective on their trauma. Along with this new outlook comes a sense of resolution and tranquility. As Martha's case underscores, this effect is due in large part to having confided to one's self: "I really know the truth and won't have to lie to myself anymore."

The depth and range of painful experiences that came pouring forth in his SMU laboratory led Pennebaker to conclude that a never-before-suspected percentage of otherwise "normal," "healthy" people harbor anguish about their pasts. They inhibit the memories and feelings associated with traumas, but with long-term destructive effects on their health and well-being. Now he seemed to have developed a relatively simple technique to help undo the damage of chronic inhibition on both spirit and body. Pennebaker's writing method revives people's ability to confide truths to themselves and others—a capacity that had become crippled by tragic circumstances and/or rigid teachings. But how did confession prevent diseases of immune dysfunction? By what mechanisms did his research subjects ward off colds, flu, allergies, autoimmune disorders, and other illnesses?

CAPACITY TO CONFIDE: AN IMMUNE POWER TRAIT

James Pennebaker is at home with people, and with computers. He seems most comfortable probing people's unconscious minds and creating ever-more ingenious experiments to quantify the results of his psychological sleuthing. He's not at home with test tubes and bodily fluids; the thought of drawing blood and sampling white cells confuses and vaguely nauseates him. But in order to prove that confession has a demonstrable effect on physical health, he'd have to show that the immune system was bolstered when people opened up. So Pennebaker joined forces with a leading team of PNI researchers: psychologist Janice Kiecolt-Glaser and immunologist Ronald Glaser. The husband-and-wife team had collaborated for years to produce evidence that the brain and immune system communicate and that emotions influence our defense against disease. Their laboratory at Ohio State University is considered one of the country's premier facilities for studying bodymind interactions.

The team decided to study confession in the lab and measure its effects on the participants' T-lymphocytes (or T-cells). To accomplish this, they would draw blood samples and separate out the T-cells. Ronald Glaser would then add to the mixture a substance known to stimulate T-cells, called a *mitogen*, and incubate the combination for two days. The mitogen Glaser used was PHA, a protein derived from red kidney beans. It causes T-cells to swell, become metabolically active, and prepare for battle. The reaction to PHA can be gauged by measuring how much of a radioactive substance the cells take up, since active T-cells will take up the most. Vigorous T-cells are one strong indicator of the potency of a person's defense against infections and cancer cells.

In the psychology lab at SMU, fifty students were randomly assigned to two groups. One group wrote their deepest thoughts and feelings about traumas; the other wrote about trivial topics. Blood was drawn from the study participants before and after the four-day writing exercise and again six weeks later. The blood samples were sent to the Glasers' immunology lab the next morning and tested for their reaction to PHA.

Compared to students in the control group, those who wrote about traumas showed a marked increase in the liveliness of their T-cells after the exercise. The PHA test showed that their defender cells had become highly active, ready to destroy invaders in their midst. (For a graphic comparison of T-cell activity between experimental and control subjects, see figure 3.1. Note that the strength of T-cells among the control members actually dropped.)

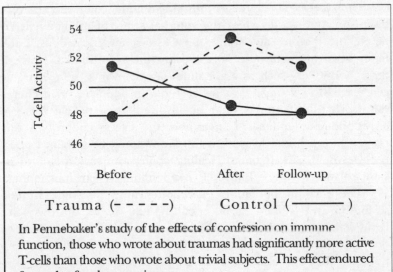

In Pennebaker's study of the effects of confession on immune function, those who wrote about traumas had significantly more active T-cells than those who wrote about trivial subjects. This effect endured for weeks after the experiment.

Figure 3.1   Immune function: response to confession.

The Immune Power benefits to students who wrote about traumas peaked soon after the weeks of writing, but they lasted over six weeks. Even at the time of the last blood test, these students' T-cell activity was stronger than it had been before the procedure. The findings were a dramatic testament to the concrete biological effects of emotional healing.

One key criticism of PNI studies is that increases in immune cell activity may not translate into real health benefits. Fortunately, Pennebaker could answer this concern, because he obtained the same health data on his research subjects that he had in all his previous studies.

The students who wrote about traumas also showed a stark drop in health center visits and reports of illness. The study helped to confirm the notion that when people confide previously inhibited thoughts and feelings, their nervous systems relax and their immune systems rally to a higher level of functioning. *When their immune systems improve, so does their overall health and ability to resist disease.*

One theory about the confession-immune connection is relatively straightforward. When the internal stress of inhibition is relieved, the person's autonomic nervous system "cools down," and fewer stress hormones are released into the bloodstream. Many of these hormones—such as adrenaline—are known to stifle immune cell reactions—*including the vigor of T-cells.* In addition, brain chemicals (such as endorphins) may be involved when people come to terms with past traumas. Conceivably, the excess endorphins that Gary Schwartz found to weaken immunity could be present in people who hold back traumas. Healing confessions may therefore restore balance to endorphin levels *and* immune system functioning.

The relationship among psychological well-being, immune strength, and vibrant good health may seem obvious. But Pennebaker and the Glasers are one of the few research teams to demonstrate a neat three-way connection among emotional, immunologic, and physical health—the tripartite relationship that is considered the gold standard of PNI research.

One other aspect of Pennebaker's collaboration with the Glasers was crucial. Among the confiding students, Pennebaker identified two groups—the "low" disclosers and the "high" disclosers. The high disclosers had chosen to write essays about experiences so upsetting that they had never before revealed them to anyone. Pennebaker hypothesized that the high disclosers, by using the writing procedure to exorcise previously held back thoughts and feelings, would benefit the most.

He was right. From the beginning to the end of the writing

procedure, the high disclosers had more vigorous T-cell responses than the low disclosers and the members of the control group. According to Pennebaker, it is no wonder that these students evidenced increases in T-cell activity. They had drawn upon the capacity we all have to acknowledge emotional truths to ourselves and work them through. The high disclosers demonstrated this Immune Power trait.

When I met Pennebaker at SMU, he described what seemed to be a groundswell of interest in his work, as more researchers discover that his writing technique is tremendously useful for people confronting past traumas, people with diseases, or just people who wish to stay healthy. Scientists at the State University of New York at Stony Brook and the University of Miami have repeated his studies and gotten similar positive results, and many clinicians report success with his techniques. I have spoken with several of these scientists, who now simply refer to the "Pennebaker method."

Why is the Pennebaker method so powerful? One reason is that so many of us have experienced devastating traumas that we've never disclosed to others. By confiding inner truths—first, to ourselves—we move away from inhibition toward expression, from incompletion to resolution. The burden lifted from the mind is also a burden lifted from the body. Our cardiovascular and immune systems begin to function with greater balance, harmony, and efficiency.

WHAT KIND OF WRITING HEALS?
ASK THE COMPUTER

Asking people what makes them healthy is an important but notoriously unscientific endeavor. James Pennebaker asked his research subjects to describe their writing experiences, and he was able to discern certain healing aspects: "letting go," expressing emotions, and gaining new insights and perspective on upsetting events. But these were not the most objective measures of experience. So to find out more about what kind of writing heals, Pennebaker turned to state-of-the-art technology.

Collaborating with Carmen Uhlmann, Pennebaker linked up computer keyboards hooked to physiological instruments. Thus, when subjects in his studies wrote confessions, the computer keys registered information from their fingertips about skin conductance (a physiologic measure of emotional arousal). This information was relayed to another computer that provided the researchers with readouts of the writer's bodily changes on a word-by-word, phrase-by-phrase basis. "The CARMEN machine, as we called it, allowed us to determine the features of language that are related to autonomic activity," commented Pennebaker.

What he found is that certain words were associated with increases in skin conductance and heart rate, which also was measured and synced to the computer. Specifically, negative emotion words—sad, hate, hurt, or guilty—were directly linked up with physiologic activation. On the other hand, positive emotion words—happy, joy, peaceful—were associated with reduced activation, a sign of physiologic relaxation. If the subjects worked through a trauma or problem, they tended to use cognitive words (such as "understand," "realize," "thought," or "knew") or causal words (such as "because," "why," or "reason"). These words, associated with reflection and insight, were linked to increases in physiologic arousal. However, if students wrote about a trauma or problem over the course of several days, telling the story over and over, Pennebaker observed a gradual decrease in physiologic activation.

What did these findings mean? They supported Pennebaker's belief that the writing process is not a thoroughly relaxing affair. It takes "work" to inhibit emotions, and it takes "work" to release those inhibitions. Confronting traumatic memories is upsetting, and this upset registers in our physiology. Even reflection and insight have a painful dimension. But in line with his earlier findings, the CARMEN machine showed that telling a story repeatedly—dealing with traumas from various angles and gleaning new insights—ultimately leads to a more relaxed state of mind.

But what about people who dwelled on the positive, and

whose physiology wasn't activated much at all? Might they not be perfectly healthy individuals who didn't need to work through any stresses or traumas? Perhaps. But the CARMEN machine couldn't answer that question. It only validated that negative emotions and cognitive insights caused physiologic arousal and that positive emotions did not.

The question was: Who got healthy? People who dealt with distressing emotions and worked through problems? Or people who maintained a positive view of upsetting events?

Pennebaker turned again to the computer, this time to analyze those narrative tales of "deceit, tragedy, and misery." Along with Martha Francis, he designed a software program called the LIWC—for Linguistic Inquiry and Word Counts. The LIWC allowed them to run their subjects' essays through the computer to determine total word counts, using the same emotional and cognitive categories. They entered the texts from 208 essays, written by subjects who participated in previous studies.

"Taken together," wrote Pennebaker, "students who evidenced the greatest improvements in physical health . . . were the ones who consistently expressed anxiety, sadness, and other negative emotion words. Expressions of happiness and enthusiasm, on the other hand, were more likely to be seen among students who did *not* evidence health improvements. . . ."

The people whose health improved used more "insight" and "causal" words as the days of writing progressed. They experienced many feelings and few insights at the beginning, but their cognitive awareness grew as they continued to write. Using this exquisitely fine analysis of linguistic content, Pennebaker had proved that people benefit most from writing when they release emotions, move toward reflection, and complete the process with greater self-awareness and understanding.

Pennebaker also had three independent "judges" rate each essay on narrative dimensions. How organized were the stories? How coherent? From day to day of writing, did the story progress and resolve, or deteriorate? Did the person become more accepting and optimistic about the trauma over time? As expected, the students whose health improved wrote essays that became progressively more coherent, organized, accepting, and optimistic. Students whose health did not improve wrote organized stories at the beginning, but they fell apart over time.

Pennebaker's computer findings—using the CARMEN machine and the LIWC program—added specificity and depth to his earlier research. He predicted the results, but the degree to which they fit his theory was "greater than I thought it would be."

Pennebaker briefly tried to translate his computer findings into a new set of guidelines for people writing about traumas. He gave subjects instructions before they wrote, emphasizing the use of negative emotion words, moving toward insight and causal words, and a coherent narrative shape. But these instructions only hindered the students' writing process and reduced the likelihood of health benefits. "People told us it was extremely hard to do this in a lock-step manner," Pennebaker commented. "It turned out to be a difficult unnatural cognitive task."

Pennebaker's computers confirmed that healing confessions are like any good stories. They have a beginning, middle, and end. They confront the anguish and ambivalence that is part of our human condition. But the best way to encourage this process was to simply create an atmosphere in which people felt free to follow their natural instinct for letting go.

IS CONFIDING A CURE FOR UNEMPLOYMENT?

One of James Pennebaker's most recent studies has special resonance, both for its psychological implications and for its relevance to our times. Over the past several years, Texas Instruments in Dallas has cut back thousands of its workers. Pennebaker and colleague Stefanie Spera decided to study a group of recently laid off male engineering executives and the effect that writing might have on their ability to bounce back and find work. All of them were in their fifties and had diligently climbed up the corporate ladder. Most had been with the company for over twenty years and had expected to retire there. As you might imagine, losing their jobs was a major life trauma for each of these men.

Pennebaker placed sixty of the laid-off workers into one of three different groups: For five days, they either (1) wrote about their deepest thoughts and feelings about the loss of their job; (2) participated in a "time-management" exercise, in which they kept a careful record, day by day, hour by hour, of their job-seeking activities; or (3) wrote about trivial subjects, as a control group.

After four months, Pennebaker had to call off the experiment. Thirty-five percent of those people who wrote about their feelings had gotten jobs as compared to 5 percent of the control group, while none of the "time-management" group had gotten work. In clinical trials of a new drug, if the investigators discover that the drug performs appreciably better than a placebo, the trial is called off and everyone gets the drug. So Pennebaker contacted the men in the control and time-management groups, explaining the good results for those who wrote about their feelings and offering to guide them through the same procedure. Only a few men signed up, a testimony to the fact that people who have not experienced the benefits of opening up are often reluctant to confront their feelings.

Would the difference in employment rates last over time? Pennebaker continued to follow these men for a total of eight months. At that point, 53 percent of the people who wrote about their loss had full-time jobs, while only 24 percent of the time-management group and 14 percent of the "trivia" writers were employed. In other words, the trauma-writers were more than twice as likely to get full-time work than the time-management people and four times more likely than the men who wrote about trivia! Moreover, the men who wrote about their feelings got jobs significantly faster than the others.

Why did so many of those who confessed get jobs? Pennebaker does not believe that the exercise increased motivation. "It was how they presented themselves in interviews. They had worked through their anger and bitterness and developed a balanced perspective. They were able to get past the trauma and get on with their lives with confidence." On the other hand, he saw the time-management exercise as a potentially destructive form of "obsessiveness training." By focusing relentlessly on their day-to-day struggles, they actually remained stuck in anger and anxiety.

Franklin was one of the men who was helped by the exercise. During the five days, he wrote exclusively about the impact his loss had on his relationship with his live-in girlfriend. After being laid off, he considered the option of seeking work in another city, and the question arose as to whether he and his girlfriend should relocate together. The issue remained unresolved and he was stymied, unable to make a decision or get a new job.

On the very first day of writing, Franklin confronted this issue head-on. The next day, he wrote about a long talk he and his girlfriend had the previous night. By the end of the week, the two of them had finally accepted a painful truth: They were simply heading in different directions. They parted as friends, and Franklin found himself a job. "Had he been in the time-management condition," Pennebaker remarked, "he would never have made this exploration, and I don't know how long it would have taken him to resolve these issues and move on."

Pennebaker is tracking down the medical records of these men to see whether confession also boosted their health. But any technique that helps people deal with the stress of job loss is bound to be health-enhancing. Pennebaker's method is powerful because many levels of behavior, consciousness, and physiology are touched by its healing effects.

"GOING WITH THE FLOW"

When people who write about traumas really allow their thoughts and feelings to flow—the process Pennebaker refers to as letting go—they seem to enter a different level of consciousness. Their physiology and mental state undergo rather startling transformations. People who spoke about traumas evidenced obvious changes in vocal tone, volume, and even accent as they let go and opened up. In the writing studies, handwriting style often changed markedly as people let go over the course of several days and sometimes even within the same day's writing. Pennebaker was astonished by samples in which people's style opened up as they opened up. One subject's handwriting changed day to day as she disclosed her feelings and achieved a sense of completion about having been sexually molested by her older brother when she was a child.

Pennebaker believes that most of us can reap the benefits of his writing technique. The motivation is manifold: We can relieve psychic tension, integrate thoughts and feelings, and deepen our self-knowledge. We also can write about traumas to prevent illness, since we may be fine-tuning our cardiovascular and immune systems in the process.

Interestingly, diary-writing or keeping a journal doesn't always foster that unique "letting go" experience. People often use diaries to record the trivia of everyday life, not to explore deeper cognitive or emotional states. Also, many of us naturally avoid such explorations. "In the back of our minds," Pennebaker said, "we think, 'I don't want to write in my journal today. It'll make me feel bad.' And you know, we're right. If we just write for one day we are going to feel worse." But all his studies demonstrate that a commitment to writing for three or four days is necessary for the shift to occur from anxiety to acceptance. Working out past traumas can't be accomplished in one sitting.

Could Pennebaker's method be used to cope with current traumas and problems, and produce similar benefits as those accrued when writing about the past? He explored this question in a study of students first coming to college. The experience amounted to a major upheaval: They'd left home and family for the first time and moved into a college dorm, where they had to fashion an entirely new network of support from a group of complete strangers. The freshmen wrote about their very deepest thoughts and feelings about coming to college, leaving parents and friends, and adjusting to a novel social environment. These students made fewer doctor visits for illness, while those who wrote about superficial topics showed a gradual increase in doctor visits. In fact, three days of writing about their difficult life transition produced health benefits that lasted four months. Apparently, said Pennebaker, writing about ongoing stressful circumstances "speeds up the coping process," thus protecting physical well-being.

Pennebaker is quick to emphasize that not everyone benefits from writing. There are roll-with-the-punches people who always seem to handle stress, no matter how intense, with graceful aplomb. But more than half of us, according to his estimate, stand to gain from applying a focused method of working through our feelings. Does this mean we should write on a daily basis? Not unless we really want to, says Pennebaker.

I think people know their own needs. I don't write in a diary every day. But I do when things are difficult, when I'm having trouble sleeping or I'm getting sick a lot.

People should pay attention to telltale signs. Look for changes in weight, feelings of depression, obsessing about a problem so much that your thoughts and dreams are filled with it. If you are ill or there's been a major life stressor, if you're having trouble with your spouse or employer, then writing can certainly help you cope more healthfully.

This balanced approach means that a rigid schedule of writing can be counterproductive. But so can a lack of awareness and commitment. Every Pennebaker study has shown that the health benefits tail off after several months. The message is simple: Sit and write for a few consecutive days when your intuition tells you that a past trauma or current problem has you by the throat. (See the writing guidelines at the end of this chapter.)

The need to confess is as much a bodymind phenomenon as the need to relax, to breathe deeply, or to rest. How do we know if we need to confide? Ask yourself: Am I continuously anxious about a current problem? Troubled by a past event? Disturbed by a present relationship and don't know why? Often, when we are anesthetized to sorrow, anger, or fear, we don't recognize the problem until it disables us. One overlap between the capacity to confide and the ACE Factor is becoming aware of the need to confront a painful issue or experience.

What if you've repressed past traumas so effectively that you have no memory of them? Can writing recover blocked memories?

Pennebaker believes it is possible, but not if you self-consciously strive for them.

> If you can get a person to sit down, really relax, and write about personal issues, he will naturally gravitate to those memories or feelings. This phenomenon emerged in a talking study I did several years ago. I call it the going-down-the-drain effect. It goes something like this: "I'm sitting in this room and the walls are brown and the carpet is gray, like the color of my socks. I've got to go back to my room when this is over to call my mother because I need her to send me a new pair of socks. We had a fight about something like this a few weeks ago and it reminds me of how uninvolved my father is." The next thing you know, the person is talking about suicidal thoughts when he began talking about socks. They spiral down toward repressed thoughts or memories until they catch themselves—"I'm not supposed to be thinking about this!" That's like putting in the stopper, but soon the going-down-the-drain effect starts all over again.

Having fully explored the possibilities of language, Pennebaker became intrigued by the work of dance therapist Anne M. Krantz, Ph.D., who suggested to him that movement was a form of expression that also could be used to confide past traumas.

Together, Krantz and Pennebaker designed a study of movement as a means of confession. Sixty-four college students were assigned to one of three groups. The first group entered a darkly lit room by themselves and were given this instruction: "For ten minutes, use any kind of movement you wish to express personally troubling feelings or thoughts about a past or present trauma that has affected, or is now affecting your life." A second group was given the same instruction, but then sent to a desk equipped with pen and paper. They were told to spend another ten minutes writing about their thoughts and feelings. A control group was instructed to do a routine of physical exercises for ten minutes. The experiment was carried out over three consecutive days.

Upon follow-up, the only people who experienced significant

health benefits belonged to the second group—those who combined movement and writing. They made fewer visits to the cam-
pus health center for several months following the experiment and
reported fewer illnesses. "The health effects were even stronger
than we usually get," Pennebaker commented. "Movement and
writing together may in fact be more potent than writing alone."
Even their grade-point averages increased.

Apparently, when we fully engage our bodies in confiding,
new dimensions of emotional experience are revealed. But we
must still use our cognitive faculties to gain new perspectives, and
writing serves that function most effectively. Emotional disclosure
is a bodymind affair, and getting our body into the act helps to
"shake loose" deeply held emotions and memories. Yet healing occurs on many levels—emotional and intellectual, intuitive and rational, heart-centered and brain-centered. When Pennebaker and
Krantz instructed students to move *and* write, they integrated these
levels into a whole experience. That brief, three-day exploration of
inner states promoted their health and well-being for the rest of
the school semester.

THE TALKING CURE:
CONFESSION, THERAPY, AND SUPPORT

With his writing method, Pennebaker proved that we don't necessarily need other people present—friends, family members, or
therapists—to confide. However, Pennebaker does acknowledge
that his subjects may have been helped by an awareness that
someone—in this case, professional psychologist(s) they barely
knew—would be reading their essays and somehow "receiving"
their expressions of anger, anguish, or resolution. At the same
time, the lack of face-to-face contact and the complete absence of
judgment allowed the "writers" to strip away their usual defenses.

Another benefit of writing is that it often helps to confide to
our selves before confiding to others. This allows us to explore
what we think and feel about a trauma privately before we take the
risky step of sharing our experience. Later, confiding in others

deepens self-understanding—we hear others' similar experiences, identify with their suffering, and get their support when we open up about our own struggles.

But there can be pitfalls when we confide in others, particularly when our motivation is to get support. For instance, you might confide an unsettling memory of early abuse to a friend, in the hopes of resolving your distress by having him show love and support. But what if he doesn't? What if he is horrified? Or anxious? Or hellbent on analyzing you to death? Then your healthy desire to work through the memory gets waylaid. (Classic problems emerge, for instance, when a victim of parental abuse confronts his or her abuser and is dismissed or condemned.) Sharing our pains with others can be healing, but it should not supplant our own efforts to resolve those feelings.

The obvious exception to this rule is psychotherapy. A good therapist enables you to make your own emotional explorations. His or her job is not to provide immediate support and instant analysis. His or her job is to facilitate your process and *then* to offer support and analysis. Group programs, such as Alcoholics Anonymous and Adult Children of Alcoholics, have strict rules about not rushing in to support or analyze people as they confide their inner truths. Indeed, the success of these groups appears to depend on their adherence to these rules.

Reliving emotions associated with past traumas is invariably a complex process. Although writing is useful for most people, it doesn't work for everyone. Moreover, writing is not a substitute for psychotherapy (although some individuals who do not otherwise need psychotherapy may get what they need from writing alone). For traumas that cause profound psychological or physical symptoms later in life, psychotherapy is recommended.

Most forms of psychotherapy elicit the capacity to confide, and Pennebaker cites a number of neglected studies demonstrating the health-promoting effects of psychotherapy. He also has observed firsthand individuals who have overcome serious illness— once they confided past traumas.

Laura is a thirty-five-year-old lawyer who suffered through the divorce of her parents when she was ten. Two years later her mother remarried a man who sexually abused Laura on and off until she was fifteen, at which time she left home to live with an aunt. She never spoke to anyone about it—including her mother. Laura recounted the anguish of that period of abuse at age twenty-four, when she was diagnosed with uterine cancer.

I had always been close to my mother. The divorce had nearly killed her and she was so happy with Jock [the stepfather]. If she had known what Jock was doing to me, it would have broken her heart. I wanted to tell her so much. Looking back on it all, the very worst thing was that I couldn't talk to my mother any more. I had to keep a wall between us. If I wasn't careful, the wall might crumble and I'd tell her everything. The same was true of my friends. I'd go out with my girlfriends and we would all giggle about boys and dating. Their giggles were real, mine weren't. If they had known what was happening in my bedroom they would have died.

Pennebaker believed that Laura's constant holding back contributed to her health problems. After her cancer diagnosis, she entered psychotherapy and used that to explore and resolve her trauma and abuse. Today, she has fully recovered from cancer. She also has been happily married for twelve years.

Could Laura's opening up to herself and her therapist have actually contributed to her recovery from cancer? Although such a possibility can never be proven in one individual case, Pennebaker's research showed that confession strengthens cells of the immune system that may be able to eliminate cancer cells spreading through the body. Psychotherapist Lawrence LeShan has long suggested that cancer patients who confide their pains, fears, and hopes in psychotherapy can invigorate their natural defense against cancer. He has documented scores of such cases.

The "raw material" that emerges in therapy forms the basis for personal transformation. We can reach that "material" in different ways—therapy, talking, writing, even movement. What matters most, however, is choosing to access that fearless part of our being that is capable of confession.

CULTURES OF CONFESSION

Many cultural institutions offer socially sanctioned vehicles for confession: Psychotherapy, the Catholic church, and the recovery movement rely, in large part, on the power of confession. In general, Pennebaker believes that we help ourselves psychologically and physically when we confess, whether to a therapist, a priest, or a twelve-step group. But he cautions against giving ourselves over completely to any institution that holds open its arms with promises of comfort and absolution in the wake of our confessions.

"If you look at different cultures," Pennebaker explained, "any institution that promotes confession is among the most powerful in that culture—whether it's the church or AA or the witch doctors in tribal societies. But one casualty might be your reality. Once you're invited to open up, the experience of the invitee is going to be structured according to the values of that institution." For that reason, Pennebaker has tried to keep his writing and talking exercises as "value-free" as possible.

Pennebaker, whose relaxed manner seems to invite trust, may be particularly successful in eliciting confessions precisely because his approach is value-free, rational, and flexible. In everyday life, people don't want or need to be told how often, how quickly, or how intensively they must express emotions.

When our capacity to confide is fully developed, the feelings we "get off our chest" don't simply float off into space. They work their way through our minds, engaging cognitive levels of awareness through which we make sense of our experiences. Thus, we come to understand how our traumas have changed our lives, relationships, and world views. These insights facilitate the healing connections I spoke about in the last chapter on the ACE Factor. In Pennebaker's view, this second phase of insight is as crucial as the first phase of unadulterated expression.

Grave psychological traumas leave our psyches in a divided state. Our mental defenses throw up walls of separation between thoughts and emotions, memories and consciousness. Talking about these events, and especially writing about them, is akin to putting back together the fragmented psychic puzzle left scattered after the experience of a disintegrating trauma. The result is greater psychological well-being *and* physical health.

By finding our own way to confide inner truths, we are taking care of ourselves in the best sense of that phrase. Whether we write or talk, confide to ourselves or others, turn to a minister, rabbi, healer, or therapist, we are engaged in a healing endeavor. Confiding to ourselves is key, but the second phase is confiding in others—few experiences are more restorative than opening up to someone who listens and empathizes. But it's important to remember that healthy confession does not require a kindly confessor. More to the point, each of us can be our own kindly confessor when we put pen to paper and work through our grief, fear, anger, and confusion.

James Pennebaker's work on confession has far-reaching ramifications for mind-body health. Those of us who wish to prevent or treat illness through drugs, diet, exercise, and stress management alone may be missing a piece. Lingering tensions, simmering angers, unspoken disappointments, current anxieties, and privately held grief can work their damage underground, where we can't see or feel their effects. Pennebaker's method offers a structured way to lure these buried feelings from their hiding place, to transfer them onto paper or speak them aloud to others, and thus to release ourselves from their inner grip. Both mind and body are thus freed from the grueling work of inhibition. Ultimately the positive effects on our spirit and our health may be immeasurable.

GUIDELINES FOR THE CAPACITY TO CONFIDE

WRITTEN CONFESSIONS

Write continuously about an upsetting or traumatic experience. Don't worry about grammar, spelling, or sentence structure; discuss your deepest thoughts and feelings about the experience. Write about any subject—ideally, one that you have kept relatively private. It is critical, however, to let go and touch your deepest emotions and thoughts. In other words, write about what happened; write how you felt about it; and write how you feel about it now.

For here-and-now traumas or ongoing stressors, write continuously about the current life problem that most troubles you. Here are additional pointers provided by Pennebaker:

- Although writing about a traumatic experience is a particularly powerful approach to healthy confessions, it is not required. Write about issues or feelings that are most relevant to your current life circumstances.
- Do not stick assiduously either to the objective experience (facts) or your reactions to it (feelings). In order to "go with the flow," write about facts *and* feelings. Explore both the objective reality of events and your emotional responses.
- Write whenever you want and feel you need to.
- Don't use writing as a substitute for action or as an avoidance strategy. A telltale sign is when you sense that you're writing *too* much.
- You may feel distressed for a short period of time after writing. These negative feelings usually will dissipate within an hour or two. Soon you will develop a sense of relief and resolution. If you are in the midst of a life crisis—such as a death or divorce—don't expect to feel instant relief. You should, however, have a better understanding of your emotions and be able to achieve a little distance and perspective.

Pennebaker's recent physiological research has led him to develop certain additional guidelines for healthy confessions. Here is how he frames these suggestions—*not* designed to be followed as mandates but as loose parameters to keep in the back of your mind.

No pain, no gain. An initial willingness to confront negative emotions and experiences is necessary before the letting go process can lead to positive emotions associated with physiologic relaxation and psychological well-being.

Allow the narrative to develop. Self-consciously striving to create a coherent narrative to explain a traumatic or unsettling experience may be unhealthy at the beginning of therapeutic writing sessions. Movement toward the development of narrative is ideal. In other words, don't try to start with a constructed story—construct one as you proceed on an organic journey of discovery.

Guide your own therapy. Writing itself is a powerful therapeutic technique. Don't allow yourself to be hamstrung by too many thoughts about how you should do this. Be aware of the above-mentioned guidelines—no pain, no gain; and the shape of healing narratives—but don't dwell on these factors when you write.

Allow yourself to be engaged on emotional and cognitive levels. Both catharsis and insight, usually in that order, are involved in the capacity to confide. Don't feel obligated to stress one over the other. Let both feelings and thoughts flow naturally, recognizing that both levels of consciousness are related to improvements in health.

GUIDELINES FOR SPOKEN CONFESSIONS

Trust. Monitor your level of trust in people to whom you wish to confide; avoid those you feel ambivalent or untrusting toward.

Nonjudgmental responses from the listener. Confiding in people who readily pass judgment can leave you feeling worse than before. If someone you otherwise trust tends to pass judgment readily, state your need before confiding: "Please do not criticize or judge what I am about to tell you."

Time and space. One of the most powerful methods for confiding, particularly with friends or spouses, is to request that they remain completely silent while you speak, not even interrupting once with an "uh-huh," or "I understand," until you complete your confession. This can last anywhere from three to thirty minutes. The experience of being heard, with no need to accommodate the listener's needs or responses, is a liberating experience—often for both individuals. If both of you need to confide, you can take turns.

Be conscious of ulterior considerations in your choice of confidant. Ask yourself why you have chosen a particular individual. Is there some secret you want the person to know? Are you trying to get a particular response—to extract sympathy or exact revenge? Don't judge your own motives harshly, but be aware of them because they could diminish the therapeutic quality of your confession.

MOVEMENT AND WRITING

James Pennebaker's research collaboration with Anne Krantz demonstrated the therapeutic value of confessions involving movement and writing. Two groups were given movement instructions, one of which also was asked to sit and write afterward. Since only the movers who wrote received significant health benefits, I recommend movement followed by writing.

In conducting the study, Dr. Krantz gave specific instructions to people regarding how to use movement to express feelings about events. You can follow the same guidelines.

Move around a free space within a room for ten minutes. Take off your shoes, make yourself comfortable, and create a private atmosphere that is most conducive for you. Concentrate completely on what you are doing. Express through movement your deepest thoughts and feelings about the issue or event that is most significant in your life. It may be a traumatic experience or one that has been problematic or upsetting. It may be a current situation or one from your past. But it should be something still very much on your mind. The important thing is to move and express that which you have never been able to say in words. Now you will say it with your body and movement. How you do this and what you do is entirely up to you. There is no right or wrong way to "move" your feelings. It's your body and only you know what you feel inside. Start with what makes sense to you. You can move on the floor, stand, or use the room in any way. You can then move slowly or quickly; roughly or softly. You might use areas of your body that you don't always use expressively, such as your spine, feet, face, or shoulders. The only requirement is to keep moving the whole time. Even if you are expressing being tired or feeling rigid, there is always a way to translate these states into movement.

4

HARDINESS: COMMITMENT, CONTROL, AND CHALLENGE

HUMAN VITALITY IS SO EXUBERANT THAT IN THE SORRIEST DES-
ERT IT STILL FINDS A PRETEXT FOR GLOWING AND TREMBLING.
                                    —JOSÉ ORTEGA Y GASSET

Suzanne C. Ouellette, Ph.D., has spent two decades reconstructing
the concept of stress. When she entered the mind-body field in the
1970s, she was among the first to question the prevailing
oversimplified notion of stress as the agent of disease. Any number
of events, many of them normal life passages such as a change in
jobs, schools, living conditions, or relationships—even joyous occasions, such as marriage and pregnancy—were being indicted as
causal factors in so-called stress-related illnesses. From the beginning, Ouellette questioned these findings. She never doubted the
scientific honesty of the stress researchers, but their conclusions
were hard to swallow. Even worse was the media's cartoon-bubble
version: "Stress kills! Avoid stress!" Ouellette did not accept that
stress and change—facts of life as unavoidable as death and
taxes—would invariably make us sick.

In her view, each of us has inner resources we can draw upon to cope with personal travails. She named a personality trait that defined our strengths in the midst of crisis: *hardiness.* Ouellette believed that hardiness was the key characteristic of people who endured stress while maintaining peak levels of mind-body health. As she saw it, hardiness was three qualities rolled into one. Often referred to as the "three Cs," they are: *commitment, control, and challenge.*

In a series of landmark studies at the University of Chicago, Ouellette went on to demonstrate the role of hardiness in human health. For over twenty years she has contributed a wealth of ideas and findings that enrich the concept of an Immune Power Personality. Today Ouellette is professor of psychology at the City University of New York, where she continues her hardiness research.

In the mid 1970s, Ouellette was completing her doctorate in psychology at the University of Chicago. She had spent two years at Yale Divinity School, studying existential philosophy. The works of Jean-Paul Sartre, Søren Kierkegaard, Martin Heidegger, and Friedrich Nietzsche, philosophers who wrote about the search for purpose and meaning in life, laid some of the philosophical groundwork for Ouellette's later scientific studies.

Another inspiration was Viktor Frankl, a survivor of Nazi concentration camps who wrote about his experiences. Frankl described how he endured such unspeakable circumstances. He later developed a form of therapy based on the search for meaning that he felt had saved him. In his book *Man's Search for Meaning,* Frankl wrote, "Even the helpless victim of a hopeless situation, facing a fate he cannot change, may rise above himself, may grow beyond himself, and by so doing change himself."

Ouellette was moved by Frankl's writings, and she embraced his philosophy. If people undergoing such experiences could survive and ultimately thrive, couldn't others in less harsh circumstances do the same? In so doing, couldn't they also protect their health and well-being? These were questions Ouellette began to pursue in 1975.

The stress studies at that time investigated whether stress caused illness, but they did not explore whether people's capacity to cope buffered the impact of stress on the body. For this reason,

Ouellette wondered whether stress *alone* could really be such a powerful predictor of ill health. She scoured the stress literature and came to the conclusion that, as stressful events accummulate, people's risks of illness do increase. But the statistical link (.30) is relatively weak. With further investigation, Ouellette found out why:

> If you look at plots of subjects' stressful life event and illness scores, you notice something interesting very quickly. Although there are a number of subjects showing a fit between stress and illness ... *there are more subjects who do not conform to this neat pattern.* Most telling for us are those that represent subjects who were given high stressful life event scores but low illness scores. Unfortunately, the stress literature tells us very little about this last group of subjects.

This was the group that interested Ouellette. Who were these people with many stressful life events and few illnesses? Did they have a sense of purpose that saw them through hard times? Did they have other personality traits that enabled them to resist illness despite their stress levels? If so, what were they?

Ouellette thought that stress could actually bring out the best in people—at least some of the time. It was a radical concept then, and it remains radical today. Truly groundbreaking was the notion that "the best in people" would not only keep their creativity and spirits afloat, it also would protect their physical health.

Ouellette referred to "the best in people" as their "resistance resources." These are social factors or personality traits that enable people to stave off the ravages of stress, including illness. In her first major study on stress and illness, she searched for resistance resources. What was that "something" possessed by people who stayed healthy under stress?

"It seemed to me that whatever that 'something' was, it would have to be multifaceted," said Ouellette.

> You would have to evaluate more than one piece of the person. Based on my evolving concepts, this personality seemed

to have three aspects. We already knew quite a bit about the value of a sense of control. That was clear in the psychological literature. The other two pieces came from different spheres, but they were applicable. Commitment was similar to the concept of engagement. Some research suggested that being engaged or involved was important for longevity. Finally, challenge was rooted in both existential philosophy and cognitive psychology. Challenge meant that people could handle sudden changes. They not only had the flexibility to cope with sudden shifts, they actively did not want life to stay the same.

The three Cs—commitment, control, and challenge—sprang from Ouellette's background in philosophy, her training in personality psychology, and her intuitive grasp of the way people roll with the punches. She also was influenced by preliminary interviews she conducted with a group of telephone company executives. Some of these businessmen were under great stress but remained superhealthy. Their sense of commitment, control, and challenge was clearly evident. Ouellette and her collaborator during the early days of her research, psychologist Salvadore R. Maddi, began to call them the "hardy" types. The term stuck. *Hardiness* would consist of three distinct but intertwined qualities: *commitment, control, and challenge.*

Ouellette designed a lengthy questionnaire that tapped all three Cs. It was a measure of each C as well as a measure of overall hardiness. Ouellette continued to observe various populations, and her understanding of how people coped with stress informed her development of this sensitive "instrument." Here is her understanding of the three Cs.

Commitment. People strong in commitment find meaning and purpose in their work and relationships. They are capable of wholehearted involvement in their activities, and choose creative pursuits and relationships based on their potential meaningfulness. By contrast, people low in commitment lack meaning and purpose. They tend to be alienated from their work and/or relationships. Such individuals shrink from commitment out of fear, uncertainty, or boredom.

Control. People who demonstrate control believe and behave as if they have influence over life circumstances. In the areas of their lives that matter most, they have a sense of mastery, confronting problems with confidence in their ability to devise and implement effective solutions. People with a healthy sense of control should be distinguished from control *freaks,* who try to manipulate others' behavior and responses. Healthy control implies empowerment; unhealthy control implies power hunger. At the other extreme, people low in control feel powerless to influence events taking place around them. Lacking self-confidence and initiative, they have a tendency to respond to extreme pressure with helpless resignation.

Challenge. Individuals high in challenge rise to the occasion because they view problems as challenges to overcome, not threats to their well-being. Whether they articulate it or not, people with challenge know that stress and change represent opportunities for growth. People who lack challenge avoid change instead of creatively adapting to change. Comfort and security are their highest values, overriding curiosity, exploration, and risk-taking.

Commitment, control, and challenge were Ouellette's building blocks of healthy coping. People who responded to loss, instability, and change by activating their inner resources would likely weather even the most trying of times.

HARDINESS AND HEALTH IN THE CORPORATE WORLD

Armed with a questionnaire to test for the three Cs, Ouellette and Maddi began to search for the ideal population to study. It had to be a group of people who were under extreme stress, so Ouellette and Maddi could test whether hardiness helped to protect them from physical afflictions.

First, they settled on a general population to investigate: corporate executives, often considered as classic stress victims. Next, they zeroed in on a specific company: Illinois Bell Telephone. After a preliminary investigation of their executives, Ouellette and Maddi realized they had struck gold. Illinois Bell had been caught in the most sweeping reorganization in corporate history, the breakup of AT&T. The upheaval at Illinois Bell would provide Ouellette and Maddi with an opportunity to test their hardiness hypothesis.

Executives at every level within the company were forced to cope with the centralization of operations and consolidation of offices and jobs. New responsibilities were thrust on many executives, and they were required to quickly learn new skills. Many jobs were threatened. When Ouellette first began interviewing middle- and upper-level executives at Illinois Bell, she instantly recognized that stress levels—and illness—were on the rise.

Ouellette's theory gained credibility as she talked with the men. (The vast majority of executives were male.) They reported a range of symptoms, from colds, to high blood pressure, to severe back pain. But other equally stressed executives were in extremely good health.

Ouellette began by conducting extensive one-on-one interviews with the executives. She had been introduced to the company's medical director, Dr. Robert Hilker, who paved the way for her seven years of research with nearly 700 Illinois Bell workers. Hilker himself had seen evidence that some workers thrived under difficult conditions, and so he was a curious and sympathetic supporter.

Some of the workers fit her hypothesis to a tee. Here from *The Healing Brain* by Robert Ornstein and David Sobel is Ouellette's tale of one such encounter with an Illinois Bell executive, as told at a research symposium:

He arrives forty-five minutes late, trench coat flying behind him, papers under his arm. Then he makes a beeline for my secretary's desk and begins calling people. He's got to call many people to let them know where he's going to be in the next forty-five minutes, while I'm in my office waiting, hearing all these phone calls. He comes in and I've prepared what's going to be a fairly difficult conversation with him about his alienation from other people, but it's difficult to do because the phone keeps ringing and every time it does he jumps up because he's convinced it's for him, and he can't talk in my office because he's so convinced he has to run out to the secretary's office. This happens three times and we're not getting anywhere.

He says to me, "Look, I really need to take all these calls, they're very crucial. But you may have something here. So why don't you talk into my tape recorder?" So he pulls out a tape recorder, puts it on my desk and says, "I'll listen to it at night when I have a chance."

[He said] "I'm thinking of a major change; I'm thinking of leaving the phone company and going to this little electronics company that's a much more risky operation, and I figure if what you're going to do is free, I'll come and get the advice. Maybe it'll be helpful." This man's protocol showed high stress and high illness. He was only in his thirties, but he had hypertension, peptic ulcer, and migraine headaches: many symptoms as well as diseases.

What stands out from his personality questionnaire is alienation, not only from himself but also from other people. He also shows some low control, but the main factor is the alienation, the lack of commitment that is striking.

Contrast this portrait to her description of a hardy individual from *The Hardy Executive*, which she co-authored with Dr. Maddi:

A small, neat man in his mid-fifties, Chuck introduced himself as someone who enjoys solving problems. In the company, his specialty is customer relations, even though he was trained as an engineer. His eyes light up as he describes the intricacies of investigating customer needs and complaints, determining the company's service capabilities and obligations, formulating possible solutions to disputes that appear fair to all parties, and persuading these parties to agree. He thinks customer relations work is more demanding as the company streamlines and approaches reorganization. Asked in a sympathetic manner whether this is making his job unmanageable, he notes an increase in stress but adds that the work is becoming all the more interesting and challenging as well. He assumes that the role he plays will become even more central as the company's reorganization accelerates. He looks forward to this and has already formulated plans for a more comprehensive approach to customer relations.

Chuck had other stresses in his life, including the death of his two-year-old grandson and his daughter's divorce, but he handled them the same way he handled the turbulence at work: with commitment, control, and challenge. He was also in excellent health, having never suffered a serious illness in his life.

Such striking cases were strong anecdotal testimony to the health-protecting aspect of hardiness. The next move for Ouellette was a systematic study of the Illinois Bell executives.

For her first investigation, Ouellette gave a large group of the businessmen the famous Holmes-Rahe stress test (a checklist of stressful life events), a checklist of symptoms and illnesses, and her new hardiness questionnaire. She was able to identify 100 highly stressed executives who got sick and another 100 equally stressed men who stayed healthy.

What distinguished these two groups? Ouellette discovered that the healthy executives were not younger, better educated, wealthier, or higher on the corporate ladder than their associates who became ill. There was only one significant difference: The healthy executives demonstrated greater hardiness.

Encouraged by these results, Ouellette and Salvadore Maddi took their research further. To prove conclusively that hardiness was a buffer against the harmful effects of stress, they had to conduct a *prospective* study, tracking their subjects over time to see who got sick and who stayed well. They evaluated 259 of the executives for stress, hardiness, and health, then retested them several times over two years.

First, they checked whether increasing stress among the executives had, in fact, been linked to greater illness. Overall, the tide of illness did rise along with levels of stress, but it was more like a ripple than a wave. They found a weak statistical relationship (0.23) between stress and illness, which left room for "many other factors influencing whether illness results."

Was one of those factors hardiness? Ouellette and Maddi wanted to know whether highly stressed men who were hardy at the beginning of the study were less likely to get sick two years down the line.

The data was unequivocal. Executives who scored high on Ouellette's hardiness measure had significantly fewer bouts with severe illness than those who lacked hardiness. In fact, *when hardy executives confronted serious stress, they were only half as likely to get sick.*

"This study provided a basis for thinking that hardiness mattered to health," says Ouellette. "We finally had a reason to take seriously the notion that people differed in how they dealt with stress, and that these differences had to do with the way they experienced themselves in the world."

HARDINESS, EXERCISE, AND SOCIAL SUPPORT

The skeptic may wonder: Was hardiness the true reason for better health among certain executives? Could they simply have maintained better health practices?

To find out, Ouellette and Maddi had the executives report on behaviors such as smoking, alcohol intake, diet, drug use, relaxation and meditation, and physical exercise. Overall, hardiness was not a reflection of the well-being that comes from a healthy diet, exercise, or relaxation regimen. Looking at exercise alone, the men who worked out reaped health benefits, but the hardy men who *also* exercised were considerably healthier.

Social support has been established as a protector of health and well-being. Ouellette and Maddi wondered if the hardy executives were healthier because they had more support. They found that the hardy executives had slightly more support from coworkers and family members, but the statistical link was "too small to raise suspicion that hardiness and social support merely reflect the same thing."

Perhaps the "unhardy" workers had more extensive family histories of illness than the hardy executives. To test this possibility, Ouellette and Maddi reviewed family histories for evidence of genetically linked diseases such as rheumatoid arthritis, heart disease, and cancer. Not surprisingly, workers with high-risk profiles for certain diseases were more likely to contract them, especially when the going got rough at work. But the hardy executives stayed healthier than the less hardy—*even if they had more extensive family histories of disease.* As Ouellette points out, "Biology is not destiny."

Apparently, we can counterbalance genetic conditions, over which we have no control, with resources we consciously bring to bear in coping with stress. In the stress wars, our controllable assets include personality hardiness, exercise, and social support.

What happened when people combined all three resources? Ouellette uncovered these remarkable findings:

- For executives with none of these resources, the likelihood of illness was 92 percent.
- For executives with one of these resources, the likelihood of illness was 72 percent.
- For executives with two of these resources, the likelihood of illness was 58 percent.
- For executives with all three of these resources—who were hardy, exercised, and got social support—the likelihood of illness *was only 8 percent.*

In a fascinating analysis, the researchers were able to discern which of the three resources was the most significant health protector. Hardiness emerged as "by far the most powerful of the three," not only in preventing current illness but in predicting health one year later.

There is no doubt about the health-promoting power of exercise and social support. But the presence of hardiness, an Immune Power trait, enabled people to reap optimal benefits from these proven promoters of health. Recent findings from PNI research help to explain this phenomenon. In many respects, hardiness is the precise opposite of helplessness. People who lack the three Cs are susceptible to feeling unmoored in the midst of change, instability, and tumult. Many animal studies have shown that helplessness suppresses the immune system.

Ouellette has an intriguing theory about why hardy people benefit more from social support. In her research, she broke down support into two categories: at work and in the family. Unsurprisingly, the executives who received support from their superiors at work developed fewer illnesses. But a peculiarity emerged regarding family support. As expected, the hardy executives who experienced more support at home had lower risks of illness. However, when hardiness was low, family support only served to *increase* illness.

Hardy individuals seek and utilize social support from their families in a healthy manner, to bolster their self-worth and self-efficacy. But people low in hardiness sometimes use support to reinforce their position of alienation, passivity, and dependence. Ouellette observed many "unhardy" workers who faced problems at work and who used their wives for ego damage control—not for discussion of potentially constructive solutions. (Such workers would rather be told how wonderful they were by their wives than engage them in an exploration of their work stresses and new strategies for coping.) The hardy workers didn't lean on their wives to distract them from their misery. They sought encouragement and engagement on relevant issues.

For Ouellette, this was the litmus test for healthy social support: Do interactions with the family encourage growth and change? Or do they reinforce fear, inaction, and dependence?

Consider the case of Andy, which was described in *The Hardy Executive.* Faced with new responsibilities, new supervisors, and continual job insecurity, he was hard hit by the changes at the company. He saw himself as a tiny link, whose placement in the larger chain was repeatedly being switched around. At times, he just wanted to retire and forget all his anxieties.

Andy took his problems home to his wife, from whom he

sought constant reassurance and support. Their relationship had begun in college, when he had finally escaped a difficult family situation. Fearful and insecure, Andy was happy to have found someone who gave him the emotional nurturance he'd never gotten at home. This set the pattern for their relationship, which became strained over many years as Andy's wife came to resent her one-way role as caretaker.

Now the strain was increasing due to Andy's fears and stresses at work. He also felt overwhelmed by the responsibilities of parenting four children. Fights with his wife erupted often, because she was tired of hearing about his problems without equal time for hers. She also knew that she could not liberate Andy from his rut. He only wanted to be nurtured; he didn't want help in solving problems and taking greater responsibility for his work and home life.

When Ouellette interviewed him, Andy's view of his future was bleak. He was disappointed with his life, and his dreams were ill defined, except for his wish to be admired and loved by people. For Andy, "everything seemed hard, and little seemed possible." In addition to his mental strain, which caused sleeplessness and appetite loss, Andy had bouts of high blood pressure and heart palpitations. Several years earlier, he had developed a stomach ulcer, for which he continued to take medication.

In contrast to Andy, Bill was a fifty-five-year-old phone company executive who scored high in hardiness. When Ouellette met him, he "had a twinkle in his eye and an easy, relaxed manner." Bill's job was to plan commercial telephone services, and he felt that this task called for innovation and creativity. The moment-to-moment activities of his day intrigued him, and he said he learned more all the time, even when the tasks seemed routine.

Bill was fully aware that the company reorganization would force many changes in his role. He couldn't predict what they would be, but he was interested in the evolutionary process and even welcomed it. "Whatever his new role turns out to be," Ouellette wrote at the time, "he is sure he will find a way to make it meaningful and worthwhile."

Seven years earlier, Bill's wife had died in an accident while they were on vacation. For a year afterward he was depressed, and when Ouellette met him, he could still evoke the grief and shock he felt at the time. But he was no longer depressed. He had sought and received the support of his two children, several grandchildren, and many friends, both men and women. He had many hobbies and activities, such as furniture-building, that enabled him to be alone without feeling lonely. Though he would consider remarriage, he felt no pressure to find a spouse in order to be fulfilled.

Despite stress at work, Bill was completely free of physical symptoms and had avoided serious illness his whole life. Bill's period of depression had not required psychiatric treatment and resolved itself over the course of a year.

The differences between Andy and Bill illustrate how people can use—or misuse—the support of others. Ouellette's research showed that the kind of support one seeks and receives is more important than the mere fact of having support. Moreover, hardy individuals procure support from friends, coworkers, and loved ones that enables them to live an exciting, meaningful life in a world perceived as being full of challenges, not threats.

HARDINESS AND IMMUNE POWER

In her research with phone company executives, and later in studies of lawyers, army officers, college students, women, and others, Ouellette has linked hardiness and physical health. Although Ouellette herself had not tested whether hardiness boosts the immune system, recent research by other scientists has directly linked the two. Psychiatrist George F. Solomon and psychologist Lydia Temoshok conducted a study of long survivors of AIDS, in which they profiled patients who outlived the expectations of medical experts. These were individuals with full-blown AIDS who were alive years after being handed a death sentence.

The long survivors were fighters who asserted their needs. They also sought meaning and purpose in their lives, whether by finding new forms of creative expression, strengthening their relationships, or helping others who were suffering with HIV or AIDS.

Not only did they possess such Immune Power traits in abundance, Solomon and Temoshok discovered direct correlations between these traits and better-functioning immune systems. Using Ouellette's hardiness questionnaire, they found that *AIDS patients with a greater sense of control lived longer and had stronger immune functions.* Conceivably, their more vigorous immune systems helped stave off opportunistic diseases, the final cause of death in AIDS.

An Italian study led by Luigi Solano followed one hundred HIV-positive individuals for one year. Using Ouellette's hardiness scale, the researchers discovered that subjects who had a greater sense of control were significantly less likely to have developed symptoms of AIDS.

Michael Antoni, Ph.D., and his colleagues at the University of Miami recently showed that HIV-infected men who participate in mind-body group therapy have improved T-helper cell counts. But Antoni has uncovered clues as to why these men show immunologic and health advantages. He ran psychological tests over several years, beginning when the men entered his therapy program. Men who showed improvements in several immune measures had become more active copers with stress. Unlike others, they did not withdraw from relationships, work, or creative pursuits. Their participation in Antoni's program—which taught coping skills—enabled them to confront their illness, take practical steps to improve their health, and remain engaged in meaningful activities. After two years of follow-ups, Antoni also found that men who demonstrated commitment to the program were less likely to have developed full-blown AIDS.

Antoni's descriptions of active copers sound like textbook definitions of commitment, control, and challenge. His work supports the view that HIV patients who develop hardy traits may demonstrably improve their immunologic health and well-being.

Despite such findings, Suzanne Ouellette emphasizes that an overriding purpose in developing hardiness is not Immune Power or even health. Many AIDS patients (or, for that matter, patients with any serious illness) who have tremendous commitment, control, and challenge do not live beyond their "expected" life spans. Their hardiness cannot and must not be questioned. Although studies are beginning to suggest that hardiness improves one's prognosis, such an Immune Power trait is only one aspect of disease recovery.

Ouellette believes hardiness is not a life-or-death issue as much as it is a quality-of-life issue. Having been faced with possibility of a shortened life span, such patients often choose to live with zest, pleasure, and meaning. On some occasions, a wondrous "side effect" of living with commitment, control, and challenge is the opportunity to live longer.

The connection between hardiness and immune functioning was strengthened by a 1988 study conducted at Arizona State University. Led by psychologist Morris A. Okun, Ph.D., the researchers evaluated thirty-three women with rheumatoid arthritis (RA), a disease in which the immune system attacks tissues in the person's joints. The inflammation that results can be excruciatingly painful and ultimately disabling.

Okun did not focus on personality in the onset of RA. He was interested in whether healthy personality traits helped women who already suffered with the disease. "Little effort," he wrote, "has been devoted to identifying positive personality profiles that contribute to successful adaptation among [patients with arthritis]." Okun would investigate whether hardiness was associated with a better-functioning immune system, and better overall health, in people struggling with RA.

He and his colleagues found that women with high hardiness had significantly higher percentages of T-cells—meaning their immune systems were more balanced. (Research has shown that RA patients who fare better have more T-cells.) At the same time, women with a greater sense of control reported better relative health and well-being. As predicted, patients who reported poorer health had more B-cells, which have been found in excess when the disease flares up. Hardiness not only balanced immunity—it fostered good health among women with a potentially disabling disease.

Research linking the three Cs to physical health suggests that hardiness is as close as science has come to capturing human resilience. Consider a study conducted in 1977 by social psychologists

Ellen Langer and Judith Rodin (now president of the University of Pennsylvania.) The two wanted to find out if nursing home residents with a sense of control would fare better psychologically and physically than a comparable group deprived of control. They recruited two groups that were evenly matched in socioeconomic levels and physical health.

All members of the first group were told by the psychologists that they were competent individuals, capable of caring for themselves and making decisions. They were then instructed to choose a plant from a large selection and told that they would be responsible for its care. Members of the control group also were given a plant, but they were told that the staff would be responsible for its care.

Within weeks, the group that was given responsibility for the plant showed a measurable improvement in mental and physical well-being. More astonishing, however, were the findings after a year and a half. Of the control group, 30 percent had died, whereas only 15 percent of the "responsibility-enhanced group" had died. Being given a plant had reduced their mortality rate by half!

Langer and Rodin believed that the real gift bestowed upon the nursing home residents was a greater sense of personal responsibility and control. Most astonishing was how little it took to engender a key aspect of hardiness: a few words from an authority figure and a potted plant. The beauty of Langer and Rodin's study, and its significance, was that a sense of control does not require massive structural changes in one's life or personal attributes. It only requires a shift in perception.

HARDINESS IS AN EQUAL OPPORTUNITY PROTECTOR

The high-powered Illinois Bell executives were perfect subjects for Suzanne Ouellette's research, but admittedly they were "mostly male, middle-class, middle-aged, married, and Protestant." Would hardiness protect people in other walks of life? Was hardiness help-ful only for certain types of stress?

Through the 1980s and early '90s, Ouellette has shown that hardiness is an equal opportunity protector. The three Cs are char-acteristic of healthy lawyers, doctors, actors, army officers, students, and bus drivers. Other researchers have discovered a hardiness-health connection among nurses, U.S. Army disaster workers, members of the Israeli Defense Force, Japanese businessmen, im-migrants, and people with serious chronic illness. And hardiness is hardly the exclusive province of men. Ouellette distributed hardi-ness questionnaires to hundreds of women in their gynecologists' offices. She discovered that women who were hardier developed fewer mental and physical illnesses.

Although hardiness cuts across economic and cultural lines, everyone has a unique way of expressing the three Cs. Ouellette has observed countless manifestations of commitment, control, and challenge. What determines whether we stay healthy under stress? According to Ouellette, the answer may lie in how our unique configuration of Cs responds to the particular demands of the world we inhabit.

Different occupations or cultural contexts call forth different configurations of the three Cs. Take, for example, Ouellette's study of army officers. She discovered that their levels of control and commitment protected them from ill health in the face of extreme stress, but a sense of challenge did not.

"The army officers did not always show the positive effects of the challenge component that executives and lawyers showed," she commented.

I believe this to be due at least in part to their work situation. Having been in Vietnam, they were now being asked to adopt a bureaucratic role. These men regarded a sense of challenge as something that might actually interfere with what their or-ganization was asking of them. They needed to put aside a sense of risk-taking and adventurousness, behaviors that might have been appropriate for their former role but that were not suitable to the one they were now playing.

Unlike army officers, high-functioning doctors need a sense of challenge. But many doctors, whom Ouellette studied extensively, downplayed the importance of commitment. Partly as a result of their medical school training, they were loath to get too involved with their patients, believing that loss and disappointment would impede their ability to function at the highest possible level. The best approach, they thought, was one of "detached concern." Despite their beliefs, Ouellette found that doctors did not benefit psychologically from their low commitment. For a doctor, removing one's self from close contact with patients was not helpful for either member of the "healing partnership." What's needed is a balance between self-protective distance and emotional involvement—a way to sustain commitment in the face of suffering.

Actors must also make adjustments in how they sustain commitment. In her studies of actors, Ouellette observed that the lack of structure in their work lives augured against commitment and control. They needed special coping strategies to keep from lapsing into helplessness and alienation. Auditions come and go, competition is fierce, and long fallow periods test the resolve of even the most talented thespians.

"Actors have to expend more energy and time structuring their lives to maintain a committed orientation," she commented.

In other occupational settings, someone having difficulty staying engaged still gets up at eight in the morning and has someplace to go. There is a setting in which the person can begin searching for something to capture his or her attention again. But if you're perpetually out of work, trying to find auditions, there is no place to go at eight in the morning. For the [hardy] actors I interviewed, it was important to set up schedules and be highly disciplined. They couldn't just wake up and see how the spirit moved them. It was very critical for them to set up appointments and lunch dates with people. For actors, it's an isolated existence, and keeping contacts was one way to stay in control and committed.

The prevailing myth about lawyers is that they thrive on stress—working endless hours, preparing briefs deep into the night, taking on caseloads that would tax the resources of mere mortals. Through it all, they remain calm, shrewd, in control. Lawyers may be granted their intermittent bouts of exhaustion, but they're assumed to maintain high-octane energy and good health as they redraw the boundaries of what most of us consider hard work.

Contrary to this myth, lawyers experience stresses and strains as much as anyone, but often ignore their effects until they're visited by serious illness. Moreover, lawyers who are committed to their work, and who avoid destructive or escapist ways of coping with stress, remain healthier than their alienated counterparts.

These were the findings in a 1982 study by Ouellette, in which she investigated stress and personality among 157 general practice lawyers. The committed lawyers reported significantly fewer symptoms of strain—such as heartburn, headaches, insomnia, irregular heartbeat, anxiety attacks, and nervousness. The "uncommitted" lawyers who engaged in "regressive coping"—handling stress by getting angry, withdrawing, drinking and smoking more, and so on—had many more symptoms of strain. Commitment was especially crucial among lawyers, not only because their workload was so heavy, but because they had to handle problems brought to them by such a wide variety of clients.

Ouellette says that one of the hardiest individuals she's ever known came from a vastly different culture from all the lawyers, executives, army officers, doctors, and actors she had studied. His name was Ignacio Martin-Baro, a Jesuit priest from El Salvador who came to this country in the late 1970s, taking on challenges that matched both his talents and his deep convictions.

Martin-Baro came to the United States to get his master's degree at the University of Chicago. He was Ouellette's first graduate student and helped to conduct her initial research on hardiness. Martin-Baro's dream was to use social science research to help his own people, who suffered immensely under the rule of a dictatorial government. Many of his compatriots lacked the basic necessities of life, living in horrendously crowded conditions without sufficient resources for economic development.

For several years, Martin-Baro traveled back and forth between the United States and El Salvador. According to Ouellette, at the University of Chicago, "It was clear to everyone that he was one of the brightest people who'd ever walked through their doors. They wanted him to stay for his Ph.D., which he did. Then he was offered a variety of prestigious positions and possibilities. But his commitment to his people in El Salvador was foremost. He was determined to go back."

Martin-Baro wanted to study the effects of crowding in his country, a massive and nearly unprecedented endeavor. He made regular trips to El Salvador to collect data, studying the psychological resources his people brought to bear against horrendous social and economic conditions. His findings showed that a sense of meaning and purpose helped many of his fellow Salvadorans survive—even those who were malnourished and crowded together in shanty shacks.

Martin-Baro kept Ouellette informed of his activities, which included his work as priest to a community of Salvadorans living a simple, spiritual life in the mountains. One aspect of his ongoing research involved interviewing citizens of El Salvador about their views of the government. His scientific investigations had political overtones, and they offended the brutal government in power. None of this stopped Martin-Baro—not even his knowledge that his life was in danger. "He lived with other priests, and their residence had been bombed a number of times," recalls Ouellette. "Friends of his had been killed, and in the mid-1970s the archbishop of El Salvador was assassinated. He knew full well that he might live only a short period of time."

On November 16, 1989, in an incident reported worldwide, Martin-Baro was one of several Jesuit priests shot and killed by right-wing terrorists in San Salvador.

Martin-Baro's commitment—to his work, his fellow citizens, his democratic ideals, and his spiritual beliefs—never waned. To Ouellette's knowledge, he remained emotionally and physically healthy throughout his ordeals. Martin-Baro's sense of control was the girding beneath his successful endeavors as a scientist and clergyman, and his thirst for challenge enabled him to confront monumental obstacles.

Ouellette recalled yet another side of Martin-Baro from his time at the university, a side that also reflected his hardiness:

Martin-Baro was someone who lived all areas of life to the fullest. Given that he was a priest, he had restrictions, and he was someone who worked remarkably hard all week. Now, Friday night was the night everyone partied. He would step out reeking of cologne, dressed to the nines, for dinner and drinking and dancing. He was a wonderful musician, with a beautiful voice, and he loved to party with people. He was someone who clearly lived life in an extraordinary way. When I talk about him to my students, they ask: "How could this person have allowed this to happen? How could he have died?" The only answer I can offer is "He had an unshakable commitment to his life's work."

Ouellette's remembrance of Martin-Baro offers insight into the Immune Power Personality. As with Gary Schwartz's ACE Factor, *flexibility* is an important facet of hardiness. While Martin-Baro's commitment was boundless, to the extent that he risked his life for his beliefs, his focus was not narrowly trained. His eyes may have been on the prize, but he never lost his peripheral vision or his capacity to enjoy life. The behavior of the person who combines commitment with challenge will never be entirely predictable.

Martin-Baro's story also illustrates that hardiness is not specific to any cultural milieu or occupational setting. "My focus then, and still now, is on the individual," Ouellette said recently. "I am interested in the way individuals make sense of who they are, the world they live in, and how they can operate in that world."

Hardiness is not only a factor in particular occupational, economic, or cultural contexts. It may protect one's health in a variety of taxing life circumstances. Consider the crisis of the woman whose pregnancy is proceeding normally, until she undergoes fetal monitoring and her obstetrician informs her that she's at high risk for a premature delivery. She's told that the life of her unborn child is threatened. She's immediately checked into the hospital, carefully monitored and injected with drugs to forestall delivery as long as possible. She is then required to lie flat on her back for weeks until her infant can be safely brought to term. Even with these stressful precautions, the risk of complications remains high. In this circumstance, in which the woman's sense of control is stripped away, could hardiness make any positive difference in the outcome?

That was the question posed by Ouellette and her colleagues at the City University of New York (CUNY) in their recent research on women with high-risk pregnancies. Ouellette was "particularly intrigued by the women who come from high-powered positions and are suddenly told that they cannot act that way anymore. It was interesting to watch them shift from making dozens of phone calls from bed, and having their staff bring in documents, to the point where they could do little more than needlepoint."

Did hardiness help these women in the face of stress and sudden loss of control? The answer is yes, with an asterisk. Preliminary results of research on sixty women with high-risk pregnancies (including many of the "high-powered" types) indicate that hardiness did not allay anxiety or depression during the period right after hospitalization. In the midst of the crisis, these women were distressed regardless of their commitment, control, and challenge. However, between one and three months later—after the immediate crisis had passed—the hardy women showed fewer residual symptoms of anxiety and depression.

Periods of anxiety and depression are understandable and perhaps unavoidable when we have no control over certain painful events. The death of a loved one, a diagnosis of severe illness, the loss of one's job, or a high-risk pregnancy all stretch our coping capacities. Ouellette's study suggests that hardiness won't anesthetize the pain accompanying such circumstances. But hardiness *will* increase resilience once a person has weathered the crisis. Ouellette believed that the hardy women openly expressed their fears and sadness during the pregnancy crisis. As a result, they bounced backed more rapidly to a homeostatic state of well-being.

ARTHUR ASHE: EXEMPLAR OF HARDINESS

One public figure who exemplified hardiness was Arthur Ashe. Few people realize that Ashe was a bona fide long survivor of AIDS. He apparently contracted the HIV virus in 1983 from a blood transfusion during open-heart surgery. (He therefore lived with HIV for nine years.) He was finally diagnosed with AIDS in 1988 after the discovery and subsequent surgical removal of toxoplasmosis, a parasitic brain infection. Dr. Henry Murray, Ashe's physician and a renowned expert in infectious diseases, was quoted as saying that his four-and-a-half-year survival after toxoplasmosis is "probably the longest in the world." According to statistics, Ashe should have died three years earlier.

These extra years of life were a gift to his family and the world. Why did Arthur Ashe, a man who had also survived multiple heart attacks and open-heart surgery, outlive every reasonable expectation concerning his survival? Certainly Ashe received the best possible medical care and, by all accounts, took excellent care of himself during the course of his illness. Yet it was probably no coincidence that a man universally known for the strength of his convictions, his courage, his grace under pressure, and his commitment to causes and people he cared deeply about should happen to be a long survivor of AIDS and perhaps the longest known survivor of toxoplasmosis.

In a December 1992 article in *Sports Illustrated,* months before his death, the following was written about Ashe:

Ashe always embodied good sportsmanship on the playing field. But if sportsmanship is also an athlete's ability to shift from being a selfish competitor to being a useful member of society, then Ashe's sportsmanship is unequalled. His gradual harvest has grown into a mountain of good.

If sportsmanship is also the ability to transform loss into fresh, competitive, creative fire, then Ashe's has been unparalleled, and his greatest transformation is his newest.

The article chronicles how Arthur Ashe turned his own tragic diagnosis into an opportunity to change society's views of AIDS, to raise hundreds of thousands of dollars for AIDS research. He had wanted to retain his privacy and "was angry at being forced to tell the public that he has the disease before he was ready." Ashe then channeled that evident anger into a cause far more worthy than media-bashing: the fight against AIDS.

It was not the first fierce battle he'd ever fought, and AIDS was not the first monumental obstacle he'd ever hurdled. Ashe overcame monumental barriers of intolerance to become the first and only black man to win championships at Wimbledon and the U.S. Open.

In these pursuits, Arthur Ashe's commitment, control, and challenge were luminously apparent. Few sports figures have so perfectly personified these traits. When it came to causes as diverse as equal justice, education, excellence in sports and academics, the eradication of racism, and the alleviation of serious illnesses such as heart disease and AIDS, his commitments were unshakable.

He confronted every obstacle—whether societal, sports-related, or medical—with a keen sense of challenge. Months before he died, he told talk-show host Charlie Rose, "The fact that I have AIDS . . . has made me much more productive. I have felt creativity like you wouldn't believe since I found this out. I've looked into it, and I've found that it is not unusual for people who think that time is short, or shorter than it normally would be, to feel like they can do just about anything."

Thus, Arthur Ashe, long survivor of AIDS and toxoplasmosis, may have been kept alive those last years—years in which he contributed so much to his family and the world—by a convergence of the wonders of medicine and the wonders of his own true nature.

HARDINESS TRAINING:
BUILDING THE THREE Cs IN YOUR OWN LIFE

Of course, looking at an extraordinary life such as Ashe's prompts the question: Can I really develop a personality trait that I don't have to begin with? In my interviews with Suzanne Ouellette, she was passionate in stating her case that personality is not a fixed entity, but rather a dynamic self-sense interacting with an ever-changing world. It is not merely genetic inheritance, early experiences, psychosocial development, here-and-now circumstances, or worldview. Personality is a reverberation among *all* of these elements—and others yet to be discovered. All of these factors continuously interact to create a more encompassing, vibrant, and unpredictable whole.

As we engage in this process of making sense of ourselves and our place in the world, we make choices. Among these choices are actions taken to enhance commitment, control, and challenge. Suzanne Ouellette and Salvadore Maddi have developed programs of hardiness education, to teach people how to make choices that build hardiness. Hardiness training programs have been carried out successfully on individual, group, and organizational levels. While the path toward hardiness is not easy, the steps can be learned, practiced, and integrated into our lifestyles.

The quiz at the end of this chapter is a short form of the questionnaire Ouellette uses in her research. Take it to determine your level of hardiness. Use the scoring system to find out your levels of commitment, control, and challenge, and your level of overall hardiness. Once you've made these determinations, you can follow the hardiness training steps with knowledge of which Cs need the most shoring up.

While Suzanne Ouellette helped develop the methods and principles of hardiness training, her current focus is research rather than therapy. Her collaborator, Salvadore Maddi, who has vast experience as a clinical psychologist, has devoted his energies to hardiness training for groups, corporations, and other organizations. In 1984 he founded the Hardiness Institute, which began by offering hardiness training to Illinois Bell Telephone. The Hardiness Institute, now headquartered in Irvine, California, offers a range of hardiness-training services to individuals and organizations of all stripes. "What happened to Illinois Bell, and the Bell System generally, is now happening in the American economy as a whole," Maddi commented. "As a result, the need for hardiness training is more evident than ever before."

Does hardiness training really improve physical health? Ouellette and Maddi led sixteen executives from Illinois Bell in a study of their hardiness training program. Half of them participated in the eight weekly sessions of hardiness training (including the four steps outlined starting on page 153), while the other half kept a stress journal and met with the researchers at the beginning and end of the program.

Although the study was small, the results were powerful. Unlike the controls, the group that received training demonstrated an increase in transformational coping and a decrease in regressive coping. Both groups were given the questionnaire before and after the course of the study. Only the hardiness-training group showed a significant increase in commitment, control, and challenge.

Finally, all subjects received blood pressure monitoring before and after the eight weeks and three months later. (High blood pressure is considered a common indicator of illness risk or strain.) Both diastolic and systolic blood pressure decreased in the hardiness-training group. Even more striking, these blood pressure drops held after three months.

Ouellette and Maddi concede that more research is needed on hardiness training to prove its health benefits. But these results underscore what common sense dictates. You can develop commitment, control, and challenge. In so doing, you buffer the negative effects of stress and create the conditions for a healthier life.

The "hardy" way of thinking and acting toward stress has a name: transformational coping. Likewise, the "unhardy" way is termed regressive coping. Let's look at what these terms mean.

TRANSFORMATIONAL VS. REGRESSIVE COPING

Transformational coping represents a healthy, hardy way of handling stress, not simply avoiding stress. By viewing stressful events as challenges, not threats, and acting decisively, we alter the stressful events themselves.

Consider the cases of two Illinois Bell executives described in

The Hardy Executive, Arthur and Edgar, who both received a negative evaluation from a superior and were thus passed up for promotion. In his response, Arthur was alternately angry and depressed. He felt cheated and had fantasies about murdering his boss. He was also depressed, ruminating about his failure and wondering if his superiors were right—that he was worthless. To quell these feelings, he drank more, especially during the days immediately after his evaluation. He took time off, went to movies with his kids, puttered around his garden, and vegged out a lot. He also looked up a woman "who always seemed interested in me" and began flirting with her. "At least I felt a little attractive," he said.

Actually, Arthur felt worthless, and his drinking, vegging out, and flirtation did not make the feeling go away. How did he deal with the supervisor at work? "I couldn't bring myself to talk to him. I'd just lower my head when I passed him in the hall."

Ouellette and Maddi described Arthur as someone who engaged in regressive coping. On a cognitive level, he viewed the stressful event pessimistically. He neither rejected the criticism as unfair nor accepted it as useful. Instead, he viewed the negative evaluation as an overall indictment of his capabilities, proving his worthlessness. Moreover, he felt there was nothing he could do about any of this. Arthur's mind-set made him feel powerless, blocking his opportunity to seize control. Instead of viewing his evaluation and missed opportunity as challenges, he saw them as threats—so much so that he spoke as if his life was over.

Arthur's anger was not the problem; how he handled his anger was. Far better than fantasies of killing his boss and subsequent drinking sprees would have been a defiant "I'll show them," followed by a commitment to himself to demonstrate more creativity and dedication on the job.

In terms of actions, taking days off and avoiding his boss would, if anything, *worsen* his situation at work. The drinking, flirtation, and other distractions were just that—distractions. In some circumstances avoidance is a useful coping strategy—particularly in the immediate aftermath of a catastrophe, such as the sudden death of a loved one. However, when you avoid concrete problems that have potential solutions, you either maintain the unhappy status quo or make matters worse. This is the essence of regressive coping.

Edgar was subjected to the same circumstances as Arthur. He too was stunned and angry. In his interview with Ouellette, he discussed his specific differences with his supervisor and his serious doubts about his future on this job. He described how he went home and talked with his wife "so that I could figure out what went wrong and what to do about it." Edgar elaborated:

After I thought this all over, it dawned on me that maybe the negative evaluation was a little understandable. . . . I hadn't been giving maximum effort. Maybe I would have given me a negative evaluation too. That really shocked me at first, but then it seemed to help. My anger [toward the supervisor] went away, and I resolved to talk this over with him, to see whether anything could be done to make it better for all of us. To tell you the truth, I also began thinking about all those doubts I had concerning the kind of job that would be best for me.

I had some talks with [the supervisor] and they went very well. I guess he was troubled about what he had done, and I was troubled about my not working up to my potential. Since then, things have been better for us both.

Edgar was a transformational coper. He did not deny his anger, or his concern over the negative evaluation, or losing out on a promotion. On a cognitive level, he perceived this event not as a tragedy but as an opportunity to reassess his job, his relationship with his supervisor, and his future plans.

Edgar was proactive in his response. First he planned a discussion with his supervisor, then he implemented his plan. He was straightforward with the supervisor, and his directness paid off in a fruitful exchange. At the same time, he began asking himself hard questions about the course of his career. Thus, his negative evaluation stimulated a reappraisal of his long-term goals. Edgar turned an upsetting event into a launch pad for self-awareness and growth.

Transformational coping is evidently healthier, from a psychological perspective, than regressive coping. In the former, we assess the event as opportunity rather than danger (challenge); devise and implement plans to change our environment or ourselves to meet the challenge (control); and follow through with conviction (commitment). In the latter, we assess the event as danger rather than opportunity (pessimism); lose ourselves in distractions and retreat from the stressful environment (helplessness); and end up feeling depressed, angry, withdrawn, or resigned (alienation).

Transformational (hardy) coping buffers the negative effects of stress on our bodies. By confronting the stressful event, we prevent a lapse into anger, depression, or helplessness—states that harm our immune and cardiovascular systems. Also, by engaging with the sources of our stress (such as Edgar's discussion with his supervisor), we transform our environment and relationships in such a way that stress levels are reduced.

Unfortunately, most corporate-sponsored stress reduction programs (which are springing up as quickly as fast-food franchises) teach employees a variety of relaxation techniques, with no mention of hardiness. This is yet another example of why mind-body techniques should be integrated into a program for the development of Immune Power traits. If Edgar, the transformational coper, had meditated to feel better *without* having taken decisive action to change his environment, he'd have remained on a relaxation treadmill for an indefinite period, battling the same tensions day in and day out.

Salvadore Maddi has developed a four-step plan for the development of transformational coping and overall hardiness. The first step involves heightened awareness of the sources of stress in one's life.

THE FOUR STEPS OF HARDINESS TRAINING

STEP 1. FOCUSING

Originally developed by psychologist Eugene Gendlin, focusing is a mental technique that paves the way for inducing hardiness.

Gendlin's approach is a simple but powerful way to tune into your bodymind, not just to relax but to locate sources of stress in your environment.

Often we skim the surface of our awareness of stress and conflict. We accept external labels (from our families, friends, or culture) for our problems, instead of looking within to define and understand our problems. Focusing helps us shift our perceptions from the conventional to the personal, which Ouellette and Maddi claim is "a prerequisite for significant personality change."

For many of us, getting in touch with our authentic creative impulses and emotions is difficult. They have been buried under layers of defense and the countless adjustments made to please and appease others. One purpose of focusing is to recover feelings and desires neglected in early life. The other purpose is to discover our essential needs, goals, and emotions in present-day stressful situations.

The practice of focusing. The first step in focusing is to find a comfortable place, retreat from daily distractions, and take your attention inward. If a particular stressful event concerns you, think about the situation and experience your bodily reactions. If no specific event concerns you, ask yourself: What stands in the way of my being happy and fulfilled? When the core event or issue arises, you should feel some physical response, such as shakiness or pressure around the temples.

Experience the physical states with as much care and sensitivity as possible. Next, find a word, phrase, or image that best captures these sensations. The word, phrase, or image should represent your mind-body state as accurately as possible. It could reflect an emotion (sadness, joy, anger); a thought (the time has come for me to assert myself with my boss); an attitude (indifferent, serious, competitive). The word, sentence, or picture (a boat sailing in choppy waters) that comes to mind should "label" the sensation.

Allow yourself to resonate back and forth between the bodily sensations and labels until you have matched the two. Reject conventional labels until you arrive at a more personal meaning. This period of mental/emotional adjustment between sensations and verbal or visual labels will involve a deepening of your awareness of a stressful problem. It also will help you begin to better understand the causes and effects of that problem.

Remember that the purpose of focusing is to integrate your deeper feelings about a situation with your attitudes, thoughts, and perspectives on that issue. Once you identify the core issue and arrive at appropriate "labels," you are likely to feel a sense of relief.

Once you have arrived at this deeper awareness and appreciation, ask yourself about your levels of commitment, control, and challenge in this specific circumstance. Use your answers as launch pads for the development of "perspective and understanding," to use Maddi's phrase. In differing ways, perspective and understanding are gained during each and every phase of hardiness training. A realistic perspective on any stressful situation—and a penetrating understanding of the dynamics involved—enables you to follow each step toward hardiness with the highest prospect of success.

STEP 2. SITUATIONAL RECONSTRUCTION

Focusing leads directly to situational reconstruction, an exercise in imagination that frees you to plan actions rooted in commitment, control, and challenge. While focusing helps you zero in on the stressful event and identify your related emotions, situational reconstruction engages your imagination and intellect to view the event objectively from several different angles and to devise specific strategies for effective coping. Situational reconstruction sets the stage for actions that not only enhance coping in a particular circumstance, but also foster a sense of meaning and purpose.

Situational reconstruction involves seven steps:

1. Identify the dominant stressful circumstance or event in your life today.
2. Imagine three ways in which the event could have been worse. Write down these three ways if it helps you to remember them.
3. Imagine three ways in which the event could have been bet-

ter. Write down these three ways if it helps you to remember them.

4. For each of the three "worse" ways, imagine (and write down, if helpful) a scenario that would explain it. What would have had to be different for these worst-case scenarios to have occurred? How would you or other "key players" have responded in these "stories"?

5. For each of the three "better" ways, imagine (and write down, if helpful) a scenario that would explain it. What would have had to be different for these best-case scenarios to have occurred? How would you or other "key players" have responded in these "stories"?

6. What specifically could you have done (or still do, if the event is ongoing) to increase the likelihood of the best-case scenarios occurring? If you have trouble coming up with possibilities, then imagine what someone you greatly admire would have done in that situation.

7. Having determined what actions would bring about a desired outcome, the final step is to carry them out. If the event is ongoing, you can implement your action plan in order to achieve success, and enhanced meaning, in the current situation. If the event is past, you can implement your action plan to prevent similar situations in the future.

Understanding the purpose of situational reconstruction is a key to its success. When you imagine three ways in which the stressful event could have been worse, you provide yourself with greater perspective and understanding. To borrow a phrase from mind-body practitioner Joan Borysenko, Ph.D., many of us "awfulize" in the face of stress. We imagine only the worst outcomes, leading inexorably to heightened stress, deteriorating self-esteem, chronic fight-or-flight, and ill health. When we take a hard, realistic look at how an event could have been worse, we don't deny our unhappiness or fear. Rather, we develop a balanced view of our circumstances. Situational reconstruction helps us to stop awfulizing, because we've imagined the absolute worst and recognize that it did not happen!

Imagining what would have had to be different in such worst-case scenarios serves a more complex purpose. It forces you to create a rich story in your mind around these scenarios, which brings them to life and, in addition, allows all the variables to be considered and the characters involved (including yourself) to show their many facets and true colors.

For instance, let's say you've been passed over for a raise at work. You feel cheated and angry at your boss, who you believe does not acknowledge your talents and hard work. In one of your worst-case scenarios, you are fired rather than cheated. You ask yourself what would have had to be different for this to occur. In your imagination, your boss would have to be far more oblivious—even cruel—to have fired you. The truth is, he may be short-sighted, but he's not malevolent. Until you practiced situational reconstruction, your anger blinded your view of your boss, making him seem entirely inflexible and unapproachable. Now you recognize that he is busy and narrowly focused. This realization enables you to plan a balanced strategy for improving relations with him, and eventually, for getting the raise you deserve.

Using your imagination in this manner—turning over the variables in your mind as if the event were a prism upon which you were shining the light of your intelligence—settles you down into a reality you can confront with clear vision.

Imagining best-case scenarios is a powerful mind-body approach to hardiness and health, not to mention success. Stephanie Simonton, Ph.D., has pioneered the use of guided imagery for cancer patients. One of her techniques is to have her patients—and others who simply wish to improve their lives and health—see themselves in stressful situations, imagining new approaches that raise self-esteem and the prospects for a desired outcome. Situational reconstruction of best-case scenarios serves a similar purpose. By having you feel and see pictures of yourself effectively solving problems, this exercise orients you toward possibilities. It anchors you in that fertile mind-state which yields the most creative solutions.

Pivotal to this technique is discovering what would have been required for the best-case scenarios to occur. Let's return to the example in which you got passed over for a raise. In one best-case scenario, you not only get a raise but also a promotion. Situational reconstruction enables you to recognize that for you to have achieved this success, you'd have had to: (a) understand your boss's limitations—and concerns—more clearly; (b) realize you've avoided him out of fear instead of making him aware of your accomplishments in a non-bragging manner; and (c) accept that your frustration has dragged you down and prevented you from reaching your potential on the job.

The beauty of situational reconstruction is how it taps both imaginal and reality-based faculties of the brain. Techniques that reach only one of these faculties are far less powerful. Imagining best-case scenarios without investigating what needs to change can become a mere exercise in wishful thinking. Exploring the nitty-gritty of what needs to change without visualizing the possibility of success can become a dry exercise in problem-solving.

The entire process of situational reconstruction leads you to identify a specific action plan. This plan stems directly from your exploration of what you can do to realize best-case scenarios. Through a careful process of deliberation, choose actions designed to increase your self-esteem, sense of meaning, and potential for success. But don't reach far beyond your grasp or attempt to live up to impossibly high standards of behavior, performance, or achievement.

STEP 3. DECISIVE ACTION AND FEEDBACK PROCESSING

"The purpose of decisive action," says Salvadore Maddi, "is to decrease the stressfulness of the circumstance. By taking action, you learn that you have more control than you thought you had." But Maddi's approach fully recognizes that action plans are not fixed programs designed to achieve fixed notions of success. Rather, they are dynamic strategies, the purpose of which is not only success but further learning—about yourself and what is meaningful to you, about others and what matters to them, and about the conditions that strengthen your hardiness.

"When you take decisive action," Maddi continues, "you get

feedback from observing yourself, from other people observing you, and from the reactions of people toward whom your decisive action is directed. In our hardiness-training groups, we use those three sources of feedback to help people deepen their sense of commitment, control, and challenge."

Let's return to the example of your quest for recognition at work and an eventual raise. The initial step in your action plan involves a discussion with your boss, in which your goals include better communication, clarification of the reasons for his denial, an opportunity to point out accomplishments you feel he has overlooked, and learning what he expects from you, to merit the recognition and raise you seek.

The results of your discussion with your boss are illuminating. You learn that he is unaware of some of your accomplishments. He finds out more about your creative contributions, and you learn more about information flow within the company. He criticizes your low profile and claims you lack initiative to match your creativity. You listen carefully and realize that he's right. He doesn't know that you keep a low profile because you fear his harshly critical response. You recognize this during the discussion, and take a two-pronged approach. First, you acknowledge that his criticism is correct, and vow to take more initiative. Second, you mention that he has been harshly critical in the past, and you worry about his reactions. He responds well to your vow, less well to your fears: "I call them as I see them," he says. The final results, however, are largely what you hoped for: better communication, some degree of mutual understanding, and greater recognition of your achievements. You tell the story to two colleagues who are friends at work. They affirm your view of what happened and applaud your courage in taking this new approach.

Now that you have taken decisive action, the next step is consideration of feedback from three sources: your boss, others, and yourself. Your boss's feedback confirmed your realization that he was more shortsighted than sadistic. You learned the extent to which your problem had been miscommunication. You discovered that information flow within the company concealed many of your contributions. Based on his positive response, you realized that your boss was open to information about your work activities. You also learned that he was *not* open to hearing about your difficulties with his management style. But you can accept this, because he responds well to other approaches.

Your feedback from others, namely two trusted co-workers, was useful in confirming your perception of events. Just as important, you feel buoyed and emotionally supported by them. You think: What a change from a few days ago, when I felt defeated, angry, and isolated.

Your feedback from yourself was also crucial. You realize that your past anger, while understandable, had blocked your clear vision and prevented necessary changes. You feel a certain relief, not shame or rage, when your boss requests greater initiative. That sense of relief is highly informative. It tells you he's right. It provides you with motivation to become more innovative on the job. And it gives you hope that greater effort will yield results, including the raise you desire.

What if the feedback from your boss had been negative? Imagine a scenario in which he ignored or berated you. What then? "The immediate feedback you get may be hostile," comments Maddi, "but the feedback you get from observing yourself or from other people observing you may not be hostile."

In this instance, feedback from others or yourself may lead you to question whether you approached him in the most appropriate manner. Or perhaps your boss holds a personal dislike of you, which you ought to recognize. You will either need to find another tack with him, or another job altogether. In either event, feedback from yourself and your colleagues will help you understand the dynamics and formulate a revised action plan.

Your decisive action, and your processing of feedback, all serve to enhance commitment, control, and challenge. Maddi comments, "Even if you're not entirely successful, taking decisive action and processing feedback builds hardiness. You notice that you're more involved. That's commitment. You feel more decisive. That's control. When you keep this going, you get a sense of the challenge that's involved in confronting stress. People are enlivened by this process."

STEP 4. COMPENSATORY SELF-IMPROVEMENT

Sometimes no amount of focusing or situational reconstruction leads to a viable action plan. Ouellette and Maddi call such a circumstance a "given." *Givens* are the cards you have been dealt in life that cannot be reshuffled. While the loss of a job or death of a loved one are clear examples, there are many other life situations that amount to brick walls. Recognizing them as brick walls is healthier than banging your head repeatedly against them. Equally important, however, is preventing the givens in our lives from becoming evidence to support a position of helplessness that leads to depression, self-pity, or self-destructiveness.

How is this possible? Ouellette and Maddi offer an approach they call *compensatory self-improvement*. Put simply, compensatory self-improvement means finding another stressful problem—ideally one associated with the given—that you can do something about and taking decisive action in that area.

Consider the case of Carter, a high-level executive in a computer software company who joined Maddi's hardiness-training program. Carter's wife, Jenny, had breast cancer. He'd done everything he could to help Jenny, procuring the best medical attention he could afford. During situational reconstruction, he realized that her surgery and chemotherapy was either going to work or it wasn't. There was nothing more he could do. This was a particularly painful given for Carter, because the uncertainty was excruciating and because he was a man whose self-image was rooted in his ability to take decisive action.

Paradoxically, the first step for Carter to regain his sense of control was to accept—in this circumstance—his lack of control. The second step was finding a related area in which he could compensate with meaningful decisive action. Maddi asked him: "In this situation, where *can* you make a difference?"

Carter realized that he could improve his relationship with Jenny, which he had neglected in the struggle simply to help her survive. Through focusing, Carter went deeper and realized that he'd lost himself in work because he was so frightened she was going to die. Jenny suffered from his withdrawal, feeling alone with her illness and sinking into depression.

In one hardiness group session, Carter realized that he'd withdrawn because he felt powerless to make Jenny's cancer go away. With the support of Maddi and the other group members, he was able to recognize that "he couldn't fix it all, he couldn't make it all better." Maddi remembered Carter's own elaboration: "I've taken the 'S' off my shirt," he said. "I've folded my cape, and I don't change in phone booths anymore."

Then Carter began to compensate. He and Jenny sat down and talked over their problems. Carter vowed to be there as a husband, not a savior. They realized they needed quality time together, so they planned a trip around the world. Carter and Jenny had a grand time with travel agents, books, brochures, and ever-changing itineraries. During this process, the old spark returned, and their relationship took on a new quality of warmth and connectedness.

Sometimes, no aspect of a given situation—even a peripheral one—offers an opportunity for exercising the three Cs. Whether you face divorce, death of a loved one, illness, or career obstacles, you still can compensate by shifting gears to another realm entirely. Choosing a new task to master, or a new creative outlet, can prevent helplessness and preserve hardiness.

HARDINESS AND MIND-BODY MEDICINE

An important recent finding of mind-body medicine is that meditation, biofeedback, visualization, and hypnosis may bolster our health *by increasing our sense of control*. Since biofeedback involves the use of monitoring equipment to enable people to alter their blood pressure, heart rate, muscular tension, or skin conductance, an inherent part of the process is learning self-control. Similarly, though without electronic instruments as a guide, meditation, visualization, and hypnosis are practices that foster a sense of control by enabling people to transform their own bodymind state. Studies conducted in the 1970s and '80s demonstrated that committed meditators have an increased "inner locus of control"—another term for what Suzanne Ouellette calls a sense of control.

Do mind-body methods change our physiology because they enhance control? Do they work by augmenting all three Cs? Common sense suggests an increase in hardiness is one facet of successful mind-body medicine. For example, people who regularly practice meditation in a disciplined fashion develop a *commitment* to their own well-being; learn a sense of *control* over mind and body; and take on the *challenge* of expanding their awareness and healing potential.

Jon Kabat-Zinn, head of the Stress Reduction Clinic at the University of Massachusetts Medical Center, whose program of mindfulness meditation was described in the last two chapters, studied a group of his patients who were taught to live fully in the moment. Kabat-Zinn's method, based on Buddhist principles, empowered patients with bodymind awareness and new ways of coping with pain, disability, and disease. Kabat-Zinn conducted a study of his participants, in which he administered Ouellette's hardiness questionnaire before and after they completed his eight-week program. He found that all three Cs were significantly increased by training in mindfulness. Many of these same patients experienced marked symptomatic relief and other health benefits, regardless of their illness.

Suzanne Ouellette believes that mind-body techniques may work (in part) by boosting hardiness. *Unless* mind-body techniques somehow help people increase their commitment, control, and challenge, they may fail to produce long-term stress reduction. "Without such an orientation," she once said, "people can collect a big bag of relaxation techniques that may not add up to anything."

Ouellette is referring to the fact that each of these mind-body techniques is a solitary expedition in self-awareness and healing. While they all may (and probably do) build the three Cs, they do so in one arena only—the inner life of the body and spirit. Unless integrated into a broader program of change, they don't transform our stressful environment or relationships. Relaxation will reduce the negative effects of stress on our bodies, but it won't change the circumstances that keep on stressing us. If, however, we *combine* meditation with hardiness training, we will be able to meet the challenges of our environments or relationships, and do so with a clear mind, relaxed body, and open heart.

A HARDINESS WRITING EXERCISE

In a 1987 interview, Suzanne Ouellette eloquently summed up her approach to hardiness development:

> In the group training that Salvadore Maddi does and in the individual counseling that I do in the offices of corporate medical directors, it becomes very clear that [hardiness] training does not depend on individual stress-reducing techniques, taken to be magic bullets. Rather, it involves a fundamental decision that one needs to make about how one's life is going. At some point, in one way or another, the people who go through this hardiness counseling are brought to that recognition. Some get there sooner than others, but the intention is to make each person realize: "My God, there are lots of things in my life that I like and lots of other things that I don't like. I am going to sit down and decide what's important and where I want to go, where I have influence, where I'm avoiding control, and where I'm keeping up my sense of being intrigued." If counseling can get a person to that point, then I think that what you're offering is a very basic kind of change. And I think that is what is fundamentally required.

Such fundamental questions can seem almost rudimentary. But, in fact, the more diligently you make such an inquiry, the more quickly you realize that the most profound changes start with the most embarrassingly simple questions.

Based on Ouellette's wonderful summation, I suggest that you sit down with pen and paper, and create three columns: one each for commitment, control, and challenge. Under the word "Commitment," write the question: "What is important and where do I want to go?" Under the word "Control," write two questions: "Where do I have influence?" and "Where am I avoiding influence?" Under the word "Challenge," write two questions: "Where am I keeping up my sense of being intrigued?" and "Where have I lost my sense of being intrigued?"

Now answer these questions by scanning your mind regarding "the many things in your life you like and the other things you don't like." Include responses about your career, job, leisure activities, creative pursuits, relationships, friendships, and family life. Note the answers in each column.

Use this writing exercise as another diagnostic tool, in addition to the questionnaire at the end of this chapter, to come to grips with your state of hardiness. Let your answers become the jumping-off point for your own hardiness induction efforts, which begin with the four steps outlined earlier. You can identify those situations that require focusing, situational reconstruction, decisive action, and compensatory self-improvement.

You also can use this writing exercise for a free-floating exploration of dreams you have deferred, memories you have lost, images you've never seen, or stories you've never told. Let your quest for commitment, control, and challenge become an adventure in self-discovery.

How Hardy Are You?

Below are 12 items similar to those that appear in the hardiness questionnaire. Evaluating someone's hardiness requires more than this quick test. But this simple exercise should give you some idea of how hardy you are.

Write down how much you agree or disagree with the following statements, using this scale:

0 = strongly disagree,
1 = mildly disagree,
2 = mildly agree,
3 = strongly agree.

A. Trying my best at work makes a difference.

B. Trusting to fate is sometimes all I can do in a relationship.

C. I often wake up eager to start on the day's projects.

D. Thinking of myself as a free person leads to great frustration and difficulty.

E. I would be willing to sacrifice financial security in my work if something really challenging came along.

F. It bothers me when I have to deviate from the routine or schedule I've set for myself.

G. An average citizen can have an impact on politics.

H. Without the right breaks, it is hard to be successful in my field.

I. I know why I am doing what I'm doing at work.

J. Getting close to people puts me at risk of being obligated to them.

K. Encountering new situations is an important priority in my life.

L. I really don't mind when I have nothing to do.

To Score Yourself: These questions measure control, commitment, and challenge. For half the questions, a high score (like 3, "strongly agree") indicates hardiness; for the other half, a low score (disagreement) does.

To get your scores on control, commitment, and challenge, first write in the number of your answers—0, 1, 2, 3—above the letter of each question on the score sheet. Then add and subtract as shown. (To get your score on "control," for example, add your answers to questions A and G; add your answers to B and H; and then subtract the second number from the first.)

Add your scores on commitment, control, and challenge together to get a score for total hardiness.

A total score of 10–18 shows a hardy personality. 0–9: moderate hardiness. Below 0: low hardiness.

_____ A	+	_____ G	=	_____	
			–		
_____ B	+	_____ H	=	_____	= Control Score
_____ C	+	_____ I	=	_____	
			–		
_____ D	+	_____ J	=	_____	= Commit- ment Score
_____ E	+	_____ K	=	_____	
			–		
_____ F	+	_____ L	=	_____	= Challenge Score

_____ Control	+	_____ Commitment	+	_____ Challenge	=	_____ Total Hardiness Score

Reprinted by permission of the publisher from "How Much Stress Can You Survive?" by Suzanne Ouellette Kobasa, Ph.D., in *American Health*, September 1984, pp. 64–77.

ASSERTIVENESS: THE HUB OF THE WHEEL

OFTEN SAILORS FIND THAT THEY HAVE TO FIGHT THE ELE-
MENTS, AS IN THE CASE OF A STORM AT SEA. WE FIND OUR FREE-
DOM AT THE JUNCTURE OF FORCES WE CANNOT CONTROL BUT
CAN ONLY ENCOUNTER—WHICH OFTEN, LIKE THE SHIP FIGHT-
ING THE STORM, TAKES ALL THE STRENGTH WE HAVE. NOW IT IS
NOT ONLY SAILING *WITH*, IT IS SAILING *AGAINST* THE SEA AND
THE STORM WINDS.

—ROLLO MAY

George F. Solomon, M.D., has been called the "father of psychoneuroimmunology." In the 1960s, the Stanford University psychiatrist blazed a trail with research on the mind-body connection. No one before him had seriously considered the influence of mental states and traits on the immune system. He and his colleague, Rudolf Moos, published a paper in 1964 called "Emotions, Immunity, and Disease." The mere title, barely understood at the time, offered a glimpse of the future of an entire new field. With an equally keen attention to the complexities of cellular behavior and human behavior, Solomon laid the foundation for PNI and modern mind-body science.

Before Solomon, few had imagined that the brain was centrally involved in regulating our biological defense network. He not only collaborated on animal experiments with an immunologist, Alfred Amkraut, to verify this, but at the same time he conducted extensive research on personality and emotions in patients with rheumatoid arthritis, a painful and sometimes crippling autoimmune disease. With a landmark paper published in 1965, George Solomon was the first American scientist to explore the notion of Immune Power traits.

However, as Solomon's research broke new ground, few in mainstream medicine took notice. Immunologists rejected the idea that the immune system "took orders" from any other system—and certainly not from the brain. Psychiatrists were skeptical of the notion that mind-states could influence cellular defenses. Although his work was published in reputable scientific journals, Solomon remained an anomaly to his own colleagues in psychiatry. He was also a man on the fringe to the immunologists, even though Amkraut, his collaborator, was a recognized member of their ranks. Procuring funds for his studies became increasingly difficult. By the early 1970s, he became frustrated in his efforts to broaden research on mind-body connections. After a decade of work, he withdrew from the field. "I left it for ten years because no one would listen," he told Steven Locke and Douglas Colligan for their book *The Healer Within*.

In the late 1970s, research by Robert Ader showed that rats could be trained to control their own immune responses. That led to a veritable explosion of research in mind-immune linkages and the formal inception of the field of PNI. Suddenly, almost every new researcher and every published paper made reference to Solomon's early work. Mind-body research gained respectability, and funding for PNI studies became more readily available. These developments heralded Solomon's return to the field. Today, Solomon is a professor of psychiatry at UCLA and chief of psychoneuroimmunology at the VA Medical Center in Sepulveda,

California. And he is back making vital contributions with new studies and connections among mind, immunity, and health.

Among the most penetrating of his new projects was a pilot study of long AIDS survivors, who were exceedingly rare in 1984, when medical treatments to prevent opportunistic infections had barely been developed. Along with Lydia Temoshok, Ph.D., of the University of California at San Francisco, Solomon identified five long survivors of AIDS who became "consultants" to their project. The consultants would provide psychological and immunological clues to common factors among AIDS patients who were beating the odds.

These five individuals were unique in their interests, life goals, and backgrounds. But they shared certain striking similarities in personality style and coping. Here is an abbreviated list of those shared traits, as observed by Solomon and Temoshok:

1. Active participation in their medical care and a sense of control over their health.
2. A sense of meaningfulness and purpose in life.
3. Being altruistically involved with other AIDS patients.
4. Acceptance of the reality of the AIDS diagnosis, alongside an adamant refusal to view the condition as a death sentence.
5. Being assertive and having the ability to say "no."
6. Being sensitive to their bodies, their physical needs, and their needs for support.

Notice that this list reflects many of the seven Immune Power traits. While each trait was apparent, the patients' assertiveness was most conspicuous. Their fighting spirit may have been prominent because AIDS is such a devastating illness, and the only way they could survive was to do battle. They had to struggle against doctors who offered little hope; a medical system that provided few answers; a society that discriminated against gay people; and a culture that viewed AIDS as an automatic death sentence.

Here is how Solomon described Randy, one of the long survivors:

Randy is feisty as hell. He seeks out treatments. He takes charge of his own care. He doesn't put up with anything. He has the fiercest determination to live that I have ever seen. He has projects; he is involved. He has a marvelous support system. Randy is now teaching in college, and his helper count is 28. [Normal is between 500 and 1,500.] This also shows that with 28 helper cells, you can still live, which shows you can't always go by the lab workup.

Solomon and Temoshok relied on the massive amount of data garnered from their feisty consultants to design a larger, systematic study of eighteen AIDS patients, including a number of long survivors. They searched for psychological factors that influenced their survival and the surprising resilience of their besieged immune systems. They conducted interviews and personality tests and drew blood samples to measure the vitality of each person's immune responses. In essence, Solomon and Temoshok were trying to verify whether Immune Power traits existed and whether they helped people stave off the onslaught of AIDS.

The commonalities among the five original survivors were no fluke. *The same personality patterns were present among the long survivors in the formal study.*

The most striking finding in the formal study was a correlation between an affirmative answer to one specific question and stronger immune functions: "Would you refuse to do a favor requested by a friend if you did not wish to?" The subtext was "Can you say 'no'?"

The long survivors answered "yes"—they would absolutely refuse the favor. *That single trait was powerfully correlated with stronger, more active immune cells.* And this effect was not limited to one type of defender cell. Refusing to do an unwanted favor was associated with stronger responses by many soldier cells—including killer Ts, virus-killing cells, and suppressor cells. All of these cell types are now considered vital in combating HIV and AIDS.

What did the ability to say "no" tell Solomon about the psychological makeup of these survivors?

"It reflects assertiveness, and the ability to resist becoming a self-sacrificing martyr. It also demonstrates the capacity to monitor and take care of your own needs, psychologically and physically. For example, a person with AIDS may not feel well. Is he going to go out and help move furniture because a friend asked him to? Or will he be able to say 'No, I don't feel up to it.' "

Susan Sontag's book *Illness as Metaphor* states that invidious metaphors about disease (such as "Cancer is the epitome of evil") are harmful to the spiritual health and well-being of people struggling with illness. But many have questioned her contention that all metaphors about illness are cruel or irrelevant. Solomon, Temoshok, and others have shown that certain metaphors about disease and health are meaningful. They help patients to find coherence and purpose in the midst of profound suffering. The psychological refusal to please for the sake of pleasing was one such healing metaphor, which appeared to have a corollary in the immune systems of patients struggling with HIV infection: Their bodies seemed to take an equally "assertive" stand against the virus.

Solomon and Temoshok uncovered several other mind-immune connections among the long survivors. Patients with the most CD4 helper T-cells—the main targets of HIV—showed less anxiety, depression, fatigue, and stress related to their illness. Patients with livelier CD8 suppressor cells, which are very important to AIDS resistance, demonstrated an ability to "withdraw to nurture the self." These patients were aware of their needs and willing to brook the disappointment of others to meet those needs. Survivors with more vigorous immune cells also had a stronger locus of control—one of the "three Cs" in Suzanne Ouellette's hardiness concept. (Figure 5.1 charts correlations between psychological factors and immune cell functions in AIDS patients.)

Solomon is quick to point out that his AIDS study, completed several years ago, was provocative but relatively small. In the past few years, he and other scientists have conducted new studies that confirm the earlier findings. We now know that surprising numbers of people who are infected with HIV stay healthy for up to a decade. Those with "fighting spirit" live longer. People with full-blown AIDS often outlive the expectations of their doctors. People

Psychological Factors and Immune-Cell Functions in AIDS Patients

| ✔ = Statistically Significant Positive Correlation

Cytotoxic "Killer" T-cells—T-cells that specifically target virus-infected cells and cancer cells

"Virucidal" cells—Immune cells that target viruses and virus-infected cells

Suppressor cells—T-cells that keep immune reactions in check, helping to prevent auto-immune disorders

Helper T-cells—T-cells that orchestrate immune responses by signaling other cells and substances to go into action

◆ —Not all psychological variables or immune cell categories included here

Increased Numbers of Immune Cells ◆

PSYCHOLOGICAL VARIABLES ◆	CYTOTOXIC "KILLER" T-CELLS	VIRUCIDAL CELLS	SUPPRESSOR CELLS	HELPER T-CELLS
Will not do an "unwanted" favor	✔	✔	✔	
Will withdraw to nurture the self	✔		✔	
Less stress from sickness	✔			✔
Less stress *other* than illness	✔	✔		
Less fatigue	✔	✔	✔	✔
Less tension/anxiety		✔		✔
More "up"		✔		

Findings derived from data in L. Temoshok et al., "Psychoimmunologic Studies of Men with AIDS and ARC," talk presented at the Fourth International Conference on AIDS, Stockholm, Sweden, June 12–16, 1988; and G. F. Solomon, M.E. Kemendy, and L. Temoshok, "Psychoneuroimmunologic Aspects of Human Immunodeficiency Virus Infection," in R. Ader, *Psychoneuroimmunology*, 2nd ed. (1991) Academy Press, New York.

Figure 5.1

with HIV who join group programs that emphasize the mind-body connection may protect their immune functions and resist the onset of AIDS for extended periods of time.

In a 1993 study, George Solomon gathered together nine of the most unusual cases he could find: individuals infected with HIV who, by all medical accounts, should have been near death. These were men with CD4 cell counts below 50.

CD4 cells, also known as T-helpers, are key players in every one of our immune responses. They activate and round up other cells and substances to do battle against disease agents. CD4 cells are also the prime targets of HIV. Therefore, CD4 counts are perhaps the most reliable index of the lethal progress of the virus: The lower they are, the more profoundly devastated the person's immune system. The average healthy person has a count between 500 and 1,500. For HIV-infected individuals, a count less than 200 now warrants a diagnosis of AIDS. Most people with counts that low suffer from opportunistic infections, from Pneumocystis Carinii pneumonia (PCP) to Kaposi's sarcoma, a recalcitrant form of cancer.

Counts below 50 are nothing short of dangerous. Yet Solomon's nine men with rapidly dwindling CD4 cells remained miraculously healthy. For an average of nineteen months, these men showed no evidence of illness. Solomon wanted to understand what was special about their immune systems and, perhaps, their personalities. He drew blood, used the latest technology to test for every critical immune function, and administered a battery of tests and interviews to thoroughly evaluate their psychological traits and states.

Solomon discovered that other parts of their immune system had become livelier, as if to compensate for the critical loss of CD4 helper cells. Their natural killer cells remained vitally active.* They had normal or elevated numbers of CD8 suppressor cells—considered crucial to defend against HIV.

These men also demonstrated remarkably healthy personality traits. Here is how Solomon described them:

---

*A number of PNI studies had already established the relationship between healthy psychological coping and the vitality of natural killer cells.

Among our nine subjects, the coping modes most often observed were interaction with the treating physician in a collaborative manner, having a sense of personal control over one's health outcome, having a future orientation to life in terms of unmet goals, acceptance of the reality of one's HIV status without its being perceived as an imminent death sentence, and an ability to withdraw from taxing involvements in order to "nurture" oneself.

All subjects reported good relationships with mother and siblings but only four with fathers; significantly, eight of nine had close friends. Strikingly, eight of nine reported being quite able to assert themselves, and seven did not feel powerless or helpless in the face of life's difficulties, including illness. Subjects most frequently described themselves as responsible, conscientious, alert, quick, and aggressive and least often as meek, bitter, and guilty.

These nine unlikely survivors evidenced extraordinary resilience in both their psychological and their immunological systems. Given what we know today about communications between these systems—mediated by a vast orchestra of messenger molecules—the connection is more than an arbitrary analogy. Through biochemical pathways, the trait of assertiveness appears to bolster and balance our immune functions.

With this foray into research on long survivors of AIDS, Solomon stepped into a realm with great potential for clinical applications. If assertiveness protected our immune defenses, then becoming assertive might prevent or slow many diseases of weakened immunity—including cancer, viral infections, chronic fatigue, arthritis, lupus, asthma, allergies, and the common cold.

Although his HIV findings were compelling, their core message was nothing new to Solomon. He'd been investigating Immune Power traits from the earliest days of his career. And assertiveness was always at the top of his list, appearing repeatedly in people who resisted autoimmune diseases, infections, and cancer. The high-tech immune studies confirmed what Solomon suspected thirty years ago, when he made his first forays into mind-body research with mice and with rheumatoid arthritis sufferers.

ON THE TRAIL OF HEALTH-PROMOTING TRAITS

Two of George Solomon's earliest studies pointed toward the concept of an Immune Power Personality. The first was with people who resisted rheumatoid arthritis (RA), a severe autoimmune disease. The second was with an unexpectedly feisty group of mice that resisted tumors.

Rheumatoid factor is an antibody found in the blood of patients with RA. It is commonly considered a genetic marker for the disease: Healthy people who have the marker are at increased risk for developing RA. Solomon wanted to know why some people with the genetic marker never got the disease.

He decided to study a group of women, all of whom had close relatives with rheumatoid arthritis. However, half of them had rheumatoid factor in their blood, while the other half did not. The women who had the genetic marker were considered high risk, yet they remained curiously free of the disease. With his colleague Rudolf Moos, Solomon conducted extensive psychological evaluations of both groups.

Among the women without rheumatoid factor, Solomon and Moos discovered a number of psychologically healthy individuals. But they also found many people with guilt feelings, somatic complaints, obsessive-compulsive behavior, low self-esteem, and neurotic behavior. In short, the women without rheumatoid factor showed some healthy and many unhealthy characteristics.

The women who had rheumatoid factor were completely different. These women demonstrated a remarkable degree of psychological health and well-being. "They lacked anxiety, depression, and alienation," Solomon remarked. "And they reported excellent, satisfying relationships and marriages. They had what we call 'ego mastery'—an ability to cope with stress. Their psychological defenses were in good shape. They liked their jobs and were happy with their lives."

What was the significance of these findings? Solomon had hand-picked a group of individuals who managed to fend off a disease to which they were vulnerable by virtue of their genes. Their unusually healthy characteristics proved Solomon's hypothesis: People who resist diseases possess traits that balance and strengthen their immune systems. The women who lacked the disease marker were "normal" in every sense; the women who had the marker yet resisted the disease were not at all "normal"—they were supremely confident and emotionally balanced!

Solomon interpreted this discovery in light of his clinical observation that many people with RA succumbed to the disease when their coping capacities were overwhelmed by stress. He'd seen many patients whose disease flared up—often disabling them—when circumstances in their lives became too much to bear. He counseled people with rheumatoid factor in their blood to seek support and professional help during periods of severe stress, in order to ward off the disease.

During this same period, Solomon and Amkraut began a series of studies on stress and immunity in mice. In one of the studies, they were using inbred mice, which are genetically identical, to evaluate their immune system's resistance to tumors caused by viruses. But a funny thing happened on the way from the animal supplier to the laboratory. Here is Solomon's rendering of the story:

The inbred mice we received for our studies had scabs, injuries, and scratches. I was annoyed with the animal supplier, who I thought was providing us with inferior merchandise. So I called him up and complained that we couldn't use them. He said, "Oh, I'm terribly sorry, you must have gotten some fighters." I said, "What do you mean, fighters?" He explained that some of the mice tend to fight, and he usually eliminates them. I said, "Some of them fight and some don't, yet they're all genetically identical?" "Yes," he said. I asked if I could come look at them, and he was happy to have me. I traveled from Palo Alto to his facility in San Jose, and sure enough, some of these mice developed spontaneous fighting behavior.

I asked him to regularly supply us with equal groups of fighters and nonfighters, so we could compare them.

What we found was significant differences between the mice in their ability to reject virally induced tumors. The fighters had much stronger resistance to cancer. It pays to get mad, even if you are a mouse!

The genetically vulnerable women who resisted RA had happy lives, strong egos, and healthy psychological defenses. The mice that resisted tumors were tough tykes that protected their turf. From two labs that were worlds apart, George Solomon was beginning to develop a case for Immune Power traits.

ASSERTIVENESS AND THE HEALTH SECRETS OF SISTERS

George Solomon questions the term "Immune Power," because a healthy immune system is not a juggernaut. It knows when to enter battle, but it also knows when to cease and desist. In people afflicted with autoimmune disease, immune cells attack their own tissues. These immune cells are insensitive to molecular signals of "selfhood" present on the surface of their own cells. The healthiest immune system is not simply the mightiest, but the most selective and strategically focused in its responses.

The mind-body literature has many terms for health-damaging personalities—Type A, Type C, coronary-prone, cancer-prone, disease-prone, "immunosuppression-prone," and so forth. Yet there is no counterpart for health-promoting personalities. The only term in the medical literature for immunologic well-being is "immune competence." Yet the term "immune-competent personality" does not connote strength *or* balance. I use "Immune Power" to indicate an immune system that is sensitive and selective as well as vigorous.

In the late 1960s, Solomon continued exploring traits in rheumatoid arthritis, this time searching for differences between people with active disease and those who were healthy. Along with

Rudolf Moos, he compared twenty women with arthritis to their healthy sisters, who had the same genetic background. They administered personality tests and recorded an hourlong interview that was later rated by two independent psychologists.

Solomon and Moos discovered a world of difference between the women suffering with RA and their healthy sisters. Here is a summary of the contrasts:

- Unlike their healthy sisters, personality tests revealed the RA patients to be masochistic, self-sacrificing, and unassertive. (They evidenced the same nice-guy pattern that researchers before and since have observed in a high percentage of cancer patients.)
- Almost all healthy sisters said they expressed their anger and provided at least one recent example. Only two of their arthritic sisters directly stated that they expressed angry feelings. There was no patient-sibling pair in which the patient said that she expressed anger more freely than her sister.
- Many of the patients complained about being trapped in bad marriages. The healthy sisters had reasonably happy and stable marriages.
- Eighty-one percent of the women with RA said they never fought with their husbands. Not a single healthy sibling said she never fought with her husband. The same arthritis sufferers who complained of bad marriages still said they never fought.
- The RA patients described themselves as tense, worried, depressed, and moody. Their healthy counterparts described themselves as active, busy, sociable, energetic, and enjoying life.
- The women with RA used terms to describe themselves that emphasized being shy, inhibited, and hard to get to know. The siblings emphasized being optimistic and easygoing.

The rich psychological data collected in this study revealed the night-and-day differences between sisters who developed autoimmune disease and those who became ill. A later, larger study using personality tests on forty-nine RA patients and fifty-three of their healthy female family members confirmed these trends. Unlike their healthy sisters, the arthritis patients evidenced depression, apathy, anxiety, masochism, self-alienation, overcompliance, and psychological rigidity.

To illustrate these stark differences, Solomon, whose memory of past cases is uncanny, told me the extraordinary story of two sisters from his original study. Both of them had proven genetic susceptibility to rheumatoid arthritis, but only one had the disease. They shared certain traits—both were high-achieving, attractive, and athletic. But their personalities and the story of their lives diverged dramatically.

The sister with arthritis had been in the air force, teaching the maintenance of military aircraft engines. One of the few women in an exclusively male enclave, she was extremely skilled and was responsible for teaching highly technical information to hundreds of men. When she got out of the service, she rushed into marriage. According to Solomon, she "tried to force herself into the conventional social role of wife and mother. She became very dutiful in those roles. That's the period when she developed rheumatoid arthritis."

Her sister was statuesque and stunning, a beauty contest winner and a superb athlete. She got pregnant at a young age, and married the father despite having had unspoken reservations about him. When he was called into action during the Korean war, she and her baby waited two years for his homecoming. Shortly after his return, she discovered that he was having affairs. Solomon recalled her rather terse remembrance of this event:

He was out on his ass before he knew what hit him. Here she was, a young woman on her own with a baby. And not too much later, she was in the Olympics. In a very difficult track event. She competed in international sports until her late twenties. Then she became a pro in another less demanding sport, one that allowed her to continue her passion later in life. She was fortunate enough to meet another guy, also a pro in the same sport, whom she married. They had a really good relationship, he became a great stepfather, and they toured together doing what they both loved to do."

At the time Solomon met the sisters, the arthritic sibling seemed to have a pressure-free life, though she admitted to frustration in her wife/mother role. She also played another role—one she appeared to relish—as her elderly father's caretaker. Despite her physical pain, she went to his house on a regular basis to clean and cook. However, it was the healthy sister who gave Solomon deeper insight into the arthritic sister's relationship with her father and what it revealed about her character.

Solomon quoted from the healthy sister's comments: "My sister and I get along great, she is a really nice person. But I simply don't understand why she continues to take care of our father. Now, I was sexually molested by this man. She refuses to talk about it, but I am virtually positive that she was too. Can you believe she is still taking care of the son of a bitch! I personally hope he rots in hell."

The sister with arthritis continued to struggle for the love of her father while denying the early abuse. She remained long-suffering and self-sacrificing. The healthy sister acknowledged the abuse of the father, was in touch with (and expressed!) her anger, and had long ago given up struggling for his love. She wasn't wallowing in bitterness or taking her anger out on others; she simply faced the truth and got on with her life. Despite her genetic vulnerability, she never contracted arthritis.

The healthy sister demonstrated many Immune Power traits: She took care of her needs, asserted herself forcefully, refused to accept abuse, hadn't the least hesitation about airing her feelings, had a supportive marriage, and was able to combine passion and play in work that was meaningful to her. Solomon still recalled how remarkably open she had been, especially considering the fact that sexual abuse simply wasn't discussed in those days. "To tell me that she hoped the father rots in hell . . . now that's open!"

Solomon's tale offers both insights and guidelines for people who inherit susceptibilities to autoimmune or even genetic diseases. There is reason for such individuals to hope that the genetic cards seemingly stacked against them do not necessarily spell disaster. How they cope with life's traumas will likely contribute to their risk profile. The healthy sister's stance over a period of decades differentiated her from her vulnerable sibling. She would not be defeated by an adulterous husband or abusive father, which appeared to make all the difference in terms of her psychological and physical health.

What about the sister who sacrificed herself for her father and succumbed to arthritis? The healthy sister's attitude toward her was not one of finger-pointing; she felt empathic outrage on her behalf. She sensed that her sister had become numb to her own pain and anger. She only wished that she'd awaken, get away from the father, and finally find her own independent path in life. Solomon shared the healthy sister's compassionate perspective.

Based on his own research findings, Solomon believes that people in situations similar to those of the arthritic sister can be told—by therapists, friends, or family members—that becoming more assertive will have positive health consequences. As long as we listen to those who are suffering, our support for transformative action will not be perceived as "blaming the victim." It will be perceived in the spirit it is intended: "I see that you are suffering, and I will support you in any changes you make to find your way out of that suffering."

THE TEST OF ASSERTIVENESS: A PSYCHODRAMA

In his study of sister pairs, Solomon also devised a clever technique to test assertiveness. He produced, directed, and starred in a "little psychodrama" with his subjects. He would play the part of a nasty, highly unreasonable department store complaint manager. The subject would come to him with a broken appliance—an iron or shaver, for instance. As the irascible manager, Solomon would absolutely refuse to take the product back under any circumstances. The unassertive, passive person would give up easily and decide she was stuck with a lemon. The assertive person would stand her ground, insisting on her rights as a consumer.

The results were striking. "We did this with twenty sibling pairs . . . and in every case the sibling was more assertive than the sister with arthritis. Apparently, assertiveness protects the immune system against stress-related damage that throws it off balance, increasing the risk of autoimmune disease.

How did the arthritic sisters react during the psychodrama? They remained polite and in control. They invariably ended the role-play with a comment along these lines: "Well, I guess I'm stuck with it . . ."

How did the healthy sisters react to Solomon's bullying? One of them decided to report him to the store's manager. Another threatened to call the Better Business Bureau. Complaints would be made to the company that manufactured the iron, and briefs would be filed in small claims court. One of the healthy subjects went over the top. "She threatened to hit me over the head with the iron," Solomon said with a laugh.

The psychodrama was so effective in the arthritic sisters study that Solomon embarked on pilot research with a small group of healthy volunteers to find out if assertiveness—or its opposite, passive compliance—is directly linked to immune functioning. His hypothesis was that people who stand up for themselves will have more balanced immune responses than people who submit to unfair treatment.

Before describing his preliminary results, one fact about stress and immunity is relevant. Natural killer (NK) cells, those freelance assassins that roam the body in search of viruses and cancer cells, are highly responsive to psychological states and traits. But the relationship between the mind and NK cells is complex. In brief, a key distinction must be made between stressful mind states that persist on a low level for long periods and those sudden, acute reactions to stress, for each has a different effect on NK cells. When we demonstrate an enduring capacity to cope with life's travails, our NKs appear to be strengthened. By contrast, when we chronically feel helpless, depressed, anxious, or stressed out, we may have weakened NK cells.

However, Solomon and other researchers have shown that acute stress in the present—say, a mugging—will stimulate our NKs. The fight-or-flight response, our nervous system's immediate response to danger, puts NK cells on notice. The reason? PNI scientists speculate that our evolutionary forefathers, who faced mortal dangers on hunting forays in the wild, would require a rise in NKs to stave off infection due to potential injury. Through brain-immune pathways, short-term danger signals a short-term increase in natural killers.

Now let's return to Solomon's assertiveness study. He believed that people who stood up for themselves in the face of psycholog-ical assault reduced their stress levels. They would not respond to an everyday exchange with a nasty stranger as if their life were threatened, because they instantly engaged in self-protective behav-ior. Hence, he predicted that they would *not* experience the rise in NK cells that occurs during acute stress.

By contrast, people who responded passively would suffer in mind and body, even if silently. The passive responders would ex-perience the role-play as stressful, because they were unable to pro-tect their own interests in the face of an interpersonal assault. Hence, Solomon predicted that they *would* experience the rise in NKs that occurs during acute stress.

For the seven volunteers, Solomon himself re-created his clas-sic role as the nasty department store complaint manager. Before each role-play, the subjects filled out questionnaires of assertiveness and blood was drawn for immune tests. Each role-play exercise was videotaped and later analyzed for nonverbal evidence of assertive-ness or passivity. Did they raise their voices? Did their expressions show defiance, confidence, anger? Or did they show resignation, reluctance, or uncertainty? Psychologists made these determina-tions through careful rating procedures. Finally, more blood was drawn immediately after the psychodrama.

The results bore out Solomon's hypothesis with uncanny accu-racy. In response to his angry stonewalling, some patients asserted their rights and others did not. The ones who rated high on assert-iveness on the video also rated high on the questionnaires. These individuals showed absolutely no change in their natural killer cells. They so effectively protected themselves against Solomon's psychological "assault" that their immune systems did not even reg-ister the event. On the other hand, the passive responders demon-strated a significant rise in NK cell activity. Solomon is now planning a larger version of this same study, an attempt to verify the link between assertiveness and immune function.

We already have evidence that people who react assertively to an existing illness are more likely to recover. A recent study reported in *Diabetes Care* compared diabetics trained to be more assertive with their doctors to a control group who received no such training. After four months, the assertive patients showed significant drops in their blood sugar and fewer physical limitations. (Although the biological mechanism of this effect is unknown, recent studies implicate immune dysfunction as one contributor to diabetes.)

A fascinating recent study conducted at Tufts University was described by Tom Ferguson, M.D.:

> In studies of people with ulcers, hypertension, or diabetes, Tufts University researchers actually taught patients a set of skills that enabled them to be more assertive with their doctors—with good results. Internist Sheldon Greenfield and social psychologist Sherrie Kaplan developed a 20-minute "assertiveness-coaching session" for patients waiting to see their physicians. Trained aides reviewed the patients' medical records with them, helped them to think of questions they wanted to ask, and urged them to take an active role. The aides also offered techniques for overcoming embarrassment and anxiety.
>
> The result: The coached patients established a much higher level of control when they saw the doctor. They directed the conversation, interrupted their doctors when necessary, and obtained a good deal more medical information. Four months later, the coached patients had missed less work, reported fewer symptoms, and rated their overall health as significantly better than patients who simply followed their doctors' orders.

The patients' improvements may have stemmed, in part, from better medical care they received as a result of their assertive behavior. But George Solomon's research suggests that their improvements also stemmed from the positive effects of assertiveness on their own bodies, including their cardiovascular and immune systems.

In a landmark study, British psychiatrist Steven Greer, M.D., showed that women with breast cancer who responded to their diagnosis with fighting spirit, as opposed to stoic acceptance or hopelessness, were twice as likely to be alive fifteen years later. Greer found that the "fighters" responded to their illness with the attitude "I am going to beat this thing." They did whatever they could to recover—seeking treatments, taking responsibility for their care, procuring emotional support, defending their needs and rights as patients and as human beings.

Thus, fighting spirit includes assertiveness, hardiness, and an ineffable dimension that can perhaps best be termed "will to live." Although assertiveness and fighting spirit are not exactly synonymous, there can be no fighting spirit without assertiveness. Standing up for themselves appears to enhance cancer patients' odds against their disease. One plausible explanation is that their feisty determination strengthens their body's defenses.

RESILIENCE AMONG THE HEALTHY ELDERLY

In recent research with healthy elderly people, Solomon uncovered new evidence that assertiveness, coping skills, and a sense of meaning enhance not only mental states but body-states as well.

He studied a group of independently living elderly individuals in their seventies, eighties, and nineties, all of whom were in excellent health. It is important to note that the immune systems of elderly people undergo natural decline. All T-cell functions suffer with aging. Solomon discovered that these healthy elderly people have fairly intact T-cell functions and stronger natural killer cells, which are capable of swift action against cancer cells and other foreign agents. As with the healthy HIV patients, their immune systems appear to either resist or compensate for their cellular losses. At the same time, Solomon found them to be "good copers" who were rarely distressed or worried. These healthy older people had that "inner locus of control," a faith in their ability to adapt to change, stress, or pain. (This concept is comparable to Ouellette's sense of control, an aspect of hardiness.)

Early in his research on long survivors of AIDS, Solomon noted that they too had an inner locus of control. They weren't control freaks, they were problem-solvers, help-seekers, and optimists—activists on their own behalf. Of course, neither the AIDS survivors nor the healthy elderly were without trouble or worry. "However," Solomon added, "when the older subjects *were* worried about something, if they were also angry about it, then they were protected from immune dysfunction. Anger protects."

Solomon speaks often about "buffers," qualities that protect us from the ravages of stress which, he points out, none of us can escape. The problem, he says, is not *stress* but rather *distress*. And we can prevent distress by getting love and support when we are alone or troubled. We can keep from falling into chronic depression when we take assertive action to change conditions that depress us. We can ease despair when we develop a sense of meaning and commitment in our relationships and our life's work. Solomon provided a personal example:

I have a ninety-three-year-old volunteer working for me, and if this were a Wednesday, you'd see him doing all my heavy Xeroxing. Here is a man who travels all over the country, all over the world. He's a remarkable man, he's been on TV as an example of a vigorous elderly fellow. He has no cognitive deficits. He does serial sevens [the mathematical stress test] like a whiz. He has no dysphoria [psychological term for distress]. Zero, zero. He has a very nice relationship with his girlfriend who is eighty-nine—they go dancing all the time and go out on dates. I've done every immune test in the world on him. Every psychological test is great and every immune test is great. I'm not saying his immune system will never go down, but he's ninety-three so the process has clearly been delayed. Maybe it'll happen when he is one hundred and three. Right now, he could pass for eighty.

The healthy elderly, resisting the pull of age on their immune systems, succeed in so doing by staying in the stream of life. They protect themselves from depression and illness with coping skills—including expression of anger. One critical aspect of assertiveness is the ability to effectively—and appropriately—express anger. The healthy elderly scored high on the control measure of hardiness. Assertiveness and a sense of control appear to be handmaidens in preventing depression *and* disease.

As with the long survivors of AIDS, Solomon set his sights on a population that conventional wisdom consigns to an inexorable march toward deteriorating health. What better way to study the Immune Power Personality? In trying to understand resilience, we all tend to focus on the young and middle-age people who ward off disease while neglecting the remarkable people who live into their seventh or eighth decades beset by few afflictions. We now have evidence from George Solomon that their mental and physical states are bound together. The implications are crystal clear: Any psychological intervention that helps elderly people to engage in meaningful activity and assert their needs will undoubtedly strengthen their resistance to illness.

THE PATCHWORK QUILT OF HEALTHY TRAITS

People who resist diseases—whether it is arthritis, lupus, cancer, AIDS, or other viruses—possess a patchwork quilt of healthy personality traits, which fit together seamlessly and serve them well as they cope with life's travails. That was George Solomon's finding in many studies and countless clinical tales over thirty years of mind-body investigations. When I asked him to summarize the health-promoting traits he had observed—cutting across many diseases and populations—he responded with this litany:

1. Being in touch with our psychological and bodily needs.
2. Being able to meet those needs by assertive action.
3. Coping skills, including a sense of control, that enable us to ward off depression.

4. Expressing emotions, including sadness and anger.
5. The willingness to ask for and accept support from loved ones.
6. A sense of meaning and purpose in our work, daily activities, and relationships.
7. The capacity for pleasure and play.

Each trait tapped a different dimension of what psychologist Abraham Maslow called "self-actualization," or realizing one's true self. Solomon views these healthy traits as potential factors in resistance to *any* disease involving deficient immunity. That includes cancer, chronic fatigue, and infectious diseases (where the immune system *under*reacts) as well as autoimmune disorders such as arthritis, lupus, asthma, and allergies (where the immune system *over*reacts).

In Solomon's studies, at least, assertiveness was the most glaring contributor to physical health. A person's assertive stance bespoke her willingness to stand up for herself, to insist on her rights—to stake a claim in this world. Assertiveness was a behavioral cue that the person was not afraid to be herself. Thus, it was a powerful indicator of psychological health and well-being. Yet Solomon believes that each of the above-listed traits play a part in physical health, and each of them can be cultivated.

Solomon also insists that people can make personality changes to fine-tune their immune systems and, thus, help to prevent or heal illnesses. He has seen patients change frequently, often because he has been the therapist who facilitated such transformation. At one of our meetings, Solomon illustrated this potential in a most vivid way. He introduced me to two women from the VA hospital staff who shared their stories with us. Frances, an occupational therapist, had suffered from scleroderma that was currently in remission. This autoimmune disease begins with a thickening of the skin, and if it progresses to internal organs, it can be fatal. She first became ill after leaving her job as a nurse—work she loved—to stay home with her children and tend to her husband. She knew that something had to change. Finally Frances went back to work and restructured her priorities.

"I had been trying to maintain the perfect family," she confessed. "It wasn't possible. Now I'm not as concerned about meeting my husband's [needs] as I am about making my life full." Her marriage improved along with her sense of personal empowerment. Soon thereafter, Frances was treated with plasmapheresis, a sometimes-effective high-tech treatment. Her disease promptly went into remission. What is really unusual about Frances is that she no longer requires any medical therapy—a remarkable response.

"I have no doubt that plasmapheresis helped her recover," Solomon exclaimed. "But what's keeping her well so that she no longer needs treatments? Could it be that she went about meeting her own needs instead of focusing on what was expected of her?"

Mara, the head nurse at the hospital, had severe rheumatoid arthritis. Both of her knees and hips had been replaced. Mara had first developed arthritis twenty-five years earlier, a few months after giving birth (a common period of onset of autoimmune disease) and while in the midst of a painful divorce. Despite the fact that her ex-husband had been unavailable and hardly supportive, she never once blew up at him. "I don't even know how to be angry," said Mara, though she was currently in therapy to rectify that problem. Mara was an extremely "nice" person who had difficulty asserting her needs.

As Mara told us her life story, a clear pattern emerged. During periods of emotional stability and satisfying work, her disease was quiescent. During periods of unexpressed grief, loneliness, dissatisfaction, or unemployment, her disease flared like wildfire. When Mara got word that her mother had died in Iran, she was unable to attend the funeral or connect with other grieving members of her family. A month later she got laid off from her job. In the aftermath of these stresses, she became crippled by pain. "I was just lost at that time. I felt totally helpless."

But Mara had a rebounding spirit. She had enough in savings and severance pay to get by, she had surgery that restored her mobility, and she got a new job at the VA Medical Center. Months later she went to Europe to see her brothers and sisters. "I was able to grieve over the death of my mother because my family was there. I went with my brothers and sisters to a bar to have a drink and we all cried. We talked as if we were at the funeral. I was there for a month, and when I returned, life went back to normal."

After her return, Mara's symptoms quickly abated. She entered psychotheraphy to learn coping strategies and acknowledge her authentic feelings. From that point on, she has remained healthy, with only minimal pain, for seven years. As I listened to her story, I recognized the elegant truth of Solomon's point that sharing and expressing emotions is a crucial buffer against the potentially debilitating and immune-imbalancing effects of stress.

Solomon, who held both Frances and Mara in high regard, resists the notion that people whose personalities play a part in their ill health are psychologically or spiritually impoverished. He believes that people can acknowledge and change their patterns without blaming themselves for their life problems or their sickness.

While Solomon doesn't think that excessive niceness is a disease, he does think that dutifulness to the point of self-neglect can compromise immunity. When we allow ourselves to be dragged into a role or activity to please others, the stress we encounter *will* lead to distress. Why? Apparently, when our work or relationship is pursued by choice rather than obligation, when it's seen as a challenge rather than a hardship, then stress will be a motivator, not a cause of anxiety and ill health.

SOLOMON'S APPROACH TO DEVELOPING IMMUNE POWER TRAITS

George Solomon and other PNI scientists are beginning to make sense of the complex biological pathways between mind and body. Solomon believes that we can enhance mind-body health by developing positive, adaptive personality traits. We can learn skills that enable us to assert ourselves without alienating people close to us.

How does he help patients develop these qualities? This section provides an overview of George Solomon's approach to transformation.

PRESCRIPTIONS FOR SELF-CARE

One of Solomon's first and simplest approaches is to give his patients permission to attend to their needs. One of his patients, a former professional baseball player, contracted arthritis soon after he quit playing. But he remained an avid fan who loved nothing more than an afternoon at the ballpark. Still, he often felt guilty about his passionate pastime. He thought he should be home working, or spending more time with his family. Solomon's response was to take out his prescription pad, on which he scribbled: *Minimum of one game per home stand.* He handed this slip to his patient and proclaimed his dead seriousness: "You tell your family that this is doctor's orders."

Solomon insists that therapists or doctors of any kind could intervene this way, if only they listened more carefully to their patients. "The patient may not need to understand why he feels guilty about going to ballgames. He just needs to get out to the damn games!" Often, once patients are given permission to honor their needs, they begin to take responsibility for meeting them and no longer require endless "prescriptions."

You can become your *own* best doctor, by writing yourself prescriptions to honor your needs. Many people prone to illness are out of touch with their needs. Solomon believes that exercise, body-based therapies (massage, the Alexander technique, or Reichian treatments), and other approaches such as meditation can make inroads for them. "I have a theory that body-based therapies help because they give you more inner somatic awareness. You monitor and tune in to your body. Self-awareness must include both psychological and physical awareness. I don't believe it's body *and* mind, I believe its *body-mind.*" Solomon's theory accurately reflects Gary Schwartz's findings on the ACE Factor—that attention to bodily states leads to connection and appropriate expressive actions that bolster health and well-being.

PSYCHOTHERAPY FOR DEEP-GOING CHANGE

For people with deeper issues, insight psychotherapy is a path for developing awareness of needs and learning the skills of assertiveness. That kind of psychotherapy is an involved process. In his studies of arthritis patients, Solomon found that their mothers were often self-sacrificing martyrs who unintentionally contributed to their children's guilt about tending to their own needs. Their fathers were perceived as overly strict. In therapy, patients with this background can shed the belief that they're "not as good a person as Mother if they don't play the martyr." What about the father's effect? "If the father was strict," Solomon commented, "the therapist can help the patient to become more permissive with himself."

Certain basic practices of psychotherapy, claims Solomon, can reap untold benefits in people who wish to prevent or overcome chronic illness. Assertiveness training, where therapists "model" more effective behaviors for patients, can turn acquiescent types who take care of others into self-protective people who take care of themselves. At the end of the chapter I provide assertiveness guidelines you can apply on your own.

First, though, consider the case of Marty, a patient who was told by his surgeon, "You have two choices. You can have a large part of your colon removed now to get rid of your ulcerative colitis, or you can try psychotherapy. Probably I'll have to take out your colon in six months no matter what." Despite his surgeon's pessimism, Marty chose therapy with Solomon. He explored issues and memories of the painful neglect by both his parents that he suffered throughout his childhood, work that freed him up considerably. "He was very successful in therapy," Solomon commented. "But he was also a remarkable person. He had a terrible family background, came from an inner city slum and worked his way through Stanford Medical School. Since therapy, he's been happily married and written a textbook on medicine. And he never had colitis again."

GETTING THE SUPPORT YOU NEED

For years mind-body scientists and doctors have been saying that social support keeps us healthy, but a useful interpretation of these findings is sorely lacking. What are we to do with this knowledge? If we recognize that our support system is lacking, is it our task to bolster our network? Certainly, but the implicit advice is so limited as to be worthless. It's like telling a friend who is lonely to go out and find new friends. Fine, but how?

Another question lies at the heart of the connection between social support and Immune Power. Studies have shown that having a large network does not necessarily confer health benefits. In terms of health, the *quality* of the relationships in our social networks is what matters most.

Solomon insists that many of us with wonderful friends and family still suffer because we don't know how to accept their support. It's important to be able to say "no" to a request for a favor; it's just as important to be able to ask for a favor. Taken together, both sides of this behavioral coin represent the essence of assertiveness. He elaborated: "If you have a good friend who asks how you're doing, and you say 'Terrific,' he's likely to say 'Great. See you next week.' On the other hand, if you say 'I'm really feeling awful,' he might say 'What can I do to help? What do you need?' If you don't communicate with your support system, then the system isn't supportive."

James, one of Solomon's patients and a long-term survivor of AIDS, had a marvelous support system that he was able to draw upon. During the seven years he lived after his diagnosis, James suffered with many opportunistic diseases. He recovered each time, and his illnesses never stopped him from living fully. In 1985, he was diagnosed with lymphoma and told he had weeks to live, even with chemotherapy. His cancer was gone within months.

During this period, James went out of his way to enlist the help of his eighty-six-year-old father. After beating lymphoma, James decided to restore a Victorian house he'd bought long ago, a task he'd put off for years. He poured his love, energy, and creativity into the project, which kept him going through all of his physical trials. His father was there for him again, doing construction work and sharing each small triumph.

James's meticulous restoration of the house to its original Victorian glory also bespoke his ability to create something beautiful—and meaningful—in the face of so much fear and stress.

"Secretly, I worried that he would soon die, having reached the goal that provided him with his sense of purpose," said Solomon, who visited the house and saw firsthand the stunning results. "Then he said to me, 'I guess I just have to find another house to restore!' And that's exactly what he did." James had begun restoring that second house when his father, his rock of support, himself became ill. It was during that stressful period that James finally succumbed to complications of AIDS.

There was no doubt in Solomon's mind that James endured for reasons beyond even his goals and his support. He was able to restore those houses because he had the requisite determination. He had the support of his father, and others, because he was unafraid to seek and accept that support. James's underlying attitude of undaunted optimism and his assertive style of coping were reasons he thrived.

Whether we are sick or well, recognizing our needs for support—and giving ourselves permission to ask for that support—is essential for any nourishing relationship. On a larger scale, these small acts of assertion—which for many of us are acts of courage—are the basis for building a rich social network. Solomon says that it's equally important to be able to refuse a favor as it is to ask for a favor—a principle that teaches us how to be assertive without being narcissistic. If we grant ourselves the human right to refuse a request for a favor—even from a beloved friend—we must respect others' rights to refuse our requests. Yet the relationship stagnates if we become so fearful of a "no" answer that we stop asking.

These essential precepts of assertiveness demonstrate that we are entitled to loving concern, but that doesn't mean we will always get it, even (especially) from those closest to us. The distinction between a healthy sense of entitlement, based on self-esteem, and an unhealthy narcissistic entitlement is the difference between being able to tolerate a negative answer or not. When we can't tolerate a "no," our woundedness leads to a spiral of anger, disillusionment, and sometimes even revenge.

A healthy reciprocity is needed for autonomous relationships, in which we grant others the same rights and feelings that we want accepted for ourselves. When this reciprocity is established, we are free enough to ask for support, smart enough to distinguish between a decline and a rejection, and strong enough to accept other people's limitations or choices. It all begins with the ability to assert our needs, rights, and emotions.

ASSERTIVENESS AND THE SEARCH FOR MEANING

Perhaps the most evanescent of Solomon's goals is to help patients find meaning in their work and relationships.

> Fulfilling the need for meaning, I believe, has psychological and physiological effects. If you have a great voice and never sing, you're frustrated. If you have wonderful coordination and never do sports, you're frustrated. If you have an inner awareness of your potentialities and don't use them, you're frustrated. Now, say a person wants to be a professional pianist and doesn't make it. That's a tough one. He must find ways to continue playing. What about teaching piano to underprivileged kids, or developing music programs in schools? Or giving free concerts? Or composing? There are many ways, but the person should be doing something in music.

If Solomon's hypothetical pianist is to find meaning, he needs an outlet for his creativity. Whether he decides to teach, develop music programs, or give free concerts, he'll have to assert himself to carve out the proper niche. Will he go out and sell himself to the head of a music program? Will he raise funds for free concerts? Whatever he does, it will require strong actions on his own behalf. Assertiveness and the quest for meaning go hand in hand.

If one were to diagram the Immune Power Personality, assertiveness would appear as the hub of a many-spoked wheel. Why? Because it is a prerequisite for a sense of meaning in work and creative pursuits. How else do we get our foot in the door of a difficult profession or artistic endeavor? Being aware of our needs is not particularly helpful if we don't take action to meet them. And of course, we need assertiveness to form healthy relationships.

One individual who personifies Solomon's notion of assertiveness as a conduit to meaning is Michael Callen, whom I described in the introduction. I met Callen at a 1984 conference entitled "Psychosocial Factors in AIDS." He was the only person with AIDS invited to participate. At that time, he was considered a long survivor, because he had been alive for three years after his diagnosis of AIDS.

With greater eloquence than most of the experts at the meeting, Callen called for more research into psychological factors in AIDS. He also spoke about his own experiences in vivid terms. The conference participants paid rapt attention as Callen rejected our culture's characterization of AIDS as an automatic and swift death sentence. He described his political battles against the established medical community, which evinced little commitment to conquer AIDS during the 1980s.

His fights on the right were counterbalanced by fights on the left. He crossed swords with established sectors of the gay community that, in his view, wished to bury their collective heads in the sands of denial vis-à-vis the dangers of bath houses and unsafe sex practices. Few people know it, but Michael Callen essentially invented the concept of "safe sex." He introduced the notion in a seminal 1982 article in a New York publication.

Callen was a warrior. In an incongruously soft-spoken manner, he expressed his outrage with clarity and his sense of purpose with specificity. His grit and determination were apparent, as were his loving concern for members of his own community and the others stricken—or about to be stricken—with HIV.

Waging battles on so many fronts would exhaust most people in most life circumstances. Yet here was Callen, fighting battles on all sides, relying on his own brand of assertiveness to accomplish these ends. He was never strident in his approach, however. He did not assault doctors or politicians at public meetings; that was not his style. But he spoke his mind and wrote with clarity and complexity.

I was certain that Callen's grace and grit had somehow contributed to his survival. He wasn't taking any antiviral drugs. (There weren't any available at that time, anyway. And when AZT and other antivirals did become available, Callen refused them.) He was taking care of himself, watching his diet, and so on, but so had countless other AIDS patients who had died in their "expected" time frame.

I continued to hear about Callen in the media for a few years. He initiated the term "person with AIDS," as an alternative to the disempowering "AIDS victim." He cofounded the Community Research Initiative on AIDS in New York, a leading AIDS organization. His approach to funding AIDS therapy research on a community basis—as a way around federal red tape—is now seen as a model for AIDS drug development. Convinced that the mind-body connection in AIDS has been ignored, he traveled across the country to interview other long survivors. Their stories, and his own remarkable history, eventually became the basis for his 1990 book, *Surviving AIDS*.

Callen died in Los Angeles in the waning days of 1993. Having lived for twelve years with full-blown AIDS, he is one of the longest survivors on record. I attended his memorial service in New York City, in which friends and family talked about him. A portrait was painted of the man I barely knew. He was quite as complex, fierce, funny, and brilliant as I had imagined. His brother told stories of their childhood together in a small town in Ohio. They had formed a "Kids Empowerment Group" when Michael was about ten years old. But that wasn't enough. He wanted the groups to spread to other neighborhoods. They started a franchise.

During the last years of his life in L.A., Callen became less active in politics, turning to his passions of cooking and music. He had a gorgeous voice, which he harmonized with four other men in the group The Flirtations. (They appeared in the movie *Philadelphia.*) Just before he died, Callen recorded a solo album, a dream he had fervently wished to fulfill.

According to George Solomon, assertiveness is more than just feistiness. As with Michael Callen, it also involves finding and following a dream. Standing up for ourselves is a health behavior, particularly when we do so in pursuit of meaning, pleasure, and creativity, while retaining our personal integrity and sense of values.

George Solomon's understanding of the psychological factors that enhance health cuts to the core of human needs and aspirations. "Freud talked about the need for fulfillment in love and work," he said, "but he didn't mention play. Play is not goal-directed behavior, it is frivolous behavior that's enjoyable for its own sake. And some people don't know how to play. I believe that people need balance among love, work, and play in order to stay healthy."

Developing an Immune Power Personality is not an overnight task—it can't be achieved through a weekend growth experience. But George Solomon's message to people who want to strengthen their immune systems is not complicated: The health-promoting personality is one who cultivates the awareness, and the assertiveness, that enables her to find meaning in love, in work, and in play.

A GUIDE TO ASSERTIVENESS

The practices of assertiveness represent an expansion of strategies I have conveyed in the last three chapters. The ACE Factor included elements of expressive action, moving awareness of bodily sensations and feelings out into the world for the purposes of redressing imbalances, and changing the environment to meet your needs. Assertiveness involves the inner states, the skills, and the conviction to make those expressive actions work.

In developing the capacity to confide, you learned how to become more aware of inner truths, work them through on paper, and confide them to others. Assertiveness encompasses the inner strength, and the outer strategies, that enable you to confide difficult truths to other people. Assertiveness is particularly important when you wish to confide truths that create potential conflict, set boundaries, or reveal needs that make you feel vulnerable.

The practices of hardiness—of focusing, situational reconstruction, and implementation of an action plan—are designed to reinforce the three Cs—commitment, control, and challenge. Assertiveness self-training provides both the emotional bulwark and the communication skills that enable you to "pull off" the action plans you set forth for furtherance of commitment, control, and challenge. Indeed, assertiveness as a practice can—by itself—bolster and expand the three Cs.

As with the other Immune Power traits, the development of assertiveness requires practice in both reflection and action. Many people confuse assertiveness with anger, aggression, or manipulation. When faced with mistreatment, injustice, neglect, or abuse, it is both functional and human for us to feel angry. But what do we do with our anger? Do we suppress it, for fear that our expression will lead to trouble? Do we repress it completely, so we don't have to suffer with bottled-up but consciously felt rage? Do we express it exactly as we feel it—even if that involves a temper tantrum of incendiary force? Or, knowing that the latter could lead to trouble, do we hatch underground schemes of retribution or revenge?

The answer, as you might imagine, is none of the above. Both suppression and repression lead to acquiescence and passivity. When we do not find effective means of expressive action, the status quo is maintained—the circumstances that prompted our initial anger never change. Whether these circumstances involve an abusive employer, a dishonest friend, or an insensitive spouse, the relationships and conditions can get worse, because the other person gets no message from us to stop.

When we let our anger explode, without a goal in mind other than sheer ventilation, no purpose is served and most often we alienate the person(s) from whom we seek redress. Verbal explosion is aggression, not assertiveness. Blaming the other person, rather than taking responsibility for our own feelings and needs, is aggressive rather than assertive. Schemes of retribution and revenge are mere forms of manipulation that have nothing to do with assertiveness.

Assertiveness is a behavioral style for effective expression and channeling of anger, honoring both our own need for honest and satisfying relationships and other people's need to be treated with fairness and respect. As such, assertiveness training has clear ramifications for mind-body health. In the book I coauthored with Lydia Temoshok, *The Type C Connection,* we discussed her model in which two behavioral extremes were associated with two different negative health outcomes. Suppression or repression of anger (the "Type C behavior pattern") was linked to immune imbalances— hence to cancer, infections, and autoimmune disorders. At the other extreme, uninhibited explosions of anger (the "Type A behavior pattern") increase the risk of cardiovascular diseases, including heart attacks and strokes.

When people heard this explanation, they often threw up their hands: "You mean, I'm damned if I do and damned if I don't?" The answer was no, because Dr. Temoshok had embraced a third option. Between the two behavioral extremes lay the Type B individual, who was able to express anger appropriately in order to meet her needs, with conscious control and a clear sense of purpose. These Type Bs relied on the third option—healthy assertiveness. This pattern was associated with reduced risk of immune dysfunction *and* heart disease.

The following guidelines for self-training in assertiveness are drawn both from George Solomon's concepts and from classic texts in the field.

STEP 1: UNDERSTANDING ASSERTION

Distinguishing assertive from passive or aggressive responses is the necessary first step, since many of us are confused by these differences. Also, a clear grasp of what is healthy assertive behavior gives you a base of legitimacy from which to operate—a sense that your imagined and soon-to-be-enacted behaviors are not only acceptable, they further the cause of your health and well-being.

The following, from behavioral scientists Edward A. Charlesworth, Ph.D., and Ronald G. Nathan, compares passive, assertive, and aggressive behaviors:

A Comparison of Passive, Assertive, and Aggressive Verbal Behaviors

Passive	*Assertive*	*Aggressive*
You avoid saying what you want, think, or feel. If you do, you speak in such a way that you put yourself down. Apologetic words with hidden meanings, a smokescreen of vague words, or silence are used frequently. Examples are "You know," "Well," "I mean," "I guess," and "I'm sorry." You allow others to choose for you.	You say what you honestly want, think, and feel in direct and helpful ways. You make your own choices. You communicate with tact and humor. You use "I" statements. Your words are clear and objective. They are few and well chosen.	You say what you want, think, and feel, but at the expense of others. You use "loaded words" and "you" statements that label or blame. You employ threats or accusations and one-upmanship. You choose for others.

STEP 2. RECOGNIZING YOUR LEGITIMATE RIGHTS

Those of us who find assertion difficult lack a healthy sense of entitlement. The reasons for this lack run deep, usually originating in early childhood experiences. While psychotherapy is one powerful tool for understanding and overturning sources of low self-esteem, a here-and-now approach to changing behavior is also essential. Often, practicing assertion in real-life situations engenders a gradual increase in self-esteem and sense of healthy entitlement.

Also, simply becoming aware of your rights—and identifying them as legitimate—fosters healthy entitlement. Here is a list of basic human rights, drawn from several sources, that are applicable

in a wide range of circumstances—including relations with doctors
and medical personnel.

You have the right to:
1. Have and express your own feelings and opinions
2. Refuse requests without having to feel guilty or selfish
3. Ask for what you want
4. Ask for information—including from professionals
5. Be heard and taken seriously
6. Have privacy
7. Make mistakes—and be responsible for them
8. Get what you pay for
9. Be independent
10. Be treated with respect, fairness, and dignity
11. Have rights—that is, to act in an assertive manner

As much as anything, these rights are reminders of your right
to *have a self* and act in accordance with your sense of your self.

Your awareness is enhanced when you take an inventory of
current life circumstances, to determine whether your needs and
rights are being met in these contexts. Figure 5.2, from Charlesworth and Nathan, lists a variety of interpersonal situations that
can occur with a range of different people in your life. These situations directly or indirectly reflect legitimate rights, such as "Refusing requests," "Expressing negative feelings," and "Making
social contacts." Within each of the boxes of this chart, rate your
assertiveness from 0 to 10. Use the table as a diagnostic tool for
pinpointing circumstances and relationships in which you need to
learn and apply assertiveness.

STEP 3. BELIEVING IN YOUR RIGHTS: A VISUALIZATION

It isn't enough to memorize your rights. You have to believe in
them, by connecting to the (sometimes buried) part of your consciousness that feels entitled to fair treatment, respect, and love.
One way to accomplish this is through a guided imagery exercise
called a "Rights Fantasy." Its purpose is to accept your basic hu-

man rights on an emotional and spiritual rather than just an intellectual level. Here, adapted from the work of Arthur J. Lange and Patricia Jakubowski, is a guide to a "Rights Fantasy." Before you proceed, refer to the eleven human rights just enumerated and select one right that you feel most *un*comfortable accepting.

"Rights Fantasy" Script

Move into a comfortable position. Close your eyes. Take a deep breath. Hold it as long as you can. Let it out slowly. Now imagine that you have the right you selected from this list. . . . Imagine how life would change as you accept this right. . . . How you would act. . . . How you would feel about yourself. . . . How you would feel about other people. . . .

Continue this fantasy for five minutes. Then . . .

Imagine that you no longer have the right. . . . Imagine how your life would change from what it was moments ago. . . . How would you now act? . . . . Feel about yourself? . . . . How would you feel about other people? . . .

Continue this fantasy for another two minutes. Now continue the fantasy for a third phase.

Imagine that you have the right again. How would your life change from what it was like when the right was missing? If you had focused on one important person or situation, how would that be different now that you had your right *back*?

Continue this fantasy for two or three minutes. Gradually return to a more outer-focused state of mind. Ask yourself these questions:

What right and circumstance did you choose for this exercise?

What images and people came to mind?

How had you been denying yourself that right?

How did it feel when you accepted that right?

How did you act differently when you had the right? When you no longer had the right?

How did others act when you had the right? When you no longer had the right?

What did you learn about yourself?

When you retrieved your right, how did it feel?

Figure 5.2 Rating Your Assertiveness in Different Situations with Different People

Directions: Fill in each of the blocks with a rating of your assertiveness from 0 to 10. A rating of 0 means you have no difficulty at all in asserting yourself. A rating of 10 means you are completely unable to assert yourself.

People: Situation:	Relatives	Friends	Strangers	Authority Figures	Subordinates	Service People	Groups
1. Refusing requests							
2. Handling criticism							
3. Receiving from others							
4. Stating your rights and needs							
5. Expressing negative feelings							
6. Giving negative feedback and confronting others							
7. Differing with others and giving opinions							
8. Making requests							
9. Expressing positive feelings							
10. Making social contacts							

How did you—and others—act this time?

When the right was returned, did it feel different?

When you finish this exercise, focus on how you have denied yourself this right in daily life, and what methods you used in fantasy to gain and regain this right. One purpose of this exercise is to help you imagine, as vividly as possible, what it would feel like to embrace a right that you and others have denied you. Visualizing how that would play out is also a useful guide to assertive actions. The purpose of imagining your newfound right taken away and returned is to sharpen your sense of the value of your right and to reinforce your belief that rights taken away can be gotten back—by you.

STEP 5. VERBAL ASSERTIVENESS

Unconscious factors play a big part in lack of assertiveness—many of us have been trained from childhood to please our parents or caretakers, to such an extent that our autonomous impulses and feelings were not validated. Fears of rejection, humiliation, or retribution remained lodged in our unconscious mind where they send us constant, nagging signals that our imagined acts of assertion will lead to disaster. Some people require psychotherapy to raise these fears to the level of consciousness and work them through, if assertive behavior is to be learned and undertaken. At the same time—for those who do and those who don't need psychotherapy—certain myths in the present also block assertiveness, and they must be addressed.

The biggest myth that plagues unassertive people is the belief that strong actions to get one's rights or needs met, or set boundaries, will invariably alienate others. The imagined end result is that we will be banished from their (whoever *they* are) world. Regardless of the origin of this myth, one way to overturn this fear is to discover in practice that you can assert your rights, needs, and feelings without alienating others. This requires awareness of certain communicative ground rules and a set of specific skills. In fact, arguably one of the biggest causes of "relapse" in people who try and fail to be assertive is the lack of these skills, which leads to some unfortunate self-fulfilling prophecies in which they do alienate others, leading them to conclude that they were right to be scared in the first place.

The biggest mistake people make when they emerge from a cocoon of past passivity is to start by blaming others for their feelings. No matter how legitimately angry you are, blame is an ineffective tool for expression—one that always results in greater conflicts and distress. Perhaps the most important skill of assertive communication is the ability to express need, anger, sadness, discontent, or frustration without blaming the other person.

In her book *The Dance of Anger,* Harriet Goldhor Lerner sets forth ground rules for effective, assertive communication. Here are key excerpts from these guidelines:

1. *Do speak up when an issue is important to you.* Obviously, you do not have to address personally every injustice and irritation that comes along . . . But it is a mistake to stay silent if the cost is to feel bitter, resentful, or unhappy . . .
2. *Don't use "below-the-belt" tactics.* These include: blaming, interpreting, diagnosing, labeling, analyzing, preaching, moralizing, ordering, warning, interrogating, ridiculing, and lecturing . . .
3. *Do speak in "I" language.* Learn to say "I think . . ." "I feel . . ." "I want . . ." instead of "You don't . . ." or "You are . . ." A true "I" statement says something about the self without criticizing or blaming the other person and without holding the other person responsible for our feelings or reactions. Watch out for the disguised "you" statements or pseudo-"I" statements . . .
4. *Don't make vague requests.* ("I want you to be more sensitive to my needs.") Let the other person know specifically what you want. ("The best way you can help me now is simply to listen. I really don't want advice at this time.") Don't expect people to anticipate your needs . . . Even those you love can't read your mind.
5. *Do recognize that each person is responsible for his or her own behavior.* Don't blame your dad's new wife because she "won't let him" be close to you. If you are angry about the distance between you and your dad, it is your responsibility to find a new way to ap-

proach the situation. Your dad's behavior is his responsibility, not his wife's.

6. *Don't tell another person what she or he thinks or feels or "should" think or feel.* If another person gets angry in reaction to a change you make, don't criticize those feelings or say the person has no right to be angry. Better to say "I understand that you're angry, and if I were in your shoes perhaps I'd be angry too. But I've thought it over and this is my decision."

The value of these ground rules is that they not only fulfill certain criteria for healthy interactions, but following them enables you to discover, in reflection and in action, that you can stand up for your rights and for yourself without alienating other people. Although on rare instances you will alienate someone despite your adherence to these guidelines, your gratifying experiences will vastly outnumber your grave disappointments. With further reflection, you'll learn that the disappointments often come in relationships in which intimacy was impossible under any circumstances. Healthy assertion is based on mutual respect.

STEP 6. FIELD-TESTING THE WORD "NO"

For some people, "no" is a four-letter word. The best way to learn it isn't is to start field-testing the use of the word. You should start in relatively "minor" circumstances, in which saying "no" is not as threatening. Refer to Figure 5.2, look along the "refusing requests" line to find a person to whom your refusal would cause some (not overwhelming) distress. At your next opportunity, give yourself permission to say "no" in the clearest, least complicated, most graceful way you possibly can. Note the other person's reactions and your own. Try to keep a certain distance, recognizing that any anxiety created in you—and the other person—is natural and, 90 percent of the time, will soon pass.

Field-test "no" in different circumstances. A good place to start is in the realm George Solomon tapped in his research: You return a defective product and must insist on a refund. Move to more difficult situations. An out-of-town relative who visited recently wants to return to your home to stay for a week. Your boss asks you to postpone your vacation to take on a new project. You and your spouse are out with friends who want to prolong the evening for a nightcap, but you're tired and want to go home. A good friend asks you for a loan even though he still owes you money. Your sense of healthy entitlement will grow in leaps and bounds if you stick with it, tolerating your own and others' anxieties while remaining clear about your desire to improve rather than damage your relationship.

STEP 7. PLANNING AND VISUALIZING SUCCESSFUL ASSERTIONS

Many people find it useful to plan and imagine assertive actions before they test the waters—it provides an anchor for their sense of entitlement and gives them greater confidence. One useful aspect of planning assertive action can be to imagine how someone else you respect would handle your circumstance, and allow him or her to be your "model."

Whether you choose a model or not, give yourself quiet time to relax and visualize the interaction. In my experience, this involves two phases. Before you embark, follow the technique of finding a quiet, comfortable place, relaxing, breathing deeply, and clearing your mind of distractions.

First, imagine the various ways the other person(s) will react and the various ways you could respond. Use this as a cognitive exercise to determine alternative strategies and countermoves—how you will deal with a variety of possible reactions. For phase two, however, select the most likely scenario, and imagine it working out exactly as you plan and hope. Stay with the image of yourself as clear, articulate, nonblaming, self-confident, and—let's not forget—successful. Your assertive act is met if not with kindness and understanding, at least with some degree of acceptance. Your purpose—even in your imagination—should not be to have the other person always agree with you or love you, but more modestly, to hear you out and respond affirmatively to your legitimate right or need.

Visualizing yourself being successful in acts of self-assertion is a crucial link in a psychodynamic chain that enables you to be assertive in reality.

STEP 8. WRITING ABOUT YOUR EXPERIENCES

Whether or not you keep a journal, you can use writing to explore your efforts to become more assertive. Refer to your experiences in reflection (the "Rights Fantasies" and visualized assertions) and action (the specific interactions you have initiated and field-tested outcomes for). Look for patterns, blocks, and underlying reasons for your difficulties. Have the utmost compassion for your own fears and difficulties—know that they are not signs of your intrinsic passivity, but rather the vestigial remnants of early experiences. For some of you, this "training" was brutal, as parents who didn't know any better caused you to fear retribution for expressing anger, needs, or rights. Exploring these roots is not a substitute but rather a parallel process with the ongoing transformations in your real-world interactions.

Also use your writing to explore how you did and how you can do better in your own eyes. In trying to develop healthy assertiveness, search for that delicate balance between the unhealthy poles of denial and self-blame—somewhere in between lies compassionate self-recognition and a true sense of responsibility.

Finally, use this journal experience to search for the sources of self-esteem, sources that should anchor every move you make toward assertiveness. Every time you succeed in establishing a healthy boundary, taking a stand of self-protection, having your feelings heard, or eliciting respect for your autonomy, you rouse the deep part of yourself that feels worthy of selfhood. These actions and reflections, George Solomon now tells us, are not only a balm for our soul, they are a boon to our health.

THE POWER OF LOVE
VS. THE LOVE
OF POWER

WHOSOEVER STUDIES TO REACH CONTEMPLATION (I.E., UNI-
TIVE KNOWLEDGE) SHOULD BEGIN BY SEARCHINGLY ENQUIRING
OF HIMSELF HOW MUCH HE LOVES. FOR LOVE IS THE MOTIVE
POWER OF THE MIND (MACHINA MENTIS) WHICH DRAWS IT OUT
OF THE WORLD AND RAISES IT ON HIGH.
                        —ST. GREGORY THE GREAT

We all believe that love is good for the soul. But is love really good
for our health? The notion makes sense, striking resonant chords
of common sense and intuition.

When we're sick, we look to loved ones for tenderness. Even
the common cold can bring out our need for caring—especially
those small acts of kindness, such as being served warm liquids and
soft foods while we remain flat on our backs in bed. We often get
better quickly when such kindness is forthcoming. When it's not,
an illness may linger interminably. The internal distress that weakens our body's defenses is intensified when we feel lonely.

"That just *feels* right," people will say, when told that loving care helps prevent or cure disease. But Yale surgeon Bernie Siegel wrote a best-selling book about the healing potential of love, aptly titled *Love, Medicine, and Miracles,* that angered some people as much as it comforted others. To skeptical scientists and physicians, simple claims about the healing power of love don't just *feel* right, since intuition is not enough for them. They won't counsel against love and support, because they know it can't hurt and perhaps it can help. (Practically speaking, the medical patient with a strong support system will take medicine more regularly, keep doctor's appointments, and so on.) But they hesitate to embrace the idea that love has a physiologically based healing influence on our hearts, our tissues, and our immune systems. Before accepting that, they require hard evidence.

What is really known about the healing influence of love? Do we stay healthy by receiving love, giving love, or both? Has anyone systematically studied these questions?

In this realm, the work of one scientist stands out. David McClelland, Ph.D., now distinguished professor of psychology at Boston University, has gone farther than any other researcher investigating love and health. McClelland has found that love is a bodymind state that occurs on levels of mind, brain, heart, hormones, immune system, and cells. Love crosses every domain that is relevant to human health. And McClelland has shown that one powerful index of our capacity to heal is our propensity to love.

Who is this scientific explorer of love's biological effects? McClelland is something of a maverick, but over the course of his forty-year career he has probably been the world's most honored and influential researcher of human motivation. As a professor of psychology at Harvard University, he authored classic texts in the field and devised standard ways of measuring people's deepest motivations.

The question coursing through McClelland's life work had been: "What drives people in their daily lives and behavior?" Put simply, he has established three primary answers: achievement, power, and affiliation, which refers to the desire for relationships. Our personalities are shaped by these motives, which exist in each of us in varying degrees and configurations.

For over a quarter century McClelland has refined his methods for measuring motives. His early research demonstrated how achievement motives predicted a person's career success; how power motives determined a person's addictions; and how affiliation motives shaped social behavior. Then, in the late 1970s, McClelland read *Type A Behavior and Your Heart,* the work of two cardiologists, Meyer Friedman and Ray Rosenman. "I was intrigued with their work," McClelland said recently, "and their descriptions of Type A individuals sounded exactly like people I had been studying for a number of years—namely, those with a high power motivation that had been stressed or inhibited."

These developments tipped off McClelland to the possibility that the motive patterns he'd been studying since the 1950s had an influence on biology—and health. He began to devote much of his time to this controversial pursuit long before the mainstream academic world addressed mind-body science. David McClelland put his formidable reputation as a psychologist and a man of science on the line as he pursued linkages between personality and health.

I recently interviewed Dr. McClelland at his office at Boston University, to learn about his fifteen years of research on love and health. As I came to understand his work, one trend was most surprising and significant: In terms of health, our desire and capacity for love may be more important than how much we are loved by others.

Understanding the precise role of love in health required David McClelland to explore shadowy scientific terrain. It was terrain in which the potential for mushiness was dangerously high. By mushiness, I mean both sentimentality and murky imprecision. McClelland avoided both when he devised studies that relied on hard measures of health—including immune functions.

Related attempts by other psychologists had fallen short, because they relied on people's rational assessments of their need and capacity for love. The problem is that love is too mysterious, too indescribable, and often too irrational for people to accurately assess their own motivations. People inspired by love may not know it; those who are not motivated by love may think they are. Many aspects of our capacity to give and receive love are simply not conscious. Scientists who poke around this terrain won't get very far with pencil-and-paper tests that ask people about their love motivations.

How, then, can scientists study love and health? McClelland refined a form of psychological testing that bypassed people's rational views of themselves. He tapped into the deeper recesses of people's minds—below the level of conscious thought—where their true motivations could be detected. He did so by getting his subjects to tell stories that sprang directly from their imaginations. These fantasies bespoke the needs, emotions, and characteristics at the person's core. Often these fantasies contradicted what the person said about his motives and feelings.

This approach had its origins in McClelland's own youth. "What people think they want, or the goals they consciously set for themselves, is certainly a part of motivation, but it may not be the most important part," he said a few years ago. "I often explain that I was the son of a minister and was well aware that people would say things on Sunday that were quite different from what they did on Monday. I learned early to distrust what people said about what they were going to do."

McClelland used the Thematic Apperception Test (TAT)— first introduced by Dr. Henry Murray in the 1930s—in which people write imaginative stories in response to ambiguous pictures of human subjects. Individuals would look briefly at the picture and write a short story about what they saw.

For example, one TAT picture shows a couple sitting on a bench by a river. Their facial expressions cannot be seen clearly. Subjects are asked to elaborate what is happening in the picture— who the people are, what each person thinks and wants, and what will happen in the future. By writing quickly after only a quick scan of the image, individuals have scant opportunity to craft a calculated story that covers up hidden motives. They are likely to project their underlying motives and characteristics onto the picture, and to create a narrative that reflects those unconscious drives. Do the man and woman love each other? Are they engaged in an argument? Does he want something from her? Does she want something from him? Is one person in the couple attempting to gain control of the other? Will one betray the other? Will they eventually come together? The story that answers these questions will spring from the respondents' imaginations, revealing sides of them that would never have been uncovered by the pencil-and-paper tests used by other psychologists to test love impulses.

McClelland became expert at analyzing people's stories in a systematic fashion. Using a sophisticated coding system, he rated their narratives for how strongly they evidenced various motivations, including: the need for achievement; the quest for power; and the desire for affiliation—close ties to family, friends, and coworkers.

How reliable was the TAT method? Beginning in the late 1950s, McClelland pioneered the use of TAT to predict people's long-term behavior with remarkable degrees of accuracy. Using these picture-story tests, he demonstrated that people's achievement motivation determined their success as entrepreneurs. He proved that people with strong power motives would be more successful managers, but they also would be prone to alcoholism. And he showed that people motivated by affiliation succeeded in jobs or school situations that called for friendly behavior.

McClelland's picture-story tests were more reliable predictors of behavior than questionnaires that asked people to report about themselves. His body of work proved that we reveal more about ourselves in fantasies that emanate from our unconscious minds than we do in self-conscious explanations of our thoughts and actions.

When PNI research emerged in the late 1970s, McClelland recognized that the lessons he'd learned about motivation could be applied to mind-body science. He posed the question: If motives of achievement, power, and affiliation influenced so many behaviors, might they not influence health? The part of the mind tapped by his TATs—the repository of deeper motives—*was the part of the mind most closely allied to the body*. Specifically, our unconscious motives are based on emotional learning, which is rooted in parts of our brains and nervous systems that also govern many physiological functions.

What makes our hearts race? Not necessarily what we say we want, but what we desperately fear or desire.

What makes our palms sweat? Not necessarily what we say upsets us, but the anxieties we dare not discuss.

What makes us distressed, run down, and vulnerable to illness? Not necessarily what we say bothers us, but the deeper disappointments we shunt from awareness.

As McClelland ventured into the realm of PNI, he would have to utilize a whole new battery of tests. McClelland's "psych" lab was supplemented by an immunology lab, and the esteemed psychologist became as adept at testing blood and saliva as he had been testing personality and motivation.

From the beginning, McClelland was interested in the influence of love on health and healing. As an expert in motivation, his point of view was unique. Other mind-body researchers had explored how much people *felt* loved, by virtue of strong support systems, a caring family, a close circle of friends, and so forth. McClelland would explore people's capacity and motivation *to love others*. His goal was to measure the seemingly immeasurable: the heart within the mind of his subjects.

STRESS, POWER, AND SICKNESS

David McClelland's first forays into mind-body research focused not on love but power. Over the years, he'd found that both love and power motivations had healthy and unhealthy expressions. Indeed, many people with strong power needs were both highly successful and happy. (The healthy side of power can be compared to Suzanne Ouellette's sense of control. Healthy power may best be captured by the term "empowerment.") But people who sought power at the expense of loving relationships would not be so healthy. Ultimately, McClelland's investigation of power would help him to grasp the physiologic effects of both power and love.

The image of the power-hungry corporate executive is indelibly imprinted on our cultural canvas. The stereotype is a bit unfair, if only because many people, from all walks of life, are obsessed with power. Today, we typically associate extreme power hunger with two different outcomes: success and sickness. We revere people who work their way to the top, even if they do so through manipulative machinations. But we also fear the ill health we believe can result. I recently read an obituary of a sneaker executive who not only started one of the biggest worldwide companies, he jumped ship and took over the helm of another. One can only imagine the stress—and the power drive—involved in such a meteoric career. He had died of a massive heart attack at the age of forty-three. Such instances reinforce our suspicion that out-of-control power drives can sometimes lead to sudden death.

In their book *Type A Behavior and Your Heart,* cardiologists Meyer Friedman and Ray Rosenman demonstrated that the cultural myth contained some truth. The vast majority of their patients with heart disease exhibited Type A behavior—a pattern of hostility, impatience, and hard-driving competitiveness. Later studies demonstrated that hostility was the "toxic core" of the Type A pattern—the trait most strongly associated with heart disease.

When McClelland came upon their work, he noted similarities between Type As and a group of subjects he had long studied. These were individuals with an intense need for power, who were constantly stressed or inhibited in their various quests. Strong power needs were not necessarily unhealthy, as long as they were expressed in an appropriate fashion and balanced by a desire for relationships. By contrast, power-motivated people who were always frustrated, or who suppressed these drives, suffered in both mind and body. These frustrated power-seekers exhibited the Type A–like behaviors—angry eruptions, a sense of time urgency, and competitive backbiting.

McClelland decided to use TAT techniques to see whether frustrated power-seekers showed evidence of heart disease. In separate studies, he analyzed the motives of college students, businessmen, and prisoners. People with a high "need for power" wrote stories about having impact on others "by aggression, persuasion . . . or by arousing emotional responses in others." In life, they tended to be argumentative, to play competitive sports, to accumulate symbols of prestige, and to assert control in their jobs or relationships.

McClelland also combed their stories for evidence of inhibited power needs. (For instance, previous studies showed that power-seekers who frequently used the word "not" actively inhibited their need for power in real life.) And he collected information about stressful events in their lives, to find out if their power needs were constantly thwarted. Whether people's power drives were inhibited on the inside, stressed on the outside, or both, the result was the same: They lived in a state of chronic tension.

David McClelland loved the fact that Meyer Friedman discovered Type A behavior when he noticed that the upholstery on the front edge of the office chairs used by his patients would become frayed in a matter of months. He kept having to reupholster these chairs, until he realized that the problem was not with his furniture but with his high-strung patients—all of whom suffered from heart disease. McClelland compared Friedman's antsy patients to his own frustrated power-seekers. "Like the Type As, they also lived on the edge of their chairs."

McClelland had previously shown that people with inhibited power drives had a tendency toward high blood pressure. But he wanted to demonstrate this linkage with airtight scientific methods. That required a long-term (prospective) study, in which subjects were tested for motivation and followed for years. It might have taken McClelland decades to produce such data, but a stroke of luck enabled him to solve the problem in a matter of weeks.

To his delight, McClelland found a collection of picture-story tests administered in 1938 by a Boston research team as part of a larger health study. The seventy-six healthy males were first studied as college seniors, and their medical progress was tracked for twenty-six years. This enabled McClelland to go back, analyze their original stories, and determine whether the motive patterns revealed had any influence on later heart problems.

The picture-story test results showed that a whopping 61 percent of the men with *inhibited power motives* went on to develop high blood pressure or die of heart disease. (Most of these men were only in their fifties when this finding was confirmed.) Among the men who did *not* show inhibited power motives, only 23 percent had developed high blood pressure or died of heart disease. The frustrated power-seekers were more than two and a half times as likely to develop hypertension or serious heart problems.

This picture emerged: Men (and perhaps women) who inhibit their strong power needs are vulnerable to a pressure-cooker effect on their cardiovascular systems. Whether the cause is internal suppression or external stress, their wish for mastery is frustrated, and they react to events with great surges of anger and anxiety. These are matched by great surges of stress hormones in the body—the fight-or-flight response of the sympathetic nervous system. Adrenaline and other endocrine secretions cause an increase in heart rate and blood pressure. When these personality types remain chronically angry and anxious, their stress hormone levels stay high and their cardiovascular systems are continuously overworked. The stage is set for serious heart disease.

Having established the role of inhibited power in heart disease, McClelland turned his sights to the immune system. He suspected that frustrated power-seekers also had weakened immunity. As it happened, the same stress hormones that overstimulate people's hearts also quash their Immune Power. Adrenaline, noradrenalin, and the corticosteroids are hormones that reduce the strength and effectiveness of our immune defender cells.

What McClelland proposed was elegant in its simplicity. People with stressed or inhibited power drives lived with chronic tension. Their anger and anxiety percolated under the surface, sometimes bubbling over, always causing the release of stress hormones. These stress hormones not only taxed their hearts, they weakened their immune systems. Frustrated power-seekers therefore are susceptible not only to heart disease but to immune disorders—infections and perhaps even cancer.

To prove his theory, however, he'd have to nail down each part of this four-pronged bodymind equation: personality pattern = stress hormone release = immune dysfunction − disease. Doing so would represent a major advance in personality-and-health research.

In a study of male college students, McClelland administered picture-story tests, urine tests for stress hormones, and saliva tests for the presence of IgA antibodies. IgA stands for immunoglobulin A—one of several different classes of antibodies. Our immune system's B-lymphocytes (B-cells) produce antibodies, which are Y-shaped protein molecules that grasp and neutralize foreign invaders. Antibodies represent our body's first line of defense against foreign substances. IgA is a particular class of antibodies that gather in the mucous membranes of our mouths and sinus cavities, where they attack the viruses that cause respiratory infections. As such, people with high levels of IgA in their saliva are more resistant to colds, flu, and bronchitis.

(PNI research has suggested the specific influence of stress on IgA antibodies. Stress hormones act as messenger molecules that tone down the activities of T- and B-cells. A B-cell that receives these "negative" messages would be less likely to produce sufficient amounts of IgA antibodies.)

McClelland used the picture-story tests to identify men with high stress and a strong need for power that was inhibited. These men also scored low in affiliation—meaning that *their need for power was stronger than their desire for human connections.* McClelland proved that these frustrated power-seekers had higher levels of the stress hormone adrenaline, lower levels of protective IgA antibodies, and more bouts of every type of illness, especially upper respiratory infections.

All the more striking was McClelland's discovery that each part of the four-pronged equation was statistically linked. He wrote:

Many studies had been carried out relating 2 to even 3 of the variables involved in this four-step process. But what seemed particularly significant to me about this study was that it showed linkages between all 4 variables theoretically involved—that is, a personality characteristic (frustrated power), hormone production (adrenaline in the urine), and an aspect of immune function (IgA antibodies) that was connected . . . with disease (reports of cold infections).

It was the type of study that PNI scientists dream about, because McClelland showed how the mind, brain, immune system, and health are absolutely interconnected.

During his investigation of power, McClelland began to suspect that its flip side—the drive for affiliation—was associated with better health. The frustrated power-seekers had forsaken human connections in favor of their struggles for ever more personal authority. His research implied that people who prioritized relationships over power had stronger hearts and immune systems. Specifically, those who scored high in affiliative motives suffered from fewer illnesses.

Was affiliation a bona fide Immune Power trait? Were people's immune systems actually strengthened by their intrinsic desire for relationships? McClelland studied college students, searching for evidence that people who prioritized relationships had more resilient immune systems. He tested their motives—and their saliva—during periods throughout the academic year associated with high and low stress. McClelland discovered that students with a *relaxed desire for affiliation* had a stronger immune defense—even during those high-stress months before exams.

What is a relaxed desire for affiliation? These were students who pursued relationships without excessive anxiety or fervor. They were more interested in people than in power, and their lives and relationships were not full of turmoil. This group showed higher IgA levels throughout the year, with only slight dips during exam time—the months of November, April, and June. Other students had lower levels throughout the year and marked drops during exam time. The frustrated power-seekers had the weakest antibodies and the sharpest decline during stressful times. (See Figure 6.1 for a graph of Immune Power among these groups during the school year.) In other research, McClelland showed that people who prioritized relationships also suffered from fewer, less severe bouts of illness.

Some immunologists questioned whether IgA antibodies are a good measure of Immune Power, accurately predicting resistance to illness. Using sophisticated statistical methods, McClelland evaluated eight studies of this connection, and he concluded that IgA

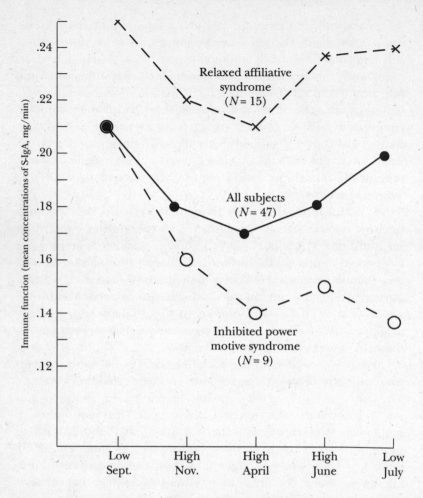

Figure 6.1   Mean concentrations of salivary immunoglobulin A (S-IgA) during periods of low stress (September and July) and high stress (November, April, and June) for 47 first-year dental students that were placed into either a high relaxed affiliativeness group or high inhibited power group. During the academic term (November, April, and June), levels of immune function in saliva are reduced for the sample as a whole. Compared with the inhibited power group, the relaxed affiliative group started with higher immune values and recovered by June (exam time!).

was a very reliable index of Immune Power—particularly of resistance to colds, flu, and bronchitis. However, he knew that IgA was only one cog in our vast immunologic enterprise. He'd have to evaluate the connection between personality and other immune defenses.

McClelland focused on the association between motive patterns and the strength of natural killer (NK) cells, which eliminate microbes and cancer cells from the body. In three studies of different populations—students, middle-class adults, and medical patients—McClelland and psychologist John Jemmott III, Ph.D., showed that people with "relaxed affiliative motives" had the most active NK cells. The frustrated power-seekers had the weakest NKs. (See Figure 6.2 for NK power in their first study with college students.)

McClelland's early findings on affiliation, immunity, and health had potentially explosive ramifications. They implied that people who were simply more interested in human connections than status and power had stronger immune systems and lower risks of illness. It did not matter if they had more extensive networks of support. It did not matter if others loved them more. It did not matter if they'd achieved great heights in their careers. What mattered was that they cared most about relationships.

MOTHER TERESA AND THE LOVE VARIABLE

McClelland came to suspect that we can increase our affiliative motivation, enhance our Immune Power, and improve our physical health. In order to prove this, he'd first have to stimulate the affiliative motivation. Could people's desire for human connections be aroused? If so, would their immune systems also be stimulated? To find out, McClelland brought a group of college students into his laboratory for a singular experiment.

His task was to devise an experimental situation that evoked people's care and concern for others. To get as uniform an effect as possible, McClelland resorted to that tried-and-true medium of emotional manipulation: the movies. He couldn't pick a classic ro-

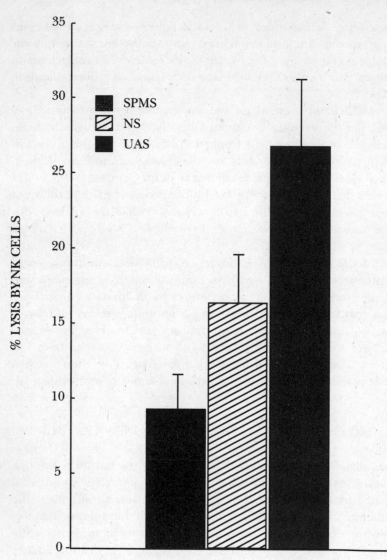

Fig. 6.2. Mean (± SE) percentage natural killer (NK) cell activity for college students characterized by the stressed power motive syndrome (SPMS), the unstressed affiliation motive syndrome (UAS), or neither syndrome (NS) in Study 1.

mance like *Casablanca,* because Humphrey Bogart or Ingrid Bergman might not be to everyone's taste. And romantic love was a terribly complicated issue unto itself. The movie's subject would have to be something or someone with relatively universal appeal. Enter Mother Teresa.

McClelland decided to show college students a documentary film about Mother Teresa, the Nobel Prize–winning nun who devoted her life to the disadvantaged of the world. The film showed vivid images of Mother Teresa's tender loving approach to the sick, starving, and dying people of the slums of Calcutta. Speaking of the film, he wrote, "It reflects faithfully her deep religious commitment to respond with love to that spark of the divine in each human being, regardless of their circumstances."

As a control, another group of students were shown a film about Nazi triumphs during World War II—a cinematic experience not likely to arouse great feelings of warmth in the average American undergraduate. Immediately before and after the films were screened, and one hour later, saliva samples were taken for IgA antibodies. Unlike students shown the Nazi film, those who watched Mother Teresa evidenced a stunning increase in protective IgA antibodies.

But there was a conspicuous problem. The first time McClelland ran this study, the students' antibody levels began to drop within an hour after the film was screened. Skeptical immunologists would snicker: These were mere blips on the radar screen of our immune system. Could such short-lived changes produce any long-term reduction of a person's susceptibility to illness?

In search of an answer, McClelland repeated the study. This time, he asked the students who watched Mother Teresa to spend the next hour "reliving in their imagination experiences in their lives in which they loved someone or were loved by someone." The students sustained their high antibody levels beyond the full hour. This finding suggests that people who normally think about love, or who change their motive pattern to emphasize love, could maintain their enhanced Immune Power. Such an increase could bolster their resistance to upper respiratory illness.

What mind-states did the movie arouse? McClelland asked the

students what they thought of Mother Teresa. Half said they were moved and inspired by her caring. A few even said that their faith in humanity had been restored. The other half had a negative view of her or the movie. They found the situation hopelessly depressing, doubted the value of her Good Samaritanism, or disapproved of her religiosity.

In one of McClelland's most intriguing findings, the students' feelings about Mother Teresa had no bearing on their antibody reactions. Even some students who couldn't stand Mother Teresa had increased Immune Power.

Why was this so? McClelland was convinced that Mother Teresa touched an unconscious chord in many students. The film's effect on their minds and bodies was deeper than their comments had indicated. To test this theory, he analyzed the picture-story tests he'd given to the students after screening the Mother Teresa film. The picture had depicted a young man and woman sitting together in the grass, and the students were asked to write a story about the couple. McClelland wondered: Having just seen a film of this magnificent woman giving open-hearted care to the disadvantaged, would they write a story of love? Or, would they write a story of fear, anger, or abandonment?

Many students wrote stories about a loving couple. Three-quarters of them showed an increase in IgA antibodies after watching the film. Another group of students wrote stories that described the couple's relationship in starkly negative terms. Only one-quarter of them showed an increase in antibodies. In other words, people's conscious reactions to the movie did not correlate with increases in Immune Power. But their imaginative stories—reflecting deeper motives of love and care—did correlate.

What, exactly, had Mother Teresa touched in people whose immune systems responded to her tenderness? To David McClelland's surprise, his old measure for affiliation—the desire for human relationships—did not provide a sufficient answer. Something more profound was going on, and he was determined to find out what it was.

AFFILIATIVE TRUST:
THE INTERFACE OF LOVE AND HEALTH

David McClelland had previously shown that affiliation motives were good for immunity and health. But the students whose Immune Power increased after watching Mother Teresa did not write stories that showed a remarkable increase in affiliation. Why not? McClelland suspected that his coding system for affiliation was not refined enough to detect the psychological change induced by the Mother Teresa movie.

More detective work was needed to find out what deeper motives were stimulated by Mother Teresa. McClelland asked James R. McKay, an industrious graduate student, to identify the students who had the biggest increases in IgA antibodies after watching the film and those who suffered the biggest drops. He then compared the picture-stories they wrote afterward and searched for differences.

McKay immediately saw night-and-day contrasts in their stories. The students whose Immune Power increased had written stories representing the couple in a positive, loving relationship. They were tales in which people shared warm feelings, helped each other out, and trusted each other. The students who suffered declines in Immune Power wrote stories in which the partners deceived, manipulated, or abandoned each other.

McKay realized why the old affiliation measure had not picked up the motive factor implicit in the positive stories. It only tapped people's *need* for relationships. It did not characterize the *type* of relationships people wanted or the reasons *why* they sought relationships. In fact, McKay discovered that some people who scored high in affiliation were more afraid of rejection—or hoping to please others—than they were openly loving.

Certainly, a strong drive for affiliation was a healthy sign for most people—which is why McClelland's earlier studies had shown its linkage to Immune Power and health. But it wasn't unambiguously healthy for everyone. Based on their findings, McKay and McClelland named a new motive pattern—*affiliative trust. It specified the desire for positive, loving relationships based on mutual respect and trust.*

McClelland and McKay twice repeated the Mother Teresa study. Both times, the students who demonstrated the sharpest rise in Immune Power showed increases in affiliative trust. Surprisingly, some students showed a precipitous drop in Immune Power after watching Mother Teresa give tender loving care! To a remarkable degree, these students wrote stories that revealed their affiliative *mis*trust.

For McClelland, Mother Teresa had become a kind of Rorschach test for a person's love motivation. Watching her compassionate behavior brought out either your warmth—or your cynical fears.

McKay explained these personality differences with a simple theory that clinical psychologists have given a technical name: *object relations*. The term is generally understood to mean "the residue within the mind of relationships with important people in the individual's life." Simply put, when our past relationships (especially early ones with parents) are characterized by love and trust, we are likely to retain positive feelings and expectations about current relationships. When our early relationships are characterized by abuse, abandonment, or dishonesty, we are likely to retain negative feelings and expectations about current relationships.

The lingering effects of early relationships strongly influence our emotional development, personalities, and behaviors for the better part of our lifetimes. Now McKay and McClelland had evidence that "the residue within the mind of relationships with important people" also influences our immune defenses.

One concern was raised about the Mother Teresa studies: IgA antibody levels can change rather rapidly in response to emotional stimuli. Perhaps a more stable measure of the immune system could be selected to reflect a person's enduring personality traits. For his next study, McKay selected such an immune measure: the ratio of T-helper to T-suppressor cells.

T-helper cells stimulate and orchestrate other parts of our immune system during an "invasion." T-suppressor cells inhibit other immune cells, so they don't overreact to an invasion and attack our own cells. We need more T-helpers than T-suppressors, and we must maintain a certain ratio to keep our immune systems balanced. If the ratio is too low—meaning that we have too few T-helpers compared to T-suppressors—our defenses won't respond vigorously to bacteria, viruses, and cancer cells. One of the hallmarks of decline in HIV-infected patients is a low T-helper/T-suppressor ratio.

James McKay gave picture-story tests and blood workups to a group of forty-eight healthy adults. He did not show them films or put them through the paces of an experimental procedure. He simply wanted to determine whether motivation influenced their immune systems under normal conditions. McKay found that people with affiliative trust had higher T-helper/T-suppressor cell ratios. People who demonstrated *mistrust* had significantly lower ratios.

McKay also had given the subjects a mood questionnaire. He discovered that their mood when the test was taken had nothing to do with their T-helper/T-suppressor cell ratios. Their immune status had not been altered by a fleeting emotion, but it had been influenced by an enduring personality trait—*affiliative trust.*

McKay's striking discovery was solidified by one additional fact: The subjects motivated by love and trust reported fewer illnesses during the previous year—including colds, flu, and bronchitis. The subjects who lacked trust reported significantly more illnesses. The evidence was clear: Personalities motivated by love and trust had stronger immune functions, which, indeed, had translated into better physical health.

Other findings over the past seven years add to the strength of their connections among love, Immune Power, and health.* McClelland, Carol Franz, and their colleagues followed a group of thirty-year-olds from 1977 to 1987. Sometime during that decade, 30 percent of the people who demonstrated affiliative trust in 1977 developed a major illness, confirmed by medical records. However,

*McClelland's work was confirmed by another scientist, Dr. Arthur Stone of the State University of New York at Stony Brook, as reported in *The New York Times,* May 11, 1994. Stone measured IgA antibodies in 100 men every day for three months. Stressful events weakened immunity and increased the risk of colds for one day. Pleasant events—mainly involving affiliation— strengthened immunity and reduced risk of colds for *two* days.

59 percent of those who evidenced *mis*trust contracted a major illness. In other words, *people motivated by love had one-half the rate of major illnesses.*

James McKay has just completed a study of affiliative trust and natural killer cells in a group of twenty-seven depressed adults undergoing psychotherapy. His preliminary, unpublished data show that people with greater affiliative trust had higher percentages of NK cells in their blood—indicating a stronger defense against viruses and cancer cells. Ten months later, people with greater degrees of trust retained their high levels of NK cells. Apparently, those of us who are depressed may prevent loss of this key immune function by maintaining or gaining affiliative trust.

In every one of his studies, James McKay has been particularly struck by the powerful negative effect of mistrust on Immune Power and health. "A significant percentage of stories written by people who had decreased immunity were terribly cynical about relationships," he commented. "They were stories in which people rejected each other or refused to become involved. The characters deceived, manipulated, or lied to each other. The attitude expressed was that people will screw you."

Redford Williams, M.D., the leading investigator of personality patterns in heart disease, has identified a similar pattern in people who suffer heart attacks. He found that "cynical hostility" is a chief characteristic among individuals who develop diseases. A famous study of 1,877 male employees of Western Electric followed them from the 1950s to the '80s. Those men with higher levels of hostility were at significantly greater risk of suffering a heart attack or dying from all causes. Such findings have added scientific weight to the long-held hypothesis that cynical hostility harms our cardiovascular systems. Now McKay and McClelland have evidence that implicates cynicism and mistrust in immune-associated diseases.

On the converse side, McClelland detected a particular quality among people high in affiliative trust, one he could not easily "code" from his picture-story tests. The love they expressed was unconditional. It was not a love that depended on returns—ego gratification, money, social status, or even self-esteem. It was a selfless, wholehearted regard for others. People with affiliative trust were not saints, who undoubtedly never sought love for ulterior reasons. But a part of their psyches came through in their stories—the part that was capable of giving and receiving unconditional love.

McClelland cited a defining moment from his favorite cinematic "Rorschach test"—the Mother Teresa movie. "She is asked in the film, How can you expend all this energy on these dying babies when you know they are going to die anyway?" he recalled. "Mother Teresa says that is irrelevant, that whether they live or die isn't important to the act of love itself."

A HEALER'S TOUCH:
AWAKENING THE LOVE MOTIVATION?

In the 1970s, even before his Mother Teresa research, David McClelland became intrigued by healers—men or women who claimed to use special powers, energies, therapeutic methods, or spiritual invocations to cure people of their afflictions. Although skeptical about their claims, he saw evidence that many healers got results. McClelland's hypothesis was that faith healers were successful when they elicited affiliative trust. To test his theory, McClelland trained his scientific curiosity on one particular healer in the Boston area.

Karmu was not your average faith healer (if there is such a thing as an average faith healer). This middle-aged African-American, whose real name was Edgar Warner, lived in a poor neighborhood and maintained the pretense of being a lower-class man of the people. In fact, he was an upper-middle-class, highly educated fellow whose background was otherwise mysterious. He claimed to be an Ethiopian Jew whose father was a famous rabbi and whose West Indian mother had taught him African mythological traditions. Karmu told an apocryphal story of his meeting with a Tibetan monk who met him, laid hands on him, bestowed upon him his new name, and pronounced him a healer of the highest order.

McClelland never knew which of Karmu's tales were authentic. But he was convinced that Karmu's healing methods often worked, because he observed remarkable remissions among patients who went to him with wide-ranging physical conditions.

Karmu's approach was decidedly eclectic. He combined light touch, massage, herbal concoctions of unknown origin, tender loving care, healing benedictions, and, according to McClelland, "the summoning of a will to live." He would not only massage people with aromatic oils, he'd also massage their egos. McClelland described Karmu as having had the best bedside manner of any faith healer he'd met, being able to buoy people's spirits with compliments, affirmations, and words of hope. That, combined with varying forms of "laying on of hands," was evidently powerful stuff.

Karmu was so charismatic and persuasive that his patients often left his office with a self-esteem makeover. He also had a sense of humor. "Karmu once told me that getting the person to laugh was half the battle."

But the sum total of Karmu's efforts appeared to raise people's affiliative trust. "There is some evidence that the tenderness he gives people is important," said McClelland. Karmu offered his patients the time and care they may not have gotten from their doctors. Sick people need to trust their physicians, and Karmu aroused that trust.

David McClelland's scientific curiosity about Karmu was piqued after his own personal experience with the healer:

I had been on an all-day trip to Washington, D.C., and upon my return I knew I had one hell of a cold coming on. I was so sick with fever, I just wanted to go home, take two aspirins, get into bed and forget everything. But on the way from the airport in a taxicab, I thought, "You believe Karmu helps people, don't you? You'd better go see him." So I stopped at his apartment.

He had a big crowd waiting for him. He saw me, and right away knew I was very sick. He was intuitive that way. Karmu put aside his other patients, took me into his office, and basically held me for thirty minutes. Now, grown-ups don't get held like that. He's a big man, I'm a big man, but he held me like a baby the whole time. When I left his office, I didn't feel any different—I still had a cold. So I went home and got into bed. The next morning I was fine, which never happens otherwise. That's when I began to think that he must be influencing the immune system.

This "healing" led McClelland to devise a controlled study to determine whether Karmu could really cure colds. The key question: Did Karmu's treatment actually raise IgA antibodies in people's saliva, thus bolstering their defense against cold viruses?

McClelland rounded up a group of Harvard students, each of whom was instructed to see Karmu within twenty-four hours of the very first symptoms of a cold. McClelland had Karmu decide, on the spot, whether to treat the student or refer him or her to a control group, in which he or she would be seen—but not really treated—by another member of his entourage. Half the students would get Karmu, and the other half would get the "placebo" treatment. (The experiment was set up to prevent the students from knowing whether they were getting the "real" treatment.) In the end, thirteen students received the "real" treatment from Karmu, while thirteen others got the "placebo" treatment from someone else.

Within forty-eight hours of each student's "treatment," McClelland monitored his or her health and took saliva samples for IgA antibodies. Here are the results:

- Eighty-five percent of the students treated by Karmu (eleven of thirteen) experienced dramatic improvements in their cold symptoms.
- Eighty-five percent of students in the control group (eleven of thirteen) contracted full-blown respiratory infections.
- Eighty-two percent of Karmu-treated students whose cold symptoms got better (nine of the eleven) also demonstrated increases in IgA antibodies.
- Zero percent of the students in the control group demonstrated increases in IgA antibodies.

The data were not hard to interpret: Karmu's cold-healing powers could be explained by a measurable boost in the antibodies that neutralize cold and flu viruses.

Apparently, when physicians at the Harvard University Health Service got wind of McClelland's unorthodox experiment, their "noses went a little out of joint." They challenged him: "Take those students with colds to health services at Harvard, tell them they'll get better and they'll *get* better."

McClelland took the doctors' bait. He repeated the experiment, this time sending half of a group of students to Karmu and the other half to the Harvard University Health Service, where the doctors promised them prompt improvement. This time none of the students treated by Karmu got sick. Most of those who went to the Harvard health clinic developed severe colds. IgA antibodies increased in many Karmu-treated patients, but *none* of the clinic-treated patients experienced a rise in their IgA antibodies.

David McClelland studied Karmu for over a decade. He died recently, so no more can be learned about his methods or their effects on mind and body. But McClelland is convinced that this unorthodox healer aroused affiliative trust in his patients. He also does not question one of Karmu's avowed precepts. "He would always say 'I'm not doing the healing. The healing power is in you; I'm only putting you in touch with it.' "

CAN THE LOVE MOTIVE BE ENHANCED FOR BETTER HEALTH?

McClelland did not intend his Karmu research as an endorsement of faith healing as the royal road to Immune Power and health. He wanted to determine whether Karmu and by implication other healers actually enhance Immune Power, and he wanted to find out the psychological secret of their success.

Ironically, McClelland's insights into Karmu led him away from faith healing, in search of other ways to stimulate the personality changes that bolster health. He realized that faith healing would never be a practical approach to mind-body medicine.

(Even if we had a faith healer in our neighborhoods, how many of us would be willing to see him or her?) Another problem with faith healing was philosophic. Must we always depend on miraculous talents from outside to trigger the healing potentialities within? If affiliative trust was an underlying principle of mind-body healing, then there must be more reliable ways to stimulate this "love variable."

These realizations led McClelland to his next phase of systematic research during the late 1980s. He wanted to find out if widely accepted mind-body therapies measurably improved physical health. If so, he wanted to know whether their success was related to their ability to raise people's affiliative trust.

Over the past two decades, mind-body medicine has flourished. Patients receiving these treatments—which include relaxation, meditation, yoga, hypnosis, guided imagery, cognitive restructuring, and group psychotherapy—have gotten relief from a vast variety of symptoms and diseases. There was also some evidence that patients undergoing mind-body treatments became less anxious, depressed, hostile, and cynical. These reports led McClelland to suspect that successful treatments also raised their affiliative trust. However, even the mind-body field had been limited by the blinders of pathology: No one had carefully investigated what healthy mind-states and traits were stimulated by mind-body therapies.

As McClelland put it, "I know hostility is bad, and the absence of bad is good. The question we keep missing in the mind-body field is 'What precisely is good?' "

For answers, McClelland turned to the field of behavioral medicine, which in the late 1970s and early '80s had spawned the new mind-body approaches to healing. To conduct this research, he didn't have to turn far. Harvard University houses arguably the leading behavioral medicine department in the country, headed by cardiologist Herbert Benson, M.D. Over two decades of research, Benson demonstrated that techniques that bring about relaxation—including meditation, yoga, and deep breathing—have demonstrably positive effects on our cardiovascular and immune systems. The "relaxation response"—Benson's term for the mental and physical changes that occur when we use these techniques—reduced the symptoms of many illnesses. During the 1980s, Benson and his colleague Joan Borysenko, Ph.D., taught relaxation in a group setting, and their approach widened to include other elements—cognitive restructuring, coping skills, nutrition, exercise, and group support.

Benson's program was not the only established mind-body treatment available in McClelland's backyard. The Harvard Community Health Plan (HCHP), a famous health maintenance organization (HMO), refers patients to Dr. Benson's Mind/Body Groups, but it also has its own behavioral medicine program, directed by physician Matthew Budd, M.D. Called Ways to Wellness, Dr. Budd's groups emphasize stress management and a novel approach to transforming moods. Budd helped his patients, who suffered from a wide variety of stress-related medical problems, to become aware of how their worldview influenced their physiology. He taught them to tune into their bodies, alter their moods, and reverse the mistrust that kept them in a continual state of anger and tension.

Along with psychologist Caroline Hellman, Ph.D, McClelland recruited eighty patients, all of whom had physical symptoms with a stress component—such as palpitations, gastrointestinal disturbances, autoimmune conditions, headaches, and sleep disorders. One-third went into Benson's Mind/Body Groups, then led by Joan Borysenko, while another third participated in Budd's Ways to Wellness groups. The final third joined a control group that only received information about stress management. Six months after the patients completed their programs, McClelland found these results:

• Patients in both mind-body programs showed significant reductions in the number of return visits to their HMO and marked relief from their physical and psychological symptoms. By contrast, people in the control group made no improvements whatsoever.
• Patients in both mind-body groups showed significantly greater increases in affiliative trust from beginning to end, as measured by TATs.

- Two additional replications of this study have turned up similar results. Participants in Dr. Budd's Ways to Wellness showed significant improvements in both affiliative trust *and* physical symptoms.

"We found that two-thirds of the people treated in mind-body groups either sustained or gained affiliative trust," said McClelland. "In the control group, only one-third sustained or gained. Furthermore, when we looked at the treated groups, the patients who sustained or gained affiliative trust had much greater physical improvement that those who did not."

McClelland's theory had been confirmed: *The mind-body groups had sustained or raised affiliative trust, and this psychological benefit was directly tied to relief from a whole range of physical symptoms.*

McClelland was building a powerful case that one secret of mind-body groups—a possible key to their healing influence—was their ability to cultivate affiliative trust. But he still wasn't sure how these groups enhanced people's love motivation.

The latter question would be difficult to answer through scientific methods. (That would require pulling apart each element—relaxation, group support, coping skills, and so on—which would be impractical and clinically hard to justify.) But McClelland observed the groups carefully, and his impressions—along with the rich clinical experience of the therapists themselves—provided insights into how mind-body therapies increase the "love variable."

His goal was not to pinpoint any one magical healing factor, but rather to characterize the combinations of mind-body practices and principles that increased people's love motivation. This focus could help doctors and patients to pursue healing modalities that opened not only people's minds, but also their hearts.

CHANGING MOODS AND MOTIVES: THE PATHWAY OF RELAXATION

The furious and fearful among us don't need lions and tigers and bears to trigger our nervous systems into fight or flight. The presumed evolutionary purpose of the fight-or-flight response was to accompany emotional signals of danger with biological changes that ready us for action in the face of danger. As if car alarms were blaring in our bodies, our sympathetic nervous systems are activated and a cascade of stress hormones are released into the bloodstream. Our hearts beat faster, our blood pressure skyrockets, certain immune cells become inactive. Although we need to be readied for some form of action, even during subtle social interplay, our bodymind responses are often out of whack. Why do we sometimes respond to a slight as if it were a threat of violence? Theorists from different camps point to various factors: repressed anger, conditioned negative thoughts, and angry behaviors reinforced from an early age.

As the debate continues, the furious and fearful among us have to find our own answers. We must look within—by cultivating attention and connection—to discover the causes of our skittery states of mind and body. As we investigate, a wonderful tool exists for immediately cooling down our bodymind systems—Dr. Benson's relaxation response.

Benson has shown that a range of mind-body techniques elicit a physiological state—the relaxation response—that counters fight or flight, calming our excitable nervous systems. His research showed that meditators evoke this response in themselves, lowering their heart rate, blood pressure, and other signs of nervous system arousal. Patients in Harvard's Mind/Body group are taught to elicit the relaxation response through meditation, mindfulness, prayer, progressive muscle relaxation, and yoga. The groups also combine elements of social support, emotional expression, and cognitive restructuring—a therapeutic method for changing negative thought patterns.

David McClelland showed that Benson's program raised many of his patients' affiliative trust and reduced their symptoms. The difficulty in determining what aspect of the groups evoked people's love motivation lies in the inseparability of their therapeutic components. Each aspect of Benson's groups appeared to play a part in raising people's love motivation and creating the conditions for healing. To McClelland, it was the whole human experience of relaxing with a group; learning new ways to cope with stress and illness; the compassion of therapists; and the care of others who share one's pain. Indeed, many programs that combine relaxation with supportive group interaction appear to put people in touch with their capacity—in fact, their profound desire—for care and human connection.

While McClelland demonstrated the health benefits of Benson's groups, other investigators have proven that mind-body group therapies specifically enhance Immune Power. UCLA psychiatrist Fawzy I. Fawzy offered group treatment to patients suffering with melanoma, a potentially lethal skin cancer. These patients sustained a significant increase in natural killer (NK) cells six months after treatment. No such increase was noted in a control group. Recently, Dr. Fawzy published a six-year follow-up: The patients who participated were *three times less likely* to have suffered a recurrence or died.

Supportive group treatments have even bolstered immunity in patients infected with HIV, the AIDS virus. Dr. Michael Antoni of the University of Miami followed HIV-positive men who participated in his mind-body groups, and he discovered that stress did not cause their CD4 helper cell counts to drop precipitously, as they had in control subjects. Two years later, Antoni and his colleague, Dr. Gail Ironson, discovered that patients who stuck with the program—attending most sessions and practicing their relaxation regularly—were less likely to have contracted AIDS.

All of these groups—Benson's, Budd's, Fawzy's, Antoni's, and others—included elements of group support, coping skills, and relaxation. McClelland was particularly interested in how relaxation might build affiliative trust. Herbert Benson may have provided an important clue: "Immediately after you elicit the relaxation response, you become calmer, less anxious, and you learn better," he said. "If you are anxious, you can't learn. It's like dropping seeds on concrete. With a quiet mind, people take things in."

Benson's calmed patients "took in" positive thoughts, self-care instructions, and stress management techniques. Perhaps people with a "quiet mind" will also "take in" the care of others with whom they share the group experience. David McClelland suspected that the group setting allows these suffering individuals, made more receptive by relaxation, to connect more deeply with each other and their own needs for human contact.

Howard Paris, a patient in Dr. Benson's Mind/Body program for people with heart disease, was one who experienced a radical shift from mistrust toward affiliative trust. Soon after he turned forty, Howard was shoveling snow when he experienced chest pain so severe that it caused him to collapse on his driveway. He soon recovered, but didn't tell anyone for fear of causing alarm. A devoted if apoplectic sports fan, Howard went to the Boston Celtics basketball game that night, and the next morning on his way to work he suffered his first heart attack.

After the heart attack, tests showed that Howard suffered advanced atherosclerosis, or clogging of the arteries. He had coronary bypass surgery, and his physician instructed him to change his habits. He cut much of the fat from his diet. He exercised regularly. His cholesterol was high at 265, so his doctor prescribed cholesterol-lowering drugs. Howard owned a hardware store, and he habitually worked over seventy hours a week. As part of his lifestyle change, he cut back somewhat on his work hours.

Despite these efforts, Howard's heart disease progressed. Over the next eighteen months, he suffered two more heart attacks. He underwent three angioplasty procedures, in which balloons were used to unblock his clogged arteries. After the third angioplasty, one of Howard's arteries collapsed and he suffered total heart block, during which his heart almost stopped beating. The surgeons were able to reinsert an angioplasty balloon, reopen his artery, and bring his heart back to normal function.

After this turn of events, Howard, who was already quick to anger, was furious. His whole life had been turned upside down. Not only did he live with mortal fear on a daily basis, but his work life and all his normal activities had been disrupted. At forty-two, he felt crippled.

"I finally said to my cardiologist, 'You need to start redirecting me, because something isn't working here,' " Howard recalled. "I told him, 'I can't keep coming back every three or four months for angioplasty. I'm not going to make it one of these times. I've done everything you and the other doctors have told me to, and I don't know what to do anymore.' "

Howard's cardiologist knew him well. He realized that he was a short-tempered fellow driven by anxiety. Despite all his health behaviors, Howard was still high-strung, and the stress of having severe heart disease only served to escalate his tension and anger. (This tendency toward anxious, hostile behavior has long been considered a contributing factor to heart disease.) As it happened, the cardiologist had collaborated with Dr. Benson in caring for other patients who joined the Mind/Body program for people with heart disease. He told Howard there was only one new avenue to consider, and that was mind-body therapy to lessen his anxiety and anger.

Howard was pleased to learn of a new approach, but skeptical about its potential value. "Having been a student of the 1960s, my concept of meditation was sitting down with my legs folded and incense burning," he said. "I wanted to know—how is this going to help my heart?"

He discovered the answer when he joined the program in September 1991. The multifaceted group, which met every week for thirteen weeks, was led by nurse practitioner Eileen Stuart. She taught group members a variety of relaxation techniques, including progressive muscle relaxation, mindfulness meditation, and yoga. She used cognitive restructuring to challenge thinking patterns that led inexorably to anxiety, hostility, or depression, and replace them with patterns that fostered tranquility, compassion, and a sense of fulfillment. Stuart created an atmosphere in which the group members felt comfortable sharing their feelings and experiences. She also led discussions of nutrition and exercise programs custom-tailored for heart patients.

The cognitive restructuring helped Howard alter his automatic responses. "I hadn't realized it, but my response to many situations was very hostile. That anger kept burning in me. I never got it out, never confronted it, never dealt with it."

Stuart helped Howard to transform his viewpoint on his daily behaviors. During the third session, he described a typical incident in his hardware store. A customer asked him a question while he was conducting inventory, interrupting his trip to the back room to store a piece of merchandise. He became enraged, and although he refrained from pitching an unrestrained fit, he let this unsuspecting individual know exactly how he felt. After telling the story to the group, Stuart asked Howard a simple question: "What if you had put that merchandise down and taken a few minutes to deal with your customer? What would have happened?" Howard thought long and hard before answering.

"Absoutely nothing. I could have done it later, or even the next day," he replied.

That was when cognitive restructuring first "clicked" for Howard. He began to apply the same simple but profound logic to all his daily, stressful interactions. Howard realized that such reactions had been so instantaneous that no logic had ever been applied. He'd been on automatic hostile pilot for as long as he could remember.

In the group, he was taught other skills for handling these moments. "As soon as a situation arose that normally triggered a hostile response, I learned that I could sift through it within seconds. I can look at the situation, take a step back, take a breath, decide what I am going to do, and then do it. Before, it would take me days to work through, and I'd be anxious and nervous and hostile the whole time. Now I can take care of these situations constructively within minutes."

After finishing the group, Howard kept up a dedicated practice of relaxation, cognitive restructuring, and behavior change. "People can't restructure the way they have been thinking for thirty or forty years in thirteen weeks. It takes time and you need to practice this constantly."

In the year after participating in the program, Howard continued to modify his daily interactions. Soon a deeper transformation took hold. Howie the competitor in sports and life became calmer all the time. His essential priorities changed. Howie the workaholic started leaving his store much earlier to spend time with his family. Ironically, he now finds that he is more effective at work even though he puts in less hours, because "I make smarter decisions that are more appropriate when I am calm.

"People wouldn't think Howie would take so much time off," he remarked. "But now, time with my family has become a priority. For example, I'm going to read a wonderful story, *The Giving Tree,* to my eight-year-old daughter's class. It's a book of hugs."

Howard's style of relating to others also changed dramatically. "I'm more tuned in to people and their feelings," he said. "I'm much better able to communicate. I'm actually hearing what they're saying to me. It's not just words. I'm taking the time to listen. Before, I already had an answer before they finished their question."

After starting the mind-body program, Howard's physical condition improved quickly. In the last two years, he has not experienced a single incident of heart malfunction. He has no more chest pain or shortness of breath. Before he could not exercise without chest discomfort. Now he maintains a rigorous exercise program without a hint of pain.

Another interesting sidelight of Howard's case involves his cholesterol count. For six months before he began the mind-body program, Howard not only dieted and exercised assiduously, he took the cholesterol-lowering drugs prescribed by his doctor. During these six months, Howard's count went down by a mere 7 points. After joining the program, his cholesterol began to plummet. Over the next fifteen months, his cholesterol dropped over 100 points. Over a two-year period, his count went from 265 to a desirably low 149. Undoubtedly, the cholesterol-lowering drugs were helpful, *but they did not appear to take effect until after Howard joined the mind-body program.*

Today Howard says he has extraordinary energy, a sense of well-being, and joy in his work and family life. His shift from stressed power motivation to affiliative trust could not be more clear. This occurred partly because he faced a life-or-death crisis and knew he had to change. It also occurred because knowledgeable mind-body practitioners, and his fellow group members, created conditions for the emergence of his innate capacity for listening, trusting, and caring for others.

ONENESS: THE URGE TO MERGE

Love is hard to catch in the scientific butterfly net, and spirituality is even harder. Yet David McClelland and his colleagues not only found a way to tap spiritual longings, they also may have forged a link between spirituality and health. This unexpected finding emerged during an investigation of ancient practices of Buddhist meditation, as applied in a modern mind-body clinic.

In the late 1980s, McClelland had joined forces with Jon Kabat-Zinn, Ph.D., head of the Stress Reduction Clinic at the University of Massachusetts Medical Center. This clinic, described in chapter 2, teaches practical approaches to mindfulness, the ancient Buddhist philosophy of living in the moment. McClelland wanted to know whether Kabat-Zinn's program improved people's health by changing their motive patterns.

Jon Kabat-Zinn emphasizes that mindfulness does not involve an overt effort to heal illness—that is, "mindfulness" is not a goal-oriented or "end-gaining" activity; just the reverse. However, the fact is that his program has treated 6,000 medical patients, and a vast majority have experienced amelioration of their physical symptoms. Living mindfully—in the moment—also happens to be good for your health.

Mindfulness grounds people so solidly in the here-and-now—and in the body—that they often become more creative, healthy, spiritual, or loving. If Kabat-Zinn's mindfulness program raised people's affiliative trust, it certainly did not set out to do so.

Aware of Kabat-Zinn's documented success in teaching mindfulness, McClelland set up a study of motive patterns among a group of medical patients entering the Stress Reduction Clinic. He evaluated twenty-seven patients, all of whom suffered from chronic conditions often associated with stress: headaches, chronic pain, autoimmune disorders, heart problems, and high blood pressure. Working with colleagues Carolyn McCleod and Joel Weinberger, Ph.D., McClelland gave all the patients picture-story tests before and after their participation in Kabat-Zinn's eight-week program. He tracked their progress for two years.

The participants experienced marked reductions in their

symptoms after completing the Stress Reduction program. More remarkable were the long-term follow-up findings. "From the end of treatment to two years later, you would expect the level of symptoms to drift back upward," said Weinberger. "But the improvements stuck. There was no difference in reported symptoms two years after they finished the mindfulness program."

Weinberger found that people's symptoms got better when their affiliative trust was raised during the course of the program. But he noticed another striking pattern in their picture-story tests. After completing the program, many patients wrote stories that reflected a sense of belonging to someone or something bigger than themselves.

Weinberger was so struck by this pattern that he gave it a name: the *oneness motive*. Jokingly referred to by McClelland as the *urge to merge* or the *longing for belonging*, the oneness motive represents the desire—and capacity—to feel that you are part of something larger than yourself. That "something" can be a group of people, family, society, nature, God, or any imaginable spiritual entity.

How did people manifest the oneness motive? Weinberger identified three specific themes in people's stories—often written after seeing a picture of a couple—that signaled *oneness:*

1. The characters in the picture have a close emotional bond, with overtones of love or empathy.
2. The character(s) are described as belonging to something larger than themselves—such as a family, organization, community, spiritual force.
3. A "softening of boundaries" between inside and outside worlds is depicted.

Weinberger used these themes to measure oneness. After a careful review, he made these discoveries about Jon Kabat-Zinn's clients:

• Most experienced significant increases in oneness motivation.
• *People whose oneness motive was enhanced through mindfulness demonstrated pronounced improvements in their medical conditions.*

- The higher people's oneness motivation by the end of the program, the greater the likelihood they would sustain physical benefits two years later.

That the oneness motive increased during Kabat-Zinn's program was not surprising either, since the Buddhist tradition of mindfulness teaches that the highest development of consciousness involves acceptance of our oneness with others, nature, the world, even the universe. "Jon's treatment is partly designed to give people a sense of being unified with the world around them," Weinberger commented. "His mindfulness meditation is a way of breaking down barriers that one might consider 'false.' He teaches patients, many of whom suffer with chronic pain, that they really are at one with the world, that their pain is part of a larger 'pain.' "

How does the oneness motive enhance health? One small study, conducted by Steven P. Kelner, a colleague of David McClelland's, showed that people who practiced a guided visualization on a theme of oneness—being connected to a larger entity or purpose—showed increases in the IgA antibodies in their saliva immediately afterward. Oneness, which overlaps affiliative trust, also may be an Immune Power trait.

The marriage of affiliative trust and oneness motivation represents the love that stems from a final dissolution of our sense of separateness. In the great spiritual traditions, this is not a love of trade-offs or stroking. It is not even a love that one *has* to *give*. It is a pure unconditioned awareness that "giver" and "receiver" both share.

In other research, Kabat-Zinn demonstrated that his program also increases hardiness and a sense of coherence. These findings speak directly to the question: Can people change their personality traits or motives to the betterment of their health? Here is Kabat-Zinn's answer, from *Full Catastrophe Living:*

These motivational characteristics have traditionally been seen as associated with deep and stable personality structures and are not usually thought to be amenable to change, particularly in a short time period. The changes we are seeing in these personality variables in the people who go through the stress clinic suggest that *training in mindfulness meditation can have a profound positive influence on one's view of oneself and of the world, including an ability to be more trusting of oneself and others.*

In a recent conversation, Jon Kabat-Zinn elaborated on what it means for a mind-body treatment—such as mindfulness—to change personality. "You're still the same person," he remarked. "But what's changing, in some way, is your model—or the deep view that you carry of what is possible and who you are. That, of course, changes attitudes and behaviors that are directly related to health."

Taken as a whole, David McClelland's research on mind-body programs shows that affiliative trust, and other healthy motives, can be enhanced, and doing so reaps psychological and physical benefits. No single technique appeared to arouse the "love variable" in health. Each program had skilled, caring clinicians who integrated relaxation, meditation, coping skills, and group support into a broader tapestry of personal transformation. Love was neither the subject nor the object of these mind-body programs. Yet each set the stage for an unfolding of affiliative trust.

Our innate affiliative trust might be comparable to the source of an artist's creativity. There's an old but true cliché about artistic ability, whether it's in music, painting, sculpture, acting, dance, or poetry: "You can't teach talent. You can only teach tradecraft. That creates the optimal conditions for an artist to allow her imagination to take root and flower." The mind-body groups taught the tradecraft of tranquility, self-acceptance, and growth. They also created optimal conditions for affiliative trust, perhaps by removing obstacles to people's natural loving capacities.

Have you ever stared directly at a shining star in a dark night sky? If you have, you've noticed that the harder you stare, the more quickly the star's light seems to fade, until it almost disappears. Soon you discover how to get it back. You need only stare off to the side, just a bit, and the same star comes sharply and sparklingly into view. Perhaps affiliative trust fades if you "stare" at it too directly, trying self-consciously to access this aspect of your personality. Perhaps by "looking off to the side"—creating conditions for its natural appearance—your affiliative trust will come sharply and sparklingly into view.

LOVE AND CARE IN THE MIND-BODY REALM

McClelland's humanistic psychology teaches that love-for-its-own-sake is more than poetic fancy—it is scientific reality. Behavioral and experimental psychologists traditionally discount people's rosy self-assessments, dismissing motives based on anything other than self-interest. But McClelland's picture-story method was not based on self-assessments; it was based on unconscious thought patterns. And it revealed that many of us naturally feel and act with care toward others, for no reward other than the warmth that alights within. This "pure" drive certainly mixes with "impure" drives (commonly called "ulterior motives"), and sometimes they alternate back and forth. This is only human, but the salient point is that many of us are motivated—at least some of the time—by unconditional love.

We know that social support protects us from illness and early death. In some studies, social support is as good for our health as smoking is destructive to our health. What do we make of these extraordinary and oft-neglected findings? Should those of us with many loving family members, friends, and social ties feel protected, while those of us who feel lonely or isolated start to worry? Although the literature on social support is impressive, it rarely scratches the surface to answer this and other critical questions: Are people without sufficient support doomed to ill health? Can people strengthen their social support to better their health? How can people solidify their networks of support?

Viewing social support as a fixed factor in our health is disempowering. Those of us who are lonely are not doomed to ill health, because we can change our circumstances. The path to change hardly depends on good fortune ("meeting the right people"). More often, it hinges on how we live out our desire for relatedness. David McClelland believes that developing affiliative trust makes us more willing and able to establish healthy relationships.

In *Care of the Soul,* psychotherapist Thomas Moore emphasizes that we don't fall into support networks, we create them by expressing our care for others:

> Loneliness can be the result of an attitude that community is something into which one is received. Many people wait for members of a community to invite them in, and until that happens they are lonely. There may be something of the child here who expects to be taken care of by the family. But a community is not a family. It is a group of people held together by feelings of belonging, and those feelings are not a birthright. "Belonging" is an active verb, something we do positively. In one of his letters Ficino makes the remark, "The one guardian of life is love, but to be loved you must love." A person oppressed by loneliness can go out into the world and simply start belonging to it, not by joining organizations, but by living through feelings of relatedness—to other people, to nature, to society, to the world as a whole. Relatedness is a signal of soul.

The term "affiliative trust" could easily replace Moore's "relatedness." Moore's vision is empowering because it eschews "waiting around to be loved." Instead, he advocates an open-hearted stance in the world as the starting point for gratifying social networks. Those of us who have been repeatedly hurt in relationships, either during childhood or in the recent past, will find it hard to remain open-hearted, but that is the challenge presented by the call for affiliative trust.

Affiliative trust is a basis for healthy relationships, and it is essential for our creative engagement in the world. Perhaps Karl Menninger understood this best when he wrote:

> To live, we say, is to love, and vice versa. If a patient is not frozen in his primary narcissism . . . he will continuously strive to

find and touch persons and things about him. He will keep reaching out first a receiving then a giving hand, making acquaintances and then friends, and finding more and more satisfactions and identifications. This is not to imply that love consists in an endless mutual hand-holding or that life is a pure culture of love. But predominantly positive relationships are ultimately productive, as well as satisfying. The production of a baby is both an example and a symbol of this, but there are other kinds of reproduction in the world. All of them require goal-seeking efforts; all of them which are really creative require the investment of love.

Studies have shown that the quality (not just quantity) of our relationships influences our health. What determines the presence in our lives of quality relationships? Here again, personality traits are pivotal. Some people motivated by inhibited power have large support networks. Often, however, their relationships are characterized by a "quid pro quo" mentality, if not an outright desire for dominance.

David McClelland would have us ask ourselves these questions about any relationship: Why do I care about this person? Am I primarily invested in what he or she can give me, whether that booty is money, sex, ego boosting, or emotional support? Or do I simply enjoy this person's qualities? Do I give in order to get? Or do I give because it is intrinsically pleasurable? Are my relationships motivated by frustrated power or unconditional love?

Of course, most relationships are not "pure," and the goal is not to "purify" them. The goal is to nonjudgmentally raise awareness of the often mixed motives we have in relationships. Once we do, we can conduct a search in our own hearts for affiliative trust. If we can find elements of unconditional love in any relationship—no matter how obscured—it is probably worth preserving *and* revitalizing. But understanding our complex motives helps us tease out the strands of affiliative trust tied up in a ball with other motives and defenses. Awareness can release the tensions that bind up our natural loving kindness.

McClelland's goal is not to extinguish power motivations and replace them with unconditional love. He encourages a balance among the many innate forces that drive us, and he seeks to lessen the internal "stress" in power and love motives. Healthy control turns into frustrated power when the ambitious person cannot tolerate setbacks in his quest. The love motive is healthy unless it turns into the neurotic search, where the person can never get or give enough love to feel satisfied. People who find themselves constantly frustrated in their expressions of power *or* love are bound to become chronically angry, depressed, or sick.

David McClelland believes that we can "de-stress" our power and achievement motives by putting them in proper perspective. One way to accomplish this is to raise affiliative trust. Some people come to this realization on their own. How often do we hear about individuals who have lost prestigious positions, or suffered terrible setbacks in their financial lives, who say: "Now I realize what's important. All I want is time with the people I love." For people who are experiencing hard times or insecurity on the job, a reshuffling of priorities toward human connections may take the sting out of setbacks at work or in financial matters. It becomes easier to roll with the punches when we allow ourselves to focus on the transcendent pleasures to be found in friendships and family.

EXERCISES IN AFFILIATIVE TRUST

The following exercises are designed to cultivate affiliative trust in a simple way. They include a loving kindness meditation and a visualization focusing on relationships. One caveat: I don't believe that any "technique" will raise affiliative trust unless it is applied alongside a searching self-examination. In *A Path with Heart*, Jack Kornfield suggests the outlines of this exploration:

In modern life we have become so busy with our daily affairs that we have forgotten the essential art of taking time to converse with our heart. When we ask it about our current path, we must look at the values we have chosen to live by. Where do we put our time, our strength, our creativity, our love? We must look at our life without sentimentality, exaggeration, or idealism. Does what we are choosing reflect what we most deeply value?

LOVING-KINDNESS MEDITATION

The following is a loving-kindness meditation, a 2,500-year-old Buddhist practice that uses repeated phrases, images, and feelings to evoke affiliative trust. Here is the version used by Jack Kornfield, a renowned teacher, psychologist, and master of meditation.

In his book *A Path with Heart,* Kornfield suggests that you begin by sitting in a comfortable position, relaxing mind and body, and letting go of plans and preoccupations. Then, inwardly recite the following phrases:

> May I be filled with loving-kindness.
> May I be well.
> May I be peaceful and at ease.
> May I be happy. . . .

Let the feelings arise with the words. Adjust the words and images so that you find the exact phrases that best open your heart of kindness. Repeat the phrases again and again, letting the feelings permeate your body and mind.

Practice this meditation repeatedly for a number of weeks until the sense of loving-kindness for yourself grows.

When you feel ready, in the same meditation period you can gradually expand the focus of your loving-kindness to include others. Choose someone in your life who has truly cared for you. Picture them and carefully recite the same phrases, *May he/she be filled with loving-kindness,* and so forth. When loving-kindness for your benefactor has developed, begin to include other people you love in the meditation, picturing them and reciting the same phrases, evoking a sense of loving-kindness for them . . .

Then you can learn to practice it anywhere. You can use this meditation in traffic jams, in buses and airplanes, in doctors' waiting rooms, and in a thousand other circumstances. As you silently practice this meditation among people, you will immediately feel a wonderful connection with them—the power of loving-kindness. It will calm your life and keep you connected to your heart.

A VISUALIZATION FOR AFFILIATIVE TRUST

Affiliative trust unfolds in our here-and-now relationships. Just as old grief clouds the open heart, current grief (and conflict) can infect our relationships, preventing development of affiliative trust. Healing current relationships with significant others is one way to open our hearts.

One approach has been suggested by Stephanie Simonton, Ph.D., who helped to develop guided imagery for cancer patients. Simonton also uses visualization for healthy individuals to help prevent illness. Most of these preventive exercises focus on the achievement of here-and-now goals, one of which is healthier relationships. The following is a visualization exercise adapted and altered for the development of affiliative trust. Take fifteen minutes to practice this every day for one week. Afterward, use this visualization when you feel "disconnected" from others and the world.

Find a comfortable place to sit or lie, and practice the relaxation method that suits you best. Take a few minutes to breathe deeply into your abdomen, and turn your focus inward.

Now turn your attention to your present life. Focus on the one significant relationship that you feel most calls for healing. Think of someone with whom there is a misunderstanding, conflict, unspoken needs or feelings, or lack of communication.

Imagine that individual in the room with you. He or she is with you in this quiet space. Take a moment to allow this image to come to life in your mind and heart.

Ask yourself: In this space, which is private and safe, what do I wish to say to this person that I have not said? What do I wish to express? Find words and expressions for your feelings. You can say or do anything you wish to convey how you feel. Imagine the other person listening but not responding.

After you have completed this part of the visualization, allow the other person to speak his or her thoughts and feelings. How would he or she respond?

After you have imagined the other person's response, allow yourself to respond again. This time, turn your attention toward healing resolution. You think: Each of us has now expressed our needs and feelings. How can we repair whatever damage has occurred? Allow yourself to build a bridge of understanding between yourself and this person.

As you imagine yourself building a bridge, pay exquisitely close attention, in word, image, and sound, to the ebb and flow of your interaction. Is there resistance? Cooperation? Continued misunderstanding? Vestigial anger? Compassionate concern? Although your goal is healing, do not force the issue. Allow whatever issues, conflicts, or leftover hurts to play themselves out. Gently direct this movie-in-your mind toward resolution, but wholeheartedly investigate that which obstructs resolution. Find it in your heart to accept the fears, angers, or conflicts that remain in either one of you or both. See if your mutual acceptance of each other leads to a new-found harmony.

Even if the visualization does not end with a complete sense of resolution, let each of you express the wish that you will find harmony and healing with the other. Wish each other peace and freedom from suffering.

The spirit of this visualization is the generation of affiliative trust. Its purpose is not to whitewash but to ever more deeply acknowledge that which obstructs the open heart. One important caveat: The visualization is *not* meant as a specific rehearsal for a life interaction, because spontaneity is quickly sacrificed if you hope to tightly control the manner in which your relationships unfold. Also, things just don't always go as planned. But the visualization is designed as an investigation of the unspoken and unfelt between you and people you care for. Thus, it can set the stage for a real-life encounter. The thrust of this exercise is to practice the courage to speak your heart and to learn more about yourself and another in relationship. What are the true blockages? What outcome do I wish for? How can we achieve harmony and healing?

HEALTHY HELPING: THE TRAIT OF ALTRUISM

A HUMAN BEING IS A PART OF THE WHOLE CALLED BY US UNIVERSE, A PART LIMITED IN TIME AND SPACE. HE EXPERIENCES HIMSELF, HIS THOUGHTS AND FEELINGS AS SOMETHING SEPARATED FROM THE REST, A KIND OF OPTICAL ILLUSION OF HIS CONSCIOUSNESS. THIS DELUSION IS A KIND OF PRISON FOR US, RESTRICTING US TO OUR PERSONAL DESIRES AND TO AFFECTION FOR A FEW PERSONS NEAREST TO US. OUR TASK MUST BE TO FREE OURSELVES FROM THIS PRISON BY WIDENING OUR CIRCLE OF COMPASSION TO EMBRACE ALL LIVING CREATURES AND THE WHOLE OF NATURE IN ITS BEAUTY.

—ALBERT EINSTEIN

Allan Luks has spent his entire adult life helping others, and now he is devoted to spreading the news: Helping is an activity that demonstrably improves the health of the helper. Luks believes that helping is our society's most underrated health behavior. Moreover, in a large-scale study he conducted of volunteers nationwide, he was able to verify his unorthodox beliefs.

Helping as a health behavior? We might think of helping as good for our moral standing or self-esteem, but not as health-promoting in the strict sense. Mainstream medical science has confirmed the value of certain behaviors that involve diet, exercise, and environmental factors. But it has neglected even to investigate the biologic value of behaviors that lend meaning, purpose, and social cohesiveness to our lives. Helping is one such behavior, and it has barely been studied for its health benefits.

Luks is currently executive director of Big Brothers/Big Sisters of New York, but his involvement in research on helping began in the mid-1980s. He had been appointed director of the Institute for the Advancement of Health, then the leading organization devoted to mind-body medicine. His own background as a civil rights and Peace Corps volunteer led him to believe that altruism—as a trait and an activity—was both emotionally and physically revitalizing.

In late 1987, Luks published an item in *Better Homes and Gardens,* soliciting people's reports of any health improvements they had experienced from helping others. It was a useful exercise in information-gathering. He conducted a line-by-line analysis of people's stories, circling words and comments that were repeated over and over. A clear pattern emerged: People who felt that their health benefited from their helping activities experienced rushes of physical pleasure and psychological well-being. After helping, they noticed sensations of warmth and energy—feelings that often were directly associated with reduced aches, pains, and other symptoms of illness.

Luks began developing a larger, more carefully structured survey on health and helping. He pursued his research with scientific rigor, collaborating with an expert in the design of behavioral studies. With the assistance of Howard Andrews, Ph.D., a biopsychologist and senior research scientist with the New York State Psychiatric Institute, Luks designed a seventeen-question survey with forty-three possible answers. The questionnaire was distributed to thousands of volunteers at more than twenty organizations nationwide. The respondents included people with a wide range of experiences, including helpers of the homeless, crime victims,

AIDS patients, medical patients in large hospitals, and runaway youths.

A total of 3,296 responses were returned to Allan Luks, and Dr. Andrews conducted a thorough and sophisticated statistical analysis of the results, which revealed striking correlations between helping and health. Of the groups surveyed, the Pilot Club International, a large volunteer organization composed mainly of women, proved to be a valuable resource. Responses included in the results came from 1,484 Pilot Club members; 1,812 members of the twenty nationwide groups; and 208 individuals from the Kansas Area Organization on Aging.

The survey asked people to rate their own health ("absolute health") and to compare their health to others their age ("relative health"). The survey of nationwide organizations also inquired about the number of doctors' visits during the previous year. In an open-ended question, everyone was asked to describe any emotional or physical effects of helping. These responses were rated and categorized by institute staff members. Finally, people were asked whether they had a physical "feel-good" sensation after their helping activities, and if so, how long it lasted.

The volunteers were queried about the frequency of their helping activities; whether they helped strangers or friends and family; and whether they mainly helped through their organizations. Luks wanted to know whether they had been influenced to become helpers by parental teachings, religious training, or "feeling part of society."

Howard Andrews tabulated the results and analyzed statistical relationships between the quantity and quality of helping, and mind-and-body health outcomes. Here are the highlights:

- Ninety-five percent of the respondents reported some "feel-good" sensations during and/or immediately after their activities. Nearly 80 percent said that these good feelings recurred long after their helping activities had ended.
- Ninety percent of those who reported feeling good as a result of helping *rated their own health as better than others their age.*
- The greater the frequency of volunteering, the greater the rela-

tive health benefits. (See figure 7.1.) There was a *ten times greater chance* that volunteers who rated their health as better than others would be weekly rather than once-yearly helpers.

- Volunteers who claimed many psychological benefits reported much better absolute physical health. Among those who reported excellent health, 30 percent indicated more than four specific psychological benefits of helping. Among those who rated their health fair or poor, only 18 percent said they experienced more than four psychological benefits.
- People who primarily helped strangers rather than friends and family reported better absolute health. (See figure 7.2.) They were also more likely to report "feel-good" sensations after helping.
- People who had personal contact with those they helped were more likely to experience "feel-good" sensations and to be more frequent—and therefore healthier—helpers.
- Eighty percent of the volunteers said the good feelings associated with helping returned, though with somewhat diminished intensity, when they remembered their acts of helping.
- The percentage of volunteers who reported many benefits from helping was much greater among those claiming parental teachings, religious training, or societal factors as strong influences on their helping behaviors.

The strength of these relationships took Allan Luks and especially Howard Andrews by surprise. This picture emerged from the data: People who frequently engaged in helping activities—especially with strangers—experienced feel-good sensations that were directly associated with better perceived physical health. Among the reports of health benefits, volunteers said that they experienced relief from chronic headaches, back pain, and stomachaches. They experienced fewer or less severe colds. They reported relief from the symptoms of chronic diseases such as asthma, arthritis, and lupus. Many volunteers said that their eating and sleeping habits had improved.

The benefits of helping were strongly related to the consistency of people's helping behaviors. As with James Pennebaker's confessions, the positive effects persisted for a while, but waned over time, unless the process was repeated. Luks now had evidence that individuals who maintained a steady "practice" of helping others were as likely to reap the benefits as people who exercised, meditated, or confided on a regular basis.

The other significant factor—the quality of helping—helped Luks to set guidelines for healthy forms of altruism. (See "Four Characteristics of Healthy Helping" on p. 282.) Volunteers who helped strangers benefited far more than those who helped friends and family. Luks recognized that helping friends and family members was wrought with potential complications. These acts of care may be motivated by obligation, guilt, or other emotional entanglements. Luks's concern was validated when he read a study by Ohio State University researchers Janice Kiecolt-Glaser and Ronald Glaser, which showed that caretakers of family members with Alzheimer's often suffered from a sense of isolation, a weakening of immunity, and a variety of illnesses.

Given these potential pitfalls, it was no wonder that the strongest relationship between health and helping involved voluntary activities with strangers. These were instances in which people freely *chose* to help others to whom they felt no long-standing obligation. The sense of social connectedness gained under these circumstances was profound, paving the way for sensations of "helper's high."

While the survey results were impressive, Howard Andrews had to weed out other variables—such as age, sex, or marital status—to make sure that the link between helping and health could not be explained by some other factor. He conducted a multiple regression analysis, which carefully controlled for demographics, to see whether Allan Luks's theory about healthy helping would stand up under more intense scrutiny.

Here are Andrews's key findings.

• *The relationship between frequent helping and positive health benefits was significant for four of the five health-related outcomes:* better absolute health, relative health, number of psychological and physical

Fig. 7.1. Relationship Between Health and Frequency of Helping.

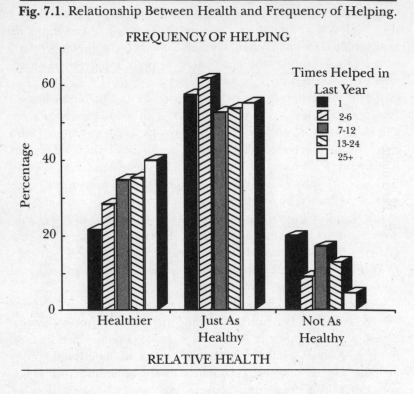

FREQUENCY OF HELPING

RELATIVE HEALTH

benefits, and a long duration of good feelings that came from helping.

• *Assisting strangers through a group was significantly linked to three of the five outcomes:* fewer visits to the doctor, the number of positive effects of helping, and the duration of good feelings resulting from helping.

As you might expect, age, sex, and marital status had strong associations with health. Health declined with age; married people had better overall health; men reported better health than women; and women reported more long-lasting good feelings as a result of helping. But here was Howard Andrews's most important finding: *The link between helping and health benefits remained strong even after age, sex, and marital status were removed from the equation.*

Fig. 7.2. Relationship Between Health and Helping Strangers.

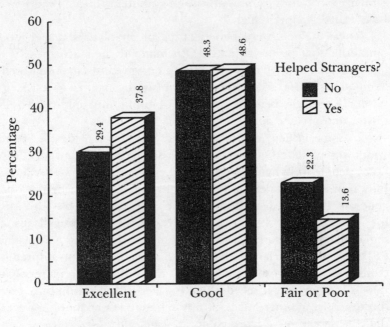

ABSOLUTE HEALTH

"My research has shown that it is the process of helping, without regard to its outcome, that is the healing factor," wrote Luks in his 1991 book written with Peggy Payne, *The Healing Power of Doing Good*. "This process can be effective to some degree for virtually every sort of human ill. Regular helping of others can diminish the effects of disabling chronic pain and lessen the symptoms of physical distress. And it can ease the tension of able-bodied people who are overworked and living in stressful times."

THE HELPER'S HIGH—PART ONE

Having demonstrated connections between helping and health, Luks set out to understand the psychological and biological mechanisms behind this effect. The key, it seemed, was the stunningly similar descriptions from hundreds of volunteers of the experience Luks called "helper's high."

These helpers were beneficiaries of characteristic feel-good sensations that occurred in the aftermath of their activities. The majority reported feelings of warmth, energy, and emotional well-being. These short-term effects disappeared, but they gave way to subtler long-term benefits: a sense of tranquility, improved self-worth, and greater optimism.

In some instances, the "rush" was directly tied to relief from symptoms of illness. Consider the case of Judy Weintraub, who helps people from her apartment in New York's Greenwich Village. Judy has multiple sclerosis (MS), a chronic condition that is now generally regarded as an autoimmune disease. In people with MS, the immune system attacks the myelin sheaths of nerve cells, causing debilitating neurological symptoms, such as pain, muscular weakness, and speech disturbances. The bane of MS is its unpredictability: One day it can brutally attack the sufferer with pain or paralysis; the next day it recedes, leaving her with no symptoms, save the dread of another attack at any moment. Over time, however, the disease can leave irreversible damage.

For Judy Weintraub, MS was more predictable than for most people. She was first diagnosed in 1975 at the age of thirty-three, after which the disease took a steady downhill course. By 1980, she could no longer walk. Since then she has generally been confined to her apartment. She has four telephones—one in each room, so she doesn't have to move from room to room to answer. One of her friends calls her a "telephone professional," because she is so superb at talking her way through bureaucratic barriers in order to assist people.

As a consultant to youth organizations, Judy develops programs that provide services to impoverished, disabled, or physically ill children and their parents. Most recently she designed a program for the children of mothers with AIDS. As much time as Judy spends on these projects, she spends an equal amount of time helping friends and strangers.

In just the past year, Judy has begun to take her first steps in over a decade. She may never be "cured," but her recent mobility is a big victory over MS. Several of her doctors did not expect her condition to show any improvement whatsoever. Judy believes that this victory is the result of many factors, not the least of which has been her helping activities. How does she know that her own helping has helped her get better?

"I don't know what the physiology of it is," said Judy. "But helping definitely gives me more energy. Which means that I can do things I otherwise could not. A kind of 'rush' comes over me." That "rush" always gives Judy a feeling of strength. It also boosts her "positive mental attitude," which she is convinced is responsible for her improvement.

Many volunteers in Luks's survey specifically compared helper's high to "runner's high"—that euphoric kick experienced by dedicated joggers. Rikki, a twenty-eight-year-old woman from Connecticut, volunteers one afternoon each week at a nursing home, where she helps wheelchair-bound patients around the premises and into the dining room. "I go home tired," she said, "but with a new spurt of energy such as one feels after a really good game of tennis."

Rikki's rush is followed by a sense of revitalization, one she remembers feeling even as a child. She said that her natural parents were abusive and neglectful, leaving her with strong needs for affection that could only be met by reaching out to strangers. "I would do the most thoughtful things for people just to hear kind words," she said. "Those words gave me that good feeling."

To Luks, the connection between helper's high and well-being was impossible to ignore. "The power of this thing is so great that sometimes I just want to shout it out," he said in *American Health*. "Even my 80-year-old father has started volunteering. My mother died, and he was very lonely. I said, 'Why don't you volunteer?' and he said no. I think he thought it was kind of a sissy thing. Finally he joined a volunteer program at his local hospital. Now he's got something to look forward to. It's given him a whole new focus."

IS HELPING AN ADDICTION?

Luks believes that the intoxicating rush reported by helpers is caused by an increase in endorphins, our brain's own painkilling chemicals. When we synthesize endorphins, our perception of pain is reduced and we may experience mild sensations of euphoria.

Studies have shown that the high experienced by inveterate joggers is undoubtedly the result of a sudden burst of endorphin production in the pituitary gland, stimulated by the "good stress" of exercise. All the signs in Luks's survey suggested that helper's high had remarkably similar biochemical and emotional features to "runner's high."

Besides the volunteers' reports, there was intriguing experimental evidence supporting the endorphin theory of helper's high. Jaak Panksepp, a professor of psychology at Bowling Green State University, has long investigated the neurobiology of bonding and altruism. In studies with dogs, rats, guinea pigs, and chicks, Panksepp showed that endorphins are released in the body when social bonding occurs.

Consider Pansksepp's study of puppies taken from their mothers. He placed the puppies in an isolation chamber, where they invariably began to cry. Panksepp then administered low doses of synthetic morphine, which immediately reduced their cries of distress. A placebo shot of saline solution did not lessen their cries. Once they had received a drug that mimics the action of body-made endorphins, their separation anxiety was quelled.

In another study, Panksepp paired rats together, administered morphine, and observed their social behavior. Compared to a control group, the rats that got morphine began to isolate from each other. Panksepp got similar results with young guinea pigs placed near a cage that housed their mothers. The animals that got morphine spent significantly less time hanging around their mothers' cages. These studies showed that providing an endorphinlike drug quenched the animals' thirst for the feel-good sensations of social contact and mothering. Their subsequent attitude seemed to be: Why bother?

For these animals, fulfillment of the need for social contact was accompanied by an endorphin rush. This rush could be re-created with synthetic drugs, quelling the animals' needs. But how is helping similar to having a bond with others, or with one's mother? Panksepp believes that helping is simply another form of social attachment. His studies of nurturing behavior suggest that giver and receiver both benefit from feel-good sensations and increases in endorphins. In human beings, the helper experiences similar feelings—warmth, increased vitality—as the person(s) being helped, because both have forged a gratifying social bond.

Even a mother's care—the primal expression of helping—may be mediated by endorphins. In one study, Panksepp gave a drug that *blocks* endorphins to the mothers of a group of puppies. Apparently, the mothers stopped receiving any pleasurable signals associated with caretaking. These mothers became less likely to play with their offspring. They were even less likely to retrieve the pups when they were picked up by a laboratory assistant and moved to another corner of their cage!

Panksepp believes that the neurobiology of bonding makes sense from an evolutionary perspective. The endorphin high is a biochemical reward for helping behaviors—the good feelings make us want to help again and again. Hence, our brains are hard-wired to reinforce the altruistic impulse. But why would a morally sound behavior such as helping be useful for evolution? Doesn't Darwin's "survival of the fittest" contradict such a notion? If we've learned anything about our evolutionary past, haven't we learned that survivors "look out for number one"?

Panksepp doesn't think so. In his view, the survival of our species depends as much (if not more) on cooperative engagement as it does on competitive infighting. Even the so-called primitive and self-serving behaviors of hunting and gathering required cooperative efforts.

Allan Luks writes, "As *Homo sapiens* evolved and brain size increased, parts of the brain contributing to the capacity to cooperate might have developed to a greater degree than others. Intrinsic helping tendencies may thus, like dominance urges, be embedded in the human brain structure, may even be part of what we think of as human nature itself."

If evolution was behind the development of brain functions that reinforce helping, the story may not end there. The helper's high would probably also be accompanied by the reward of better health. Here, perhaps, is an evolutionary ethos that parallels "survival of the fittest." Might there be a parallel principle of "survival of the most compassionate"?

The answer is a tentative yes. Studies have shown that runners, whose endorphin levels jump, experience increases in Immune Power and balance. Regular exercise can stimulate immune functions—especially natural killer (NK) cell activity. As I detailed in chapter 2 on Gary Schwartz's research, people who are chronically stressed or repressed may produce a constant overload of endorphins that *suppresses* immune functions. But the brief burst of endorphins associated with "good stress"—such as exercise or creative challenges at work—appears to *boost* the immune system.

With Allan Luks's reports from hundreds of helpers, whose high is strikingly similar to runner's high, it is reasonable to infer that helper's high is also associated with increases in Immune Power. This would explain why regular helpers tend to be healthier; their immune defenses benefit from those brief surges of endorphins. The fact that so many helpers reported fewer symptoms from colds, allergies, asthma, and autoimmune diseases suggests that their immune systems were indeed balanced and bolstered by helping activities. More research on the immunologic effects of helping is needed to identify specific functions that are influenced by altruism.

What explains the relief of pain symptoms experienced by so many helpers? Clearly, pain relief—whether it is backache, headache, or any other chronic pain—could result directly from an increase in painkilling endorphins.

If Jaak Pansksepp and Allan Luks are right, and there is an evolutionary principle of "survival of the most compassionate"— one that is anchored in our biochemistry—then we have yet to harness its potential to promote our health and well-being, as individuals and as a civilization.

WOMEN VOLUNTEERS:
STRONG EVIDENCE FOR HEALTHY HELPING

Although Allan Luks's survey was strong evidence, he knew it was not the final word on healthy helping. One criticism of his research was that most of the health measures were people's own self-reports. A study that used more objective health criteria (medical records) would produce more definitive results. Also, the strongest evidence on mind-health linkages comes from long-term studies, in which healthy people are followed for years to see who gets sick and who stays well. In such a study, would regular helpers remain healthier for decades?

A study by Phyllis Moen, Ph.D., the Ferris Family Professor of Life Course Studies at Cornell University in New York, reports the results of a thirty-year investigation of 427 married women with children who lived in upstate New York. These women, who ranged from twenty-five to fifty years old at the outset, were first interviewed in 1956. The same group was located and interviewed again in 1986. Called the Women's Roles and Well-Being Project, the study offered "the rare opportunity to examine the long-term effects of multiple roles."

Dr. Moen wanted to find out whether certain roles or social conditions increased women's longevity. Moen and her colleagues, Donna Dempster-McClain and Robin M. Williams, Jr., tested various theories about which women would live longer. Would women who occupied many different roles, in addition to wife and mother, live longer? Did women who played particular roles achieve life extension? One theory was that women who were employed, and therefore not consigned to a constricting homemaker role, would live longer. Another was that women with more children would be stressed by their heavier caretaking burden. In toto, Moen and her colleagues examined six different roles: worker, church member, friend, neighbor, relative, and member of volunteer clubs/organizations.

The researchers discovered that women who lived longer could be characterized by only two factors: *They engaged in multiple roles and they were members of volunteer organizations.*

No other theories were borne out. Being employed did not help them live longer, contrary to the popular opinion of many social scientists. Women with more children did not die sooner. Moen and her colleagues controlled for education, levels of social support, husband's occupational status, social class, number of children, general life satisfaction, self-esteem, and gender role traditionalism. None of these factors explained away the connection between multiple roles, volunteering, and a longer life for these women.

According to Moen, the women with multiple roles or who volunteered were more "socially integrated"—hence, less isolated. We know that social isolation leads to early mortality, while social integration is related to a longer life span. Also, women ensconced in the culture and society of the 1950s had fewer opportunities to break out of an isolated homemaker role. One can imagine that women who found ways to do so benefited psychologically and physically. But there is more here than meets the eye. These women *did* have more social support and higher self-esteem—but these factors were *not* directly linked to longer life. There was something special about having multiple roles and helping activities that enabled these women to live longer.

In 1992, Moen published a revealing follow-up study of 313 of the 427 women whom she interviewed. This time she showed that multiple roles and helping activities not only predicted longevity, they also predicted better health. To demonstrate this, she and her colleagues used *three* different measures: the time lapse before onset of a serious disease, the woman's own appraisal of her health, and a careful review of the woman's medical history.

"I now have a third study, showing that multiple roles and volunteering also promotes psychological well-being," Moen recently said. "Thus, I have looked at three different outcomes—longevity, health, and psychological well-being—and I have gotten the same results for each. I'm very excited about this, because the findings are quite robust."

Other salient findings from Moen's research include:

- Fifty-two percent of the women who did not belong to volunteer clubs or organizations in 1956 had experienced a major illness by 1986, compared with only 36 percent of women who had been active in their communities.
- Women who were active in 1956 showed significantly higher self-esteem thirty years later than did women who had not been active.
- In contrast to Luks's findings, the duration and timing of volunteer work/membership was not significant in predicting health or well-being. Specifically, a woman who volunteered at various times during the thirty years had the same health/longevity benefits as women who volunteered continuously.

Since Moen's research involved women exclusively, the question arises as to whether men receive similar benefits from helping. Allan Luks's survey suggests that they do. But so does a seldom-recognized finding from one of the most famous long-term studies of social relationships and health ever conducted. In 1982, University of Michigan epidemiologist Dr. James House published his data from the Tecumseh Community Health Study, in which 2,754 adults were followed for a decade. After adjusting for age and other demographic factors, House discovered that men reporting a higher level of social relationships were significantly less likely to die during the follow-up. When one reads the study's fine print, however, one discovers that *volunteering activities were among the most powerful predictors of reduced mortality rates.* Men also may lower their risks of illness by finding ways to help others.

I asked Moen why she thought that women who volunteered were healthier over the course of thirty years. "One thing is that volunteering is voluntary," she replied. "It's the fact that choice is involved. This week I spoke with a retired man who started driving for the Red Cross, but he decided he didn't like it. With volunteer work, if you don't enjoy it, you stop. With certain other roles, such as caregiving or paid work, you often have no choice. In these instances, you don't have the sense that you're in control."

Allan Luks also has found that helpers have more perceived control over their lives and well-being. They choose activities that yield the greatest sense of meaning, affiliation, and connection to something larger than themselves—whether it is a cause, a person, a group, or a belief. This choice reflects commitment *and* control.

"I believe that altruism also is an important part of this," said Moen. "I just can't say how much. The literature suggests that people who are altruistic in terms of time also donate money. I don't think it's either time or money, it's both. Altruism involves a mind-set of wanting to make the world a better place."

Moen's research has received little fanfare in the press or the mind-body community. Nonetheless, in a study design that meets the gold standard for social science research, Moen demonstrated powerful associations between altruism, health, and longevity.

IS THERE AN ALTRUISTIC PERSONALITY?

In recent years, psychologists have confirmed the existence of an altruistic personality—someone who naturally helps people in need. Ultimately, it may be impossible to separate the contribution to health of altruistic traits and helping behaviors. Helping flows directly from the altruist within ourselves who feels compassion and chooses to act on those feelings.

Therefore, helping should not be viewed as a behavior that can be prescribed like a pill. All of us have our own complex set of feelings about helping, which are rooted in our upbringing and personality. Nevertheless, there is reason to believe that everyone can be motivated to help. It may simply require soul-searching to find the altruist within.

Altruism is an Immune Power trait that drives a behavior— helping—which is directly associated with improved health and well-being. Therefore, we improve our health in two ways: by discovering the altruist within and by helping. The two reinforce each other, and they cannot be pried apart.

The late Norman Cousins understood the inseparability of altruism and helping. Allan Luks told me about a conversation he once had with Cousins, author of *The Anatomy of an Illness* and *Head First: The Biology of Hope,* and an early supporter of PNI research. Soon after Luks began his investigation of healthy helping, Cousins encouraged him.

"Don't you understand what you're coming up with?" he asked Luks. "You're proving what people already know." Cousins continued, "They simply don't realize they know it. When Carl Jung [the great psychoanalyst] talked about our collective unconscious, he meant that we as a people have a collective wisdom, which for a variety of reasons does not manifest itself. Altruism and its benefits are part of that wisdom."

Cousins convinced Luks that people had lost touch with their native empathy. They needed an encouraging "push" to engage in activities that would remind them of the pleasures of giving. Teaching people about the health benefits was one approach; giving them practical advice on helping was another. But Cousins strongly believed that everyone possessed traits of compassion, no matter how buried.

"Altruism is like a muscle," Cousins said. "It must be used, or it atrophies." To Cousins, using our altruistic "muscle" meant getting out there, helping others, and learning from experience that our labors are as healing for us as they are for the people we've helped.

Is the altruistic personality rooted in biology, learned during childhood, reinforced by social environment, or all of the above? The answer is important, because if there is no biological basis for altruism, then perhaps some people simply have this capability and others do not—in which case no one can develop this Immune Power trait.

As with most current questions of personality, it appears as if genes, biology, learning, and environmental factors all play a part. However, only in the past decade have psychologists recognized that empathy has a biological basis. Jean Piaget, the renowned Swiss psychologist, contended that children did not feel empathy until their brains were sufficiently developed to make sense of other people's experiences—around age seven or eight. That point of view was psychological doctrine until research in the 1970s and '80s proved otherwise. Among several psychologists who overturned the old dogma was Martin L. Hoffman of New York University. Hoffman showed that newborn babies will cry in response to the cries of another infant. Moreover, they barely respond to equally loud computer simulations of babies' cries or even to tape-recordings of their own cries.

"Virtually from the day they are born, there is something particularly disturbing to infants about the sound of another infant's cry," Dr. Hoffman told Daniel Goleman of the *New York Times.* "The innate predisposition to cry to that sound seems to be the earliest precursor of empathy."

Empathy researchers have created some tricky psychodramas to demonstrate just how empathic babies can be. Dr. Carolyn Zahn-Waxler, a developmental psychologist at the National Institute of Mental Health, gathered mothers and their infants or toddlers into her lab to observe the children's responses when the mothers or other children were distressed. She often had adults drop materials or bump their heads to see if the children would comfort them. In "naturalistic" studies carried out in the home, Zahn-Waxler would train mothers to simulate pain, fake a cough, act angry or cry, and then rate their own children's reactions. In all these instances, children demonstrated their own upset and, with sounds and gestures, tried to comfort their distressed parents.

"We couldn't be sure whether the one-year-old was giving reassurance or seeking it, or both," commented Zahn-Waxler. "But in children only a few months older we'd see unmistakable expressions of concern for the other person. The floodgates of altruism open along with the development of language."

What begins in infancy as a reflex develops into the fully formed response we call empathy—a complex cluster of feelings, thoughts, and actions. Zahn-Waxler found that by the second year of life, children demonstrate not only empathy but the altruistic behavior that follows. After age two, children begin to show wide differences in their capacity to respond empathically. Some develop altruism sooner than others. At each developmental stage, some children show more altruistic behavior than others.

But Zahn-Waxler insists that altruism is not the psychic province of any select group. "I see altruism developing almost universally and showing up in predictable forms at relatively predictable stages and ages. That suggests to me that whatever part experience plays, the organism is 'hard-wired' with a tendency to respond empathetically and, based on that, to develop altruistic behavior."

Today, neuroscientists are mapping that hard-wiring. Leslie Brothers, a psychiatrist at the California Institute of Technology, has honed in on the visual cortex, the area of the brain that processes the meaning of what has been seen, and its connections to the amygdala, a brain structure centrally involved in emotional responses. When we mammals see another in trouble or pain, as evidenced largely by his or her facial expression, this visual information is translated by the brain in a manner that arouses conscious feelings of vicarious fear, sadness, and concern. "The evidence suggests that there are specific brain circuits for social response to emotional signals," said Dr. Brothers. "This is the type of neural activity that should lie at the base of empathy."

Thus, the altruistic personality is one whose upbringing, social environment, and life experience has nourished his or her native empathy. The work of the above-mentioned scientists proves that all of us have the potential to feel others' pain and to help accordingly. What blocks us from becoming the altruists we can be? Dr. Marion Radke-Yarrow, chief of the National Institute of Mental Health's Laboratory of Developmental Psychology, has collaborated with Zahn-Waxler to chart the later stages in the development of empathy. Their work has enriched our understanding of how empathy is either stunted or encouraged by parents and other caretakers.

Differences from child to child in the expression of empathy show themselves at age two or three. Radke-Yarrow and Zahn-Waxler found that children whose empathic responses grew and matured were those whose parents demonstrated the distressing effects their behavior could have on others. Such parents would say, "Look how sad you've made her feel." Their research did not suggest that blaming or shaming children made them more empathic. Rather, focusing their awareness on another's hurt feelings would keep alive the native empathy of their babyhood, while adding more sophisticated cognitive levels of understanding. Their work echoes Norman Cousins's remark that altruism is a muscle that must be used, lest it atrophy.

For those of us whose altruistic muscles have become weakened, Cousins has one simple prescription: Go out and exercise them. Allan Luks agrees, and he preaches that the best way to become empathic is to start helping people now. The mere act of helping often stirs empathy in people who seem to have lost that facility.

AWAKENING THE ALTRUIST WITHIN

Western science has less to offer in terms of awakening the altruist within than do the great spiritual and wisdom traditions of East and West. In these traditions, the source of altruism, or "service"— the term preferred by spiritualists—is an awareness of self as an entity undivided from others, the world outside, the cosmos. Indeed, the highest expression of this "unity consciousness," as it is sometimes called, is no separate sense of self whatsoever.

Albert Einstein said that our common "delusion" is that we are all separate selves. He called upon us to "free ourselves from this prison by widening our circle of compassion to embrace all living creatures and the whole of nature in its beauty."

In their book *How Can I Help?* Ram Dass and Paul Gorman refer to Einstein's commentary: "It is to ourselves, then, that we must first look in our effort to see what limits the spontaneous expression of helping instincts. How does who we think we are affect what we have to give? How does this 'delusion of consciousness' that 'separates us from the rest' narrow the range of our compassion? What different understanding of our being might nourish and deepen what we have to offer one another?"

The paradox in calling us to look to "ourselves" is that our sense of ourselves as separate is precisely what prevents us from helping. But the perspective of the spiritual traditions can encompass such seeming contradictions. The deeper we look into ourselves, the closer we come to an absolute widening of our self-sense, until our "identity" is so broad that no distinctions are made between self and other, self and world.

Every great spiritual tradition teaches that our true self—the subtle essence of who we are—cannot be distinguished from Spirit or God, as defined in that particular tradition. That is the basis of *The Perennial Philosophy*, elaborated by Aldous Huxley in his 1944 book of the same name. Huxley found this philosophy at the heart of Hinduism, Buddhism, Taoism, Judaism, Christianity, and Islam. Each religion has a conceptual version of unity consciousness—the indivisibility of the individual soul and the universe or divine spirit.

Each of these traditions teaches that our small "selves" are part of a bigger "SELF"—an all-encompassing being, energy, spiritual entity, or God. We become spiritually enlightened when our small self is subsumed by an awareness of the big SELF. Achieving this state of enlightenment can require a dedicated growth process over the course of a lifetime. And yet this awareness can occur in a quicksilver moment, since we are always at one with the big SELF. We just don't always know it.

Sometimes, that quicksilver moment can occur during the act of helping. Bridging the gap between self and other can spark our sense of being connected to something larger than ourselves. The following excerpt from *How Can I Help?* is one woman's story depicting such a moment. Although the spiritual aspect is implicit, the sense of transcending boundaries is luminously apparent.

Marie, the helper, worked in a social welfare office. Her job was to "size people up" and direct them to the appropriate departments within her division of Family Services. Marie felt uncomfortable sizing people up, and tried to change her approach to better help her clients. One of these clients, Viola, not only transformed her approach to work, she touched her heart in a transformative way. Marie wrote this about her experience:

> There was this woman who was living on the street, one I used to pass on my way to the bus. She was homeless, alcoholic; later it developed she had had a cancer diagnosis. For some reason I decided to take up with her. I liked her smile. Enough of sending everyone elsewhere. I knew the whole

maze of social services; I'd take her around myself—clinics, shelters, Medicare, whatever. I guess I wanted to know you could help one person yourself. She was very uncomplaining. Viola. She was willing, even funny about it. "Well, Marie," she'd say, "what are you going to do for me today?"

Oh, the scenes we went through! They called me once from the Women's Shelter. Somehow she'd brought in three pints of Seagram's Seven that night, and a group had gotten drunk. That was against the rules, and I had to take her out. "You told me you'd be good," I said. "You were warm there." She said, "Well, we got warmer."

Or I set her up once with a counselor. After a while he called. "Look, she shows up irregularly, and she always wants to argue with me when she does. What's she here for?" And I'd tell Viola, and she'd say, "Sure, I love to argue with these people. He wants to talk about my childhood all the time. But he doesn't even remember what childhood was like himself. Trust me, Marie."

And I did. I'd have to laugh. She was so insightful and honest. Oh, I really did love her, that one—I really did. But the problems went on for months. Nothing seemed to work out. She kept going back on the street, drinking, getting sicker, all the rest. The more helpless I felt, the more I just loved her; what else could I do? And I'd try again. "Look. Viola," I'd say. "Look where, Marie?" she'd reply. It became a kind of joke between us: "Look." "Look where?"

She moved to a park near my house, and there she started to really go downhill. One evening I went to see her and she was sitting under a tree. She looked awful. I had this powerful feeling that she was getting very close to death. So I went through everything with her one more time: her drinking, her health, her eating, her shelter. She could come live with me. I'd reached that point of willingness.

She just listened, and finally she said, "You know, dear, there's nothing you can do for me anymore." And I saw she was right, I just saw that. And I heaved this big sigh, just let go.

About then, it started raining lightly. I finally said, "Well, it's getting late and wet. Shall we go get some coffee?"

She said, "Yeah . . . well . . . I'll see you later then." But somehow it felt to both of us like I wouldn't.

I went to the bus, and I was crying on the bus. I felt just brokenhearted. I felt there was something else, I didn't know what. Then this thought came to me that she was out there alone in the rain. Just that. So I got off and took the other bus back and went into the park with a newspaper on my head. I must have looked pretty funny.

She was under the tree. She looked up at me. I sat down. She said, "What are you doing here?" I said, "Nothing, really. I just felt like being with you a little more." She said, "Okay."

So we sat in the rain. There we were. It was relatively dry, because this was a big sycamore tree. I told her about how my father taught me to identify trees by their bark and how I loved trees and nature and felt happiest there. She told me about the desert. She used to live in Arizona. Her favorite place was the desert; it was so peaceful there.

We watched the rain. We watched how the squirrels ran around and the last few people scurrying out. We watched how the park looked with no one in it: some birds, a stray dog . . . some mist beginning to appear. And I felt finally at peace, and we stayed silent a long time. I felt such love.

She walked me to the bus. She said, "Thanks." I said, "For what?" She said, "For nothing." We laughed. "You've been very good to me," she added. We were teary. We hugged. Then I got on the bus, and we waved good-bye. I never saw her again. I'll always love her."*

In Marie's story, the distinction between helper and helped begins to blur. Although it is Marie who reaches out, there is an indelible sense that Marie and Viola meet in a time and place where healing is reciprocal. Because Marie had taken Viola's pain into

---

*Marie's story is excerpted from Ram Dass and Paul Gorman's book, *How Can I Help?* (1986; Knopf, New York.) Used by permission.

her heart, she was able to sit with her and give her what she needed most—simple companionship. Marie was also able to side-step all-too-common helping traps—the feelings of emptiness, in-sufficiency, or powerlessness that come when people realize that they can never magically vanquish other people's pains and problems.

Perhaps the most profound statement in Marie's tale is "The more helpless I felt, the more I just loved her; what else could I do?" When Marie's helping effort, which began with certain fixed intentions and goals, went by the wayside, there were two alterna-tives left. She could have thrown up her hands, saying "This woman won't even let me help her! I give up." But Marie saw a deeper truth—that in her remaining days, Viola was not about to give up the freedom that was her dignity. Marie could embrace the only other alternative: to accept the inevitability of Viola's choices, and her death, and to simply *be* with her. In so doing, Marie left her ego behind and found a place by Viola's side.

Recognizing the possibility of leaving one's ego behind can be the first step toward altruism that lifts the spirit. This entails a frame of reference that is not automatic or even comfortable for many of us. But a spiritual orientation is certainly one basis for au-thentically healthy helping.

There is no trick to spiritual awareness, although a committed practice of meditation or devotion to the principles of a particular spiritual tradition is a "path" to enlightenment. *The Perennial Philos-ophy* implies that spiritual awareness leads ineluctably to empathy, charity, and service. As the Hindu spiritual leader Srimad Bhagavatam once said, "Learn to look with an equal eye upon all beings, seeing the one Self in all."

Ken Wilber put it this way:

True enlightenment is said to issue in social action driven by mercy, compassion and skillful means, in an attempt to help all beings attain the supreme liberation. Enlightened activity is simply selfless service. Since we are all one in the same Self, or the same mystical body of Christ, or the same Dharmakaya, then in serving others I am serving my own Self. I think when

Christ said, "Love your neighbor as yourself," he must have meant "Love your neighbor as your Self."

Wilber's comment clarifies that the motivation for helping is not always "clean" of self-interest. Thus, no helping impulse must be proven to be "pure." Certainly, when we engage in helping that is *exclusively* reward-driven—with no genuine human contact or understanding—it simply feeds our egos. But if *any* element of our giving is based on empathy—the reflex that comes so naturally that no conscious thoughts intervene—then the gulf between self and the other is bridged. The good news here is that we don't have to strive toward some perfectionistic ideal of helping. Motivations are invariably mixed, and recognizing them as such is a healthy form of self-acceptance. Finding the altruist within does not mean rooting out every vestige of self-interest. It only means contacting the deeper sources of our compassion.

The broad streams of personality psychology and spirituality meet in poorly charted waters, but the mind-body-spirit connection has forced many open-minded scientists to swim in them. For those who have—mainly the transpersonal psychologists—the two streams converge to form a river of understanding. With regard to altruism, the convergent understanding is that compassion is part of our true nature, whether we define that nature in the language of biochemistry, psychodynamics, or spirituality.

THE HELPER'S HIGH—PART TWO

"Highs" are usually followed by a slippery slide into fatigue, achiness, or general torpor. The aftermath of helper's high is an exception to that trend. As Allan Luks has shown, the second phase of helper's high—which follows after the immediate feelings of euphoria—often includes a long-lasting emotional tranquility, enhanced self-esteem, fewer symptoms of distress or depression, and a sense of optimism. This second phase occurs, however, only when people engage in a relatively regular routine of helping activities.

Consider eighty-three-year-old Blanche Goebel of Louisville, Ohio, a helper whose long-term sense of well-being has kept her in tiptop shape. Blanche visits people at the nursing home where her husband was a patient before he died. She plays cards with them and writes letters to people who are going through hard times. Here's how Blanche described the benefits she received from helping:

> Depression goes along with old age, but even earlier on, when I was really down, I could snap out of it by doing something nice for someone. It leaves a glow that will see me through the bad period. I heard of one old gentleman who parks on the edge of the lot so that busier people can park closer. It makes him feel good, even though it's a small thing. I notice when others shyly tell me of their little helpful acts that they are always smiling and pleased with themselves. I've noticed that the unhappy and unhealthy ones are the selfish ones, the ones too concerned about self.

Unlike friends her age, Blanche has no high blood pressure, no chronic aches and pains, and no need for medication.

In Luks's survey, 57 percent of the volunteers indicated that their self-esteem was raised by their ongoing activities, and 53 percent reported such gains as greater optimism and decreased depression and helplessness. Helping's long-term effects may be even more impressive than the euphoria of the short-term high. An enduring enhancement of self-worth and reduced symptoms of psychological distress are the goals of long-term psychotherapy, meditation, and other mind-body approaches. The fact that volunteer activities produce such powerful psychological changes over time demands further study.

How helping promotes health also requires more study. Right now it appears as if endorphins—and perhaps other brain chemicals—serve to bolster the immune systems of regular helpers. But these biochemical changes are inextricably tied to the psychological uplift experienced by helpers.

Thus, the mind-body benefits of helping cannot be separated.

Presumably, both phases of helper's high involve emotional changes (euphoria, reduced depression, increased self-esteem, and so on) that are accompanied by biochemical changes (increased endorphins), which, in turn, stimulate immune functions. Though teasing apart these relationships is important, it seems unlikely that healthy helping could influence the body without affecting the mind, and vice versa. Suffice it to say that people who are emotionally untouched by helping probably won't receive the physical benefits. The people in our survey who said that their self-esteem increased were more likely to report better health," Luks commented.

As with people who regularly meditate, helping activities lead to an emotional calm that continues as long as some regimen is maintained. Also like exercise and meditation, the frequency of helping is a key factor.

The meditation/helping connection is particularly telling. Many meditative techniques involve forgetting one's small self for a period by concentrating on one's breath or focusing on a mantra or counting exercise. For meditators from many traditions, calming the mind allows for the building of a psychic bridge to a higher (or deeper) reality. Their practice clears the psychic space necessary for the ascent of a more encompassing awareness, one that allows for connectedness with "something larger than ourselves." Helping yields strikingly similar effects. Committed helpers temporarily forget their egoistic concerns and "give themselves over" to another person or higher cause. It is no wonder, then, that helpers report physiologic states similar to those evidenced by meditators: a sense of pleasure followed by relaxation and well-being.

You may recall the experiment conducted by David McClelland's colleague Steven Kelner. Dr. Kelner had a group of subjects relax and visualize themselves in a circumstance in which they felt a "oneness with something larger than themselves." Immune tests conducted before and after this guided exercise showed that the subjects experienced an increase in IgA antibodies—a reliable index of resistance to upper respiratory illnesses. Helpers who feel connected to someone or something larger than themselves may experience such increases in Immune Power on a consistent basis.

"For millennia, people have been describing techniques on

how to forget oneself, to experience decreased metabolic rates and blood pressure, heart rate, and other health benefits," said Harvard cardiologist Herbert Benson. "Altruism works this way, just as do yoga, spirituality, and meditation." Today, Benson often prescribes helping—in addition to relaxation and other medical treatments—for patients who suffer from intractable physical conditions.

FOUR CHARACTERISTICS OF HEALTHY HELPING

From his survey, Allan Luks was able to identify the specific elements of helping among those who reported psychological and physical improvements. These four critical factors provide strong guidance for people who want to help, but wish to avoid the pitfalls and maximize the potential benefits to themselves and the subjects of their care.

PERSONAL CONTACT

People who reported both phases of helper's high, as well as long-term mental and physical benefits, were far more likely to have spent time with the people they helped. Writing checks, raising funds, or collecting clothes and canned goods for the poor did not produce the same effects, presumably because they lacked this crucial element of personal contact.

Allan Luks understood these findings from his own personal helping experiences. "For me, the difference between working with someone and helping without that contact is astonishing," said Luks. "When there was no person to connect with, the feeling of sheer euphoria never occurred, nor did I get the relaxed, calm feeling that follows the initial high."

Contact with the person(s) being helped is the invaluable aspect of helping. Public attention, acclaim, awards, and letters of gratitude don't seem to do the trick. The psychospiritual component of altruism depends, ultimately, on the relationship formed with others in need. When you choose helping activities, don't eschew philanthropic donations or phone calls made on behalf of voluntary organizations—these are certainly meaningful forms of help. But if you wish to experience the health and spiritual benefits of helping, personal contact is essential.

FREQUENCY

Weekly helpers reported significantly better health than once-yearly helpers. "The ideal frequency," says Luks, "is about the same weekly amount of time recommended for getting the best benefits from either meditation or exercise—about two hours a week."

While there should be no rules about the amount of time devoted to helping, a regular schedule that meets your needs makes good sense. As with meditation, exercise, or nutritional programs, it's best not to allow lapses to create a vicious cycle of guilt, in which the inevitable end result is abandonment of your commitment.

HELPING STRANGERS

Another clear trend in the volunteer survey was that people who predominantly helped members of their family or close friends were less likely to report helper's high and health benefits. Luks believes that we exercise greater freedom of choice in helping strangers than loved ones. Often we help family members and friends out of obligation, codependence, proximity, or impossible circumstances. When our young children or elderly parents become ill, we have no choice but to caretake them. Dutiful helping can reduce our sense of control and exacerbate stress. While these helping experiences don't *have* to be unhealthy, they are often muddied by the complex relationships involved.

By contrast, helping strangers—one on one, in a volunteer organization, or professionally—is more likely to create opportunities for bonding, and therefore to heal our sense of isolation and extinguish our false separations between self and other, self and world.

LETTING GO OF RESULTS

"If you are determined that the recipient of your efforts will benefit from what you do," writes Allan Luks, "you will probably emerge from the experience frustrated and unhappy. You must simply enjoy the feeling of closeness to the person you are trying to assist."

Judy Weintraub made this same point from her own helping experience. "It's not important to be able to say 'I turned this person's life around.' I prefer, 'I helped this person in pain at a particular time.' And if that particular time happened to be one instant, well, then it was just one instant. The point is, you're not tied to the end result."

Jon Kabat-Zinn embraces the Buddhist paradox that the harder we push, the less we reap. The same can be said for service. We hold ourselves, and the other being helped, in mutual regard and acceptance. We do what we can for others, expecting no gratitude, no success, no reward. The dignity of this relationship is its own intrinsic reward.

Allan Luks makes one simple but crucial point about healthy helping. It is a practice that can be easily woven into daily life. "To be helpful to others does not necessarily mean a change of careers or a move to the inner city," he writes. "What it does mean is a change in perspective." Although becoming part of an organized volunteer effort is the best path, even the "smallest" acts of kindness toward others in daily life can contribute to a sense of calm, self-esteem, and connectedness. Helping someone across the street, offering specialized knowledge to a friend in trouble, holding the door for a stranger—these efforts can be made more frequently, more consciously, and with more loving intent.

HEALTHY VS. UNHEALTHY HELPING

Altruism gone awry can sap the spirit as profoundly as healthy helping uplifts the spirit. People who help primarily for ego gratification feel powerless and angry when their charges aren't sufficiently gracious, or when their actions don't produce the hoped-for results. The medical patient who isn't cured, the homeless person who isn't housed, the friend whose life remains chaos, the alcoholic who falls off the wagon, all indicate to the ego-centered helper that his efforts have gone for naught. He comes to one of two conclusions: "Why should I keep extending myself when these people can't get it together?" or: "It's too painful to help when I end up feeling helpless."

Does this mean that healthy helping must forsake goals altogether? Allan Luks's research indicates that goals—such as getting successful drug treatment for an addict, talking a friend through depression—are good guiding lights for helpers. But they should never be the light at the end of the tunnel. Fixing everything is the worst possible goal orientation for any helper. When goal attainment becomes the overriding reason for helping, sooner or later the helper will lose her sense of control. Things just don't always turn out as we wish them!

Allan Luks sets forth certain common-sense guidelines for burnout prevention:

1. Pace yourself.
2. Get plenty of support, encouragement, and company for yourself.
3. It's not necessary to rescue the whole world; in fact, don't kid yourself that you have the total responsibility for even one other person.
4. Explore what kind of helping is comfortable for you.
5. Go ahead and do what you comfortably can.
6. Feel free to give up on a particular effort when you get into a situation that isn't right for you.
7. Don't quit helping because of one rejection or disappointment or bad experience.
8. Recognize that even when you see other volunteers around you having a wonderful experience—while you're not—it does not mean you are not suited for helping.

EXERCISING ALTRUISM

Although every spiritual tradition teaches compassion, not every one has specific practices for cultivation of compassion. Tibetan Buddhism is one that does. The spiritual path set forth in Tibetan Buddhism is divided into three broad streams, each of which has several tributaries: the Hinayana, the Mahayana, and the Vajrayana. The Mahayana, which is the path of compassion, entails practices for the development of empathy in mind and heart. The most important of these is called *Tonglen,* which means "taking and sending." Tonglen is a guided meditation in which you visualize someone you know and love who is suffering. You take his or her suffering into your own being in the form of an image, literally breathing it in and holding it in your heart. On the outbreath, you send all your own strength, health, and energy out to that person. You continue that practice, then expand it to include all the suffering of people in that town. Gradually, you extend your willingness to take on suffering and transmit healing to include the entire state, then the country, then the planet, then the universe.

Tonglen undercuts the sense of separateness between self and other that all spiritual traditions teach are illusory. By embracing others' pains as our own, we find peace in the knowledge that none of us is alone in our suffering.

Use this practice of Tonglen to develop the part of yourself that feels connected to all other beings. In a recent book, Ken Wilber fully described Tonglen:

In meditation, picture or visualize someone you know and love who is going through much suffering—an illness, a loss, depression, pain, anxiety, fear. As you breathe in, imagine all of that person's suffering—in the form of dark, black, smoke-like, tarlike, thick, and heavy clouds—entering your nostrils and traveling down into your heart. Hold that suffering in your heart. Then, on the outbreath, take all of your peace, freedom, health, goodness, and virtue, and send it out to the person in the form of healing, liberating light. Imagine they take it all in, and feel completely free, released, and happy. Do that for several breaths. Then imagine the town that the person is in, and, on the inbreath, take in all of the suffering of that town, and send back all of your health and happiness to everyone in it. Then do that for the entire state, then the entire country, the universe. You are taking in all the suffering of beings everywhere and sending them back health and happiness and virtue.

Wilber points out that no one actually gets ill doing this exercise. The point is to go beyond thinking about helping, to actually feeling the pain of others we wish to help. "Tonglen ... exchanges self for other, and thus it profoundly undercuts the subject/object dualism," he writes. "It asks us to undermine the self/other dualism at exactly the point we are most afraid: getting hurt ourselves. Not just talking about having compassion for others' suffering, but being willing to take it into our own heart and release them in exchange. This is true compassion, the path of Mahayana."

WRITING PRACTICE OF ALTRUISM

As you engage in helping activities, you may wish to keep a journal in which you explore the specifics and meaning of your service to others. Become aware of the state of mind and heart with which you approach helping others. Be completely open not only to your altruism but to your selfishness, your resentments, your disagreeable feelings and sensations. Use your altruism entries to explore the self/other duality—how you experience it and whether you overcome it. Do not write these entries as an extension of your good deeds; if you do, you will feel subtly obligated to accentuate the positive. The helper's high will happen, and I suggest that you record every pleasurable sensation. You can go back and be reminded of the joy you brought to others and yourself. But have compassion for yourself even—especially—when your heart is closed to others. That investigation is as worthwhile for developing altruism as more direct efforts to contact your compassion. Notice changes in your health and well-being and the health and well-being of those you have served.

SELF-COMPLEXITY: THE HEALTHY HYDRA

IN EVERY CORNER OF MY SOUL THERE IS AN ALTAR TO A DIFFER-
ENT GOD.

—FERNANDO PESSOA

One reason that the Greek myth of Hercules inspired so many Hol-
lywood incarnations was its central plot, which had the muscular
hero undertake twelve "labors." These labors required Hercules to
conquer creatures ranging from horrific man-eating birds to three-
headed dogs. The second labor called upon him to slay a gigantic
nine-headed monster known as the Hydra, which possessed one
central, immortal head. In mortal combat, Hercules used his sword
to cut off one of the Hydra's heads, only to discover that two more
heads quickly grew to replace the one severed. Finally, with the
help of Iolanus, Hercules burned out the roots of these decapita-
tions, severed the immortal head, and buried it under a rock.

   Consider, for the moment, the positive aspect of the Hydra's
power. Although this mythological monster went down to defeat,
its strength—and its survival before confronting Hercules—had

been its ability to swiftly replace losses to its own being. With nine heads and the capacity to replace one lost with two, the Hydra was a formidable opponent whose resilience was rooted in its regenerative powers.

In this sense, the Hydra is a compelling model of mind-body health. According to Patricia Linville, Ph.D., professor of psychology at Duke University and the Fuqua School of Business, we may have one immortal self, but in our daily lives and consciousness we have multiple "selves"—like the Hydra's nine heads. Each "self" represents a facet of our personalities—a role, relationship, activity, or identity. To withstand the impact of stress on mind and body, we require the Hydra-like capacity to replace lost or harmed selves with other selves. Simply put, if one "self" is under constant stress or is wounded in some way, we need other selves to fall back on.

Linville believes that we buttress our physical health when we have many vital selves we can call upon to sustain our energy, well-being, and sense of purpose when we suffer inevitable losses over the course of our lifetime.

She calls this trait "self-complexity." Based on tenets of cognitive psychology, she developed the theory that our sense of self is based on various mental "representations" that involve roles, activities, relationships, and identities. She calls these mental representations "self-aspects." People high in self-complexity have many self-aspects that are both well developed and highly distinct. For instance, a complex woman could think of herself in terms of various roles (lawyer, friend, mother), kinds of relationships (colleague, competitor, nurturer), types of activities (running, playing tennis, writing), overarching traits (hardworking, creative), goals (career success), and so forth.

Linville believed that people with many self-aspects were better protected against profound inner distress when they suffered a loss. Consider the plight of a woman going through a divorce who has only two significant self-aspects—wife and lawyer. Moreover, these two self-aspects are closely linked in memory, because her husband is also an attorney with whom she has shared many professional experiences. Her anguish, and any negative thoughts and emotions she has about herself as a wife, spill over and affect her feelings about herself as a lawyer. She becomes vulnerable to clinical depression and physical illness.

By contrast, a woman with more developed and distinct self-aspects would have a different response. Let's say she identifies herself as a wife, lawyer, tennis player, theater buff, and friend. Also, her wife self-aspect does not share features or memory traces with her other self-aspects. In her case, the negative feelings and self-judgments associated with her divorce do not spill over and blacken her feelings about other parts of herself. Her other self-aspects also buffer the stress of her divorce. She continues to see herself as an effective lawyer, fine tennis player, avid theater buff, and caring friend, since those self-aspects are not totally tied to her wife aspect.

"In this case," said Linville, "the thoughts and feelings associated with the divorce are confined to a smaller part of her self-representation, and what's more, she has these relatively uncontaminated parts of herself to help her cope better with the divorce."

Her uninvolved aspects become even more important to her, partially compensating for her loss and reducing her stress. Like the Hydra's heads that grow in place of the severed one, these other "selves" sustain emotional well-being after a stressful assault.

When Patricia Linville realized that multiple selves protected people from undue suffering, she saw the potential for a mind-body connection. She was aware of mind-body research linking depression, hopelessness, and hostility with immune dysfunction, heart disease, and other physical illnesses. If self-complexity prevented people from lapsing into depression, hostility, or hopelessness, might it also prevent them from getting sick? Could self-complexity buffer the body from the ravages of stress, the way it buffered the mind?

In 1987, Patricia Linville discovered that people with self-complexity were indeed physically healthier under stress. But she did not reach this realization overnight. It took several years for her to define and measure self-complexity, to understand its potential influence on health, and to create a study that did justice to her own complex thinking.

DON'T PUT ALL YOUR EGGS IN
ONE COGNITIVE BASKET

Linville's initial interest in complexity had nothing to do with health. In fact, it had nothing to do with the self. Her doctoral dissertation was an exploration of the complexity of people's views of other social groups. She discovered that people in different demographic categories—old or young, black or white, male or female, and so on—viewed their own group with great complexity. Put differently, they saw many different sides, shades, and characteristics among people like themselves. Their characterizations of others tended toward the simplistic and stereotypic—"they" were "good" or "bad" in this or that area.

"People often lacked a complex view of other groups," Linville commented. "This led them to make very quick, very strong, and very emotionally extreme evaluations of other groups."

Linville recalled her presentation of these findings to her dissertation committee, an experience that is invariably stressful. One moment stuck in her mind. A clinical psychologist said to her, "Do you think this has anything to do with the self?" Linville had never even pondered the question, so she was caught off guard.

"All I could do was mumble," she remembered. "And this was the middle of my dissertation. I'm sure I said nothing very intelligent."

But his question stayed with her long after she completed her doctorate. How might her theory of complexity relate to the self?

Linville already knew that people with a greater depth and breadth of knowledge in any area—whether it is art, music, politics, food, or ethnic/racial groups—have a more complex understanding. Such individuals demonstrate balance and perspective in their viewpoints, rather than hot-headed emotionalism or quick judgments.

For instance, a teenager who has never heard the Rolling Stones or the Beatles may argue that the current favorite Pearl Jam is the greatest hard rock band ever. His baby-boomer father has never listened to Pearl Jam, but he scoffs at his son's claims. Both lack complex knowledge, and their emotional reactions are therefore extreme. The father has a friend, however, who not only knows every Stones and Beatles album, he stays current with rock and roll and knows Pearl Jam inside out. He gives his friend and his friend's son a thoughtful comparison of the older bands and the latest grunge-rock sensation.

Perhaps, Linville thought, this same principle did apply to the self. For instance, did people with simplistic views of themselves have more extreme emotional reactions under stress? They might judge themselves harshly unless they saw many sides of their own behavior. (Just as the person with a simplistic view of an ethnic group might judge members of that group harshly.) Such harshness could lower self-esteem and put them at risk for depression. By contrast, people with more complex views of themselves might have more balanced reactions to stress. Perhaps they'd be kinder toward themselves and less volatile under pressure.

The more Linville thought about her advisor's comment, the more it made sense. Complex people, she surmised, would also have many "selves" to compensate—in terms of emotional investments and real-life activities—when one "self" had been wounded or destroyed. Such an individual is less likely to be overcome by fear, despair, anxiety, and other extreme emotional reactions to stress. This idea became the primary focus of Linville's work at Yale University, where she was assistant professor of psychology during the late 1980s.

Before she could test this theory, Linville had to measure self-complexity. She settled on a playful procedure that would spark people's imaginations as they thought about themselves. First, she developed a list of thirty-three traits, chosen to represent a wide range of characteristics that students used to think about themselves. (such as "relaxed," "lazy," "outgoing," "rebellious," and "affectionate"). Each trait was placed on an index card, and the packet of thirty-three cards was handed to each participating student.

Linville told the students to use the cards to describe themselves. They were instructed to make piles of these traits that belonged together in a particular category of selfhood. The traits could be grouped in any way that was meaningful—under head-

Table 8.1

SELF-COMPLEXITY

Examples of Two Subjects' Feature Sorts

Subject 1

Relationship with men	Relationship with friends	Relationship with family	Studies	Physically	At parties
Outgoing	Humorous	Emotional	Quiet	Individualistic	Humorous
Playful	Relaxed	Playful	Studious	Affectionate	Playful
Reflective	Assertive	Reflective	Organized	Industrious	Outgoing
Mature	Outgoing	Mature	Mature	Quiet	Sophisticated
Emotional	Mature	Assertive	Reserved	Organized	Affectionate
Assertive	Emotional	Humorous	Industrious		Competitive
Competitive	Reflective	Outgoing	Individualistic		Imaginative
Relaxed	Soft-hearted	Individualistic			Impulsive
Humorous	Not studious	Unconventional			Mature
Affectionate	Affectionate				
Soft-hearted	Individualistic				
Individualistic					
Sophisticated					

Subject 2

Dorm life	Home life	School	Social life	Work (dining hall worker)	Activities
Playful	Lazy	Reflective	Outgoing	Industrious	Imaginative
Relaxed	Emotional	Reserved	Humorous	Rebellious	Relaxed
Outgoing	Relaxed	Unorganized	Quiet	Playful	Quiet
Assertive	Humorous	Lazy	Relaxed	Outgoing	Outgoing
Competitive	Playful	Insecure	Playful	Assertive	Assertive
Affectionate	Affectionate		Insecure	Relaxed	Unorganized
Humorous	Unorganized		Impulsive		Affectionate
Soft-hearted	Soft-hearted		Not studious		Soft-hearted
Unorganized	Not studious		Conformist		
Lazy	Irresponsible				
Imaginative					
Individualistic					

293

ings such as "Dorm Life," "School Life," "Relationships with Family," "Relationships with Men," and so forth. The student could use the same trait in more than one pile, and they were given blank cards to repeat traits as many times as they desired. (See table 8.1 for two examples of subject's trait sortings.)

To determine a final "self-complexity" score for the students, Linville did not simply count the number of categories or traits used in their piles. That would indicate the number of self-aspects, but Linville was after something more refined. She also wanted to know how *distinct* each self-aspect was.

One way to determine the distinctness of each self-aspect was to count the number of times a trait was shared among different "piles." For instance, a man who used a "quiet" card in his professional, recreational, and family "piles" had self-aspects that melded together (thus lowering his self-complexity score). A man who used "outgoing" in his professional pile, "raucous," in his recreational pile, and "quiet" in his family pile would be more complex.

Linville developed a mathematical formula (based on recognized statistical methods) to calculate self-complexity. She fed each student's card sorting lists into a computer programmed with the formula, and it spit back a final score for each student. This "self-complexity score" was based equally on two factors: the number *and* the distinctness of the person's self-aspects.

With her measurement in hand, Linville wanted to know whether self-complexity reduced the extremity of people's emotional reactions to events. To find out, she designed a rather tricky experiment. She tested a group of male students for self-complexity, then exposed them to experiences that evoked feelings of failure or success. Would their emotional responses be influenced by how complex they were?

Linville and her colleagues gave fifty-nine men a phony analytical task to perform, after which a psychologist explained what they had accomplished. Half were told they had failed; the other half were told they succeeded. After the experiment, Linville discovered that more complex people experienced fewer highs in their self-esteem and mood after "success." But they also experienced fewer lows after "failure." By contrast, people low in self-complexity had more severe swings of mood and self-esteem in both directions. Her theory was confirmed: Self-complexity prevented people from having extreme emotional reactions to highly charged events.

"People who lacked self-complexity were not happier in general, nor were they sadder," Linville commented. "But they were more variable. Their emotional states changed a great deal in response to success or failure."

Since complex people had less severe reactions, I wondered if they were emotionally "flat." Perhaps they experienced neither valleys nor peaks, and their lives lacked color and vitality because they had spread themselves thin among so many self-aspects. But Linville has found that complex people were no less capable of passion and intensity. They simply did not hang so much of their self-esteem on isolated experiences of success or failure. In short, complex people had that rare and properly celebrated quality of mind-body health: *a sense of balance.*

In her next study, Linville followed a group of thirty-one women, asking them to graph their emotional states on a day-by-day basis. Over a two-week period, the women with high self-complexity were less likely to experience extreme variations in their emotions. Linville's findings suggested that complex people were less vulnerable to anxiety and depression when times got tough.

Linville's concept of complexity had one ironically simple interpretation. It was implied by the subtitle of her first paper on the subject: "Don't Put All of Your Eggs in One Cognitive Basket." (Here, "cognitive" refers to conscious awareness of an aspect of self.) People who made such an investment were easily overwhelmed by stress on their one self-aspect. Just as we should avoid putting all our eggs in one basket when we pursue a job, a deal, or a romantic relationship, we should avoid pouring all of our hopes, dreams, and identifications in one aspect of our selves. Doing so is a risky endeavor, leaving us vulnerable to low self-esteem, anxiety, and depression.

Linville's next hunch was that self-complexity must influence physical health. If investing in many different self-aspects prevented low self-esteem, anxiety, and depression, then perhaps it also prevented illness.

"I had been teaching Health Psychology at Yale," she recalled. "And I was getting more familiar with the literature on stress and illness. I saw the evidence that stress reactions could influence health through neuroendocrine pathways connected to the immune system. If self-complexity altered your emotional reactions to stress, then it made sense that self-complexity would have an effect on health and illness."

SELF-COMPLEXITY AND PHYSICAL HEALTH

One way that Immune Power traits promote health is by buffering the negative effects of stress on the body. In Patricia Linville's view, self-complexity is a perfect example of the "buffering" theory. People with many distinct self-aspects rely on them when one part of themselves has been traumatized—as in a divorce. Their many other selves guard against overwhelming distress or depression, keeping them emotionally and physically well.

A classic example of a vulnerable person who lacks self-complexity is the widower whose life is entirely bound up in his spouse before her death. He has few interests, activities, or relationships apart from her, and her passing leaves him emotionally bereft and physically at risk. On the other hand, many of us know elderly people with self-complexity, whose many vital, independent activities keep them vigorous and healthy. They suffer when their spouses die, but the loss does not destroy their lives or decimate their health. Within months they bounce back—emotionally, spiritually, and physically.

But could the health-protecting power of self-complexity be proven? In 1987, Linville set out to do just that. She recruited 109 undergraduate students, roughly half men and half women, to participate in her study. All of them carried out the card-sorting task (exactly the same as described earlier) to determine self-complexity. They also completed a battery of tests on recent and current life stresses (in their academic life, home life, social life, and so forth), depression, physical symptoms, and illnesses. Linville had them repeat these procedures two weeks later, because she wanted to know if stresses reported at the first session led to illnesses within a relatively short time frame. After the two weeks, 67 percent reported at least one type of illness; most were colds, flu, backaches, and cramps.

She discovered that students who reported more stressful life events at the beginning of the study were more depressed two weeks later. They also were beset by more physical symptoms and illnesses. But Linville's key finding was this: *People high in self-complexity who had been subjected to high levels of stress were less prone to depression, physical symptoms, and other illnesses.*

By contrast, people who lacked self-complexity suffered more instances of depression, physical symptoms, flu, and other illness when exposed to stress.

Self-complexity not only buffered the negative effects of stress in general, it specifically prevented stress-related illnesses, such as colds, bouts of the flu, aches, and cramps. This finding strongly suggested that self-complexity prevented immune system breakdowns, since our immune defenses are responsible for warding off colds and flu.

DO WE HAVE MANY SELF-ESTEEMS?

Linville became fascinated with the idea that each of our various self-aspects has a life of its own. Among complex people, these individual "lives" are more distinct. For instance, the healthy woman who undergoes a divorce has self-aspects—gardener, friend, and volunteer—that were fully developed and had few connections to her marriage. Or the healthy businessman who loses his biggest account has self-aspects—father, dancer, and fisherman—that are totally separate from his corporate identity.

Patricia Linville wanted to know: "Does each self-aspect have its own self-esteem?"

She offered a hypothesis. "Let's say I have a different self-esteem about my research, my teaching, my friendships, my physical self, my parenting, and so on. Then it is perfectly possible for me to feel good about myself as a researcher, competent as a teacher, and bad about my physical self. If I feel terrible about one part, does self-complexity keep me from feeling worse overall?"

Linville decided to test whether: (1) people with self-complexity would have different self-esteems for each self-aspect; (2) people with high self-esteem in other areas of life would be less likely to feel bad when one "self" suffered from low self-esteem; and (3) these same complex individuals would be less prone to depression and stress-related illnesses.

To answer these questions, she conducted a study with 155 male and female students. Linville tested not only their self-complexity, but also their self-esteem in various areas of their lives, including mental abilities, social skills, physical self, and leadership capabilities. She also tested their overall (global) self-esteem: How good did they feel about their whole selves?

Here are Linville's key results:

- People did indeed have different self-esteems for different areas (such as mental abilities, social skills, physical self, and leadership capabilities).
- People with greater self-complexity had more distinctions among their various "self-esteems."
- People with greater self-complexity suffered a less severe drop in overall self-esteem when one self-aspect suffered.
- *People with greater self-complexity suffered fewer bouts of depression and illness when self-esteem in one part of their lives dropped.*

People with low self-esteem *did* have more physical symptoms, mental health problems, and illnesses. However, if they also had self-complexity, *they were prone to far fewer mental and physical disorders.* As Linville predicted, having many distinct selves protected people against the ravages of stress in any one area of their lives.

DO COMPLEX WOMEN LIVE LONGER?

How persuasive was Linville's data regarding physical health? Though she did not test immune responses, the lower incidence of respiratory infections was strong evidence that self-complexity protected immunity. Her studies had one other strength and one weakness: She did measure self-complexity first and health later, removing the biases that occur when people evaluate mind-body states in retrospect. But she followed people for only two weeks, not long enough to observe whether self-complexity helped to maintain long-term health.

However, the long-lasting health benefits of self-complexity were confirmed in another scientist's research. In chapter 7, I described the Women's Roles and Health Study led by Phyllis Moen, Ph.D., of Cornell University. Her study showed that women who were active volunteers were healthier over the course of thirty years. But Moen also had investigated the health effects of multiple roles—a concept that overlaps self-complexity.

Moen's study involved 313 women, all of whom were wives and mothers. Their health and psychological well-being was evaluated in 1956 and again in 1986. Moen wanted to know whether women with multiple roles, beyond that of wife and mother, lived longer and aged more successfully. Indeed, *women who occupied multiple roles lived longer. They also had better psychological profiles, better health, and fewer illnesses over the course of thirty years.*

Moen's health measures were not only based on self-reports, but also on objective medical histories. The fact that multiple roles in 1956 predicted health and longevity in 1986 was astonishing evidence that women with many facets and activities are protected against severe illnesses and early death.

Although multiple roles is not the exact same concept as self-complexity, Linville thinks they are close enough: People with multiple roles are likely to be more complex. Moen also believes that multiple roles reflected women's vivacity and social involvement. She writes:

Occupying multiple roles within society augments an individual's social network, power, prestige, resources, and emotional gratifications. Bronfenbrenner [a famous sociologist] hypothesizes that an ever-broadening role repertoire promotes human development, in part by facilitating interactions with persons occupying a variety of roles. He notes that "roles have a magic-like power to alter how a person is treated, how she acts, what she does, and thereby even what she thinks and feels." But particular roles can also be detrimental to health, as we found in the case of caregiving. This suggests that preference and choice, as well as level of autonomy, may be important elements in linking role attachments to health. And satisfaction in a role, rather than simply role occupancy, may be key.

For women in the 1950s, opportunities for self-development and social integration were often limited. Apparently, the conscious choice to take on activities in the world buffered the potential distress of limited options and isolated existences. Finding ways to express and adopt multiple roles in a cultural environment often hostile to women's autonomy was a sign of self-complexity. It was probably also a sign of Ouellette's three Cs—commitment, control, and challenge.

SELF-COMPLEXITY, GRIEVING, AND BODYMIND WELLNESS

The test of our strength and self-esteem is how we generally respond to loss and failure. Do we become chronically hopeless and forlorn? Maintain a stiff upper lip and move on? Or do we grieve the loss or failure, grasp its meaning, and make changes to ensure a brighter future?

As a response to stress or trauma, chronic hopelessness is fraught with mind-body peril. Relentless cheerfulness looks good from the outside but stunts growth on the inside. A process of grieving and transformation represents the healthiest mind-body approach. What is involved in grieving a loss, grasping its meaning, and transforming ourselves for a brighter future?

As Patricia Linville's work has shown, self-complexity gives us perspective. Our self-aspects are like protective cushions, softening the blow of trauma so that we don't lapse into despair. Despair, I must emphasize, is not the same as grief. In despair, we resign ourselves to a terrible fate—the loss of hope. In that sense, despair is static. Grieving, on the other hand, is a dynamic process. When we grieve, we experience the profound sorrow of a loss. Almost by definition, grieving is a mind-state we expect to enter and we expect to leave behind. We "bottom out," as people in the recovery movement say.

Self-complexity doesn't block the grieving process; it prevents a collapse into hopelessness. By helping us maintain our sense of ourselves as whole, worthwhile beings, it confines our negative feelings to the wounded part. Consider the middle-age man whose self-aspects include engineer, coworker, and golfer. If he loses his twenty-year engineering job, the loss will be devastating under any circumstances. But he is in danger of becoming emotionally overwhelmed, because his coworker self completely intertwines with his engineer self. Since most of his friends are fellow workers, he feels embarrassed about the firing, jealous that they still have their jobs, and ripped out of the social fabric of his work life. That leaves him with golfer—not enough to fall back on. It's hard to go through a healthy grieving process when your life seems to be in tatters.

If the same man also had reader, tinkerer, friend, and volunteer self-aspects, he'd have a range of activities to keep him vitally involved with other people and the world. These other selves give him the strength and equilibrium necessary to grieve and then find perspective on his so-called failure. He feels hurt by the firing, but that pain does not "infect" the other selves. They have an independent life of their own.

We might imagine the different parts of ourselves as intrapsychic "friends" we turn to for support and solace when we are in trouble. These "friends" remind us that life goes on despite our current anguish or confusion, and that reminder keeps us going. When trauma or failure occurs, we need our "friends" more than ever. Our varied self-aspects are indeed like friends that get us through the hard times.

THE DYNAMIC SELF

Self-complexity may be a more encompassing quality than the Hydra metaphor suggests. Certainly, compensating for lost or harmed self-aspects with other self-aspects is a powerful healing capability. But Linville also captured the dynamism of people who "let a thousand flowers bloom" in their characters and hence their lives.

A person with self-complexity appears to be developing and expressing his or her authentic self. Our authentic selves can never be monotonous, one-dimensional entities. In our essences, we are prismatic configurations of many traits, talents, longings, emotional proclivities, deep-seated goals. Our authentic selves are hardly reducible to one set of traits. We are multifaceted, sometimes contradictory characters whose lives are enriched when we allow those facets full expression.

Lawrence LeShan believes that becoming our authentic selves directly supports our biological healing systems. He therefore helps his cancer patients find their own unique "song to sing." He encourages them to develop their individuality in work, creative pursuits, and relationships. If one accepts that the authentic self is invariably multifaceted, then LeShan's prescription requires only the slightest amendment: We must find our own *songs* to sing.

Complex people have many traits and facets that, described individually, may seem to contradict one another. But they coexist in relative harmony, and the person is richer for them.

Perhaps our times, characterized by continual change and flux, call upon us to become many different, seemingly contradictory selves. In his most recent book, *The Protean Self*, the eminent psychiatrist Robert J. Lifton, M.D., expresses the view that people have developed the capacity to change shapes as a remarkably healthy adaptation to our times. Indeed, Lifton defines resilience as the ability to "evolve a self of many possibilities."

The "protean self" refers to the Greek myth of Proteus, the prophetic old man of the sea. Proteus knew all things, past and present, but he did not wish to divulge his knowledge. When captors tried to force him to prophesize, he would try to escape by assuming all sorts of shapes—that of a leopard, a serpent, a lion, a tree, fire, water. If a captor held him fast, however, the Greek god would return to his original shape, give the answer, and plunge back into the sea. Over time, mystics came to regard the shape-shifting man as a symbol of the original matter from which the world was created.

Lifton sees Proteus as a metaphor for the adaptive self in the latter stages of the twentieth century. As in the myth, the protean self is not a collection of disconnected parts with no center. The person has an "original shape" that is coherent.

"Though variation is the essence of the protean self," writes Lifton, "that self has certain relatively consistent features. Central to its function is a capacity for bringing together disparate and seemingly incompatible elements of identity and involvement in what I call 'odd combinations,' and for continuous transformation of these elements."

The protean self is quite reminiscent of Patricia Linville's self-complexity. Her research subjects displayed many distinct selves—as evidenced by "odd combinations" of cards with differing traits—and they were healthier as a result. Although Robert Lifton did not discuss health per se, he argues throughout his book that complex personalities are more resilient.

Psychoanalyst Stephen A. Mitchell has identified two broad streams of thought in psychology. One stream views the self as something that people do and experience over time. Using this "temporal metaphor," the self is considered multiple and discontinuous—constantly shifting and changing in different relationships and circumstances. Others view the self as something that exists in space. Using this "spatial metaphor," the self is considered singular and continuous—a complete entity with different layers and structures (the "true" self, the "core" self, the "ego," the "id," and so on). From this perspective, there is something about ourselves that never changes, an essential "I" that is substantial, integrated—whole.

Which stream of thought is right? According to Mitchell, they both are. He concludes that part of what lends dynamism to our lives is the tension between our multiples selves in time and our unitary Self in space. He uses metaphor to show how these two views can be integrated:

Think of self as operating like cinematic film, composed of discrete, discontinuous pictures that, when run together, create something very much continuous and integral. Of course, with both film and selfhood, in a literal sense the experience of "motion" and continuity is an illusion. Yet this is an extremely dull and misleading literalness. The "illusion" creates an experience that has a powerful subjective richness of its own, creating a larger, "moving" picture, very different from (and much more than) the simple sum of the discrete pictures. Each frame is both a discrete, discontinuous image and a subunit of a larger, continuous process that takes on a life of its own.

In our own lives, attention to each "frame" means developing color, texture, and composition for each part of ourselves. In "motion" these "frames" flow together in a seamless whole, creating an experience of life that is continuous despite the shifts from frame to frame, scene to scene, reel to reel.

Mitchell describes his own approach to psychoanalysis as one that encourages development of both multiple selves *and* a central self that organizes them into a whole. "One of the great benefits of the analytic process," he writes, "is that the more the analysand can tolerate experiencing multiple versions of himself, the stronger, more resilient, and durable he experiences himself to be. Conversely, the more the analysand can find continuities across his various experiences, the more he can tolerate the identity diffusion entailed by containing multiple versions of self." Translation: When we know and strengthen our central, organizing self, we can live out our multifaceted qualities without losing our sense of who we are. As a result, we become "stronger, more resilient, and durable."

Thus, we need a balance between too much continuity, which can lead to stagnation and paralysis, and too much discontinuity, which can lead to fragmentation. For this reason, Patricia Linville believes it is important for us to have many distinct self-aspects that, like the film frames, nevertheless flow together in a continuous fashion.

How does the balance between multiple selves and one unitary self appear in people with self-complexity?

"When I talk to people in our experiments, they don't feel uncomfortable or disjointed by the fact that they have different parts to their lives," said Linville. "They are quite comfortable with the fact that it's all part of themselves, that something is tying it all together. They don't feel they have to be the same identical person, in thought or in action, in each of these areas of their lives."

"Differentiation" is a good term for fully developing our distinct self-aspects. When we become well differentiated, we learn that we can be both loving *and* assertive; open *and* self-protective; tuned into others *and* the self; able to say no to friends *and* still be empathic helpers. The key is flexibility and the recognition that our authentic selves can never be pigeonholed.

Is there a downside to such highly differentiated self-aspects? If each self is so distinct, is it *harder* to experience a sense of continuity? The extreme example is multiple personality disorder (MPD), in which people have such distinct selves that they lose their central self completely. The result is a form of psychosis. These individuals can only shuttle from one entirely self-contained personality to another, with no apparent unifying thread. Case histories of MPD are notoriously dramatic and sometimes downright unbelievable. One such case was depicted in the movie *The Three Faces of Eve*, in which Joanne Woodward played a woman who had fragmented into three separate personalities with no shared gestures, expressions, habits, vocal qualities, or even memory banks. All they seemed to have in common was the same body. Where does self-complexity end and *The Three Faces of Eve* begin?

In response, Dr. Linville made a useful distinction. The person with MPD (or another form of personality disintegration, schizophrenia) has selves that are totally compartmentalized—walled off from other parts of the self. When one self is activated, the person has no awareness of other parts or, indeed, of one central, organizing self.

Healthy people with self-complexity shift between self-aspects, depending on social circumstances or relationships. But they never lose their sense of wholeness. Their selves are highly distinct but overlapping. Such individuals perceive links between selves, not rigid walls. Their ability to move gingerly from self to self is a nimble quality made possible by the strength of their "core." Like the Hydra, they have a central, "immortal" head without which they cannot exist. Their other "heads" give them options, flexibility, and a more diverse character.

In fact, complex people have such a strong sense of their central selves that they can tolerate the dissonance between selves that seem completely at odds. Robert Lifton answered critics who claimed that the complex personality has no coherent self. "I would claim the opposite," he wrote. "Proteanism involves a quest for authenticity and meaning, a form-seeking assertion of self. The recognition of complexity and ambiguity may well represent a certain maturation in our concept of self. The protean self seeks to be both fluid and grounded. . . ."

In his book *The Evolving Self,* psychologist Mihaly Csikszentmihalyi celebrates complexity on every level—biological, psychological, societal, cultural, planetary, even cosmic. He believes that complexity is needed for any system to remain resilient. Complexity is "the direction in which evolution proceeds," and we enhance development of our species by encouraging complexity.

Although Dr. Csikszentmihalyi does not discuss personal health as an outgrowth of complexity, his views dovetail with Linville's when he argues that self-complexity requires both differentiation and integration. "A person is differentiated to the extent that he or she has many different interests, abilities, and goals," he writes. "He or she is integrated in proportion to the harmony that exists between various goals, and between thoughts, feelings, and action."

Differentation without integration, and vice versa, is problematic. A highly differentiated person who is not integrated could be either a psychotic or a genius who suffers with terrible inner conflicts. An integrated person who is not well differentiated may be vulnerable to stress or illness, and won't live up to his or her potential for meaning and creativity.

Csikszentmihalyi describes exemplars of complexity. "These are individuals whose actions demonstrate what a life dedicated to complexity could be like," he writes. "But they cannot be reduced to a type, for there cannot be a single path for reaching personal harmony. Because differentiation is one-half of a complex consciousness, each person must follow his or her own bent, find ways to realize his or her unique individuality."

One of Csikszentmihalyi's exemplars is Linus Pauling, the Nobel Prize–winning chemist who, at the age of ninety-three, was still making vital contributions to medicine and humanity. Here is Csikszentmihalyi's assessment of Pauling's complexity:

> When we talked to Pauling he was over ninety years of age. Straight as a pine sapling, sharp as a tack, he sat for two hours reminiscing about his life and work. He could remember the dates on which he wrote various papers over sixty years ago, and the circumstances that led up to them; he recalled with a smile the boys he used to play with in Portland, Oregon, over eighty years ago, and the street addresses at which they lived. More than any single impression, what was so striking in Pauling's account is how much he seemed to enjoy every day of those ninety years, and how much of a piece his entire life was.
>
> Pauling's biography is a textbook case of complexity. In his youth he was able to visualize the relationship between quantum mechanics at the subatomic level and the molecular structure of chemical elements; having been able to demonstrate the nature of that relationship, he earned a Nobel Prize in chemistry. In a sense, this part of his life was dedicated primarily to a process of highly specialized intellectual differentiation. Later Pauling turned his energies toward society and toward nature. He put his body as well as his reputation on the line to protest against heedless nuclear development, organized scientists against nuclear armament, and for a while became involved in national politics. For these activities, he earned the Nobel Peace Prize.

Linus Pauling was the only person to win two Nobel prizes, each for a completely different field of accomplishment. (Talk about differentiation!) Csikszentmihalyi did not mention that Pauling came within a hairsbreadth of discovering the spiraling structure of DNA, the molecular coding for every aspect of our lives, before Francis Crick and James Watson did. Nor did he mention the work that probably made Pauling a household name: his championing of Vitamin C for prevention and treatment of diseases ranging from colds to cancer. Relentless in his scientific endeavors, stalwart in his beliefs, but never less than even-handed and respectful in his presentations, Pauling's "textbook" personification of complexity was apparent over four decades.

And Pauling's good health was legendary. He attributed much of that to his vitamin regime, but his self-complexity was undoubtedly a contributor. After turning ninety, he developed prostate cancer, which is practically epidemic among older men, but he continued to conduct research, write, and live life to the fullest until his death in 1994.

The dynamic self is like a tightly knit tapestry of interlocking patterns that appear seamless. To create such a tapestry, we need attention to detail—our individual self-aspects—and attention to the larger pattern. We can let our many aspects flourish, as long as they are integrated into a whole that makes sense—a life that is livable. If we try to experience more than our bodies can handle, then our multiple selves are not well integrated. If we lead double lives in our relationships, betraying the trust of people we love, then our multiple selves are not well integrated. However, if we retain our bodymind integrity, nurturing that indelible aspect of self that transcends all our roles and activities, we can pursue the diverse possibilities of life with abandon. Doing so manifests care for our souls, and our health.

COMPLEXITY, TRANSFORMATION, AND HEALING

Patricia Linville recommends certain commonsense strategies that people can follow to enhance their awareness and differentiation of various self-aspects. "Exploring and Cultivating Self-Aspects" on pp. 319 to 321, is an exercise based on her suggestions.

However, a particular form of psychotherapy, which has

evolved over forty years, also builds self-complexity. It is called *psychosynthesis,* and was first developed by the Italian analyst Roberto Assagioli, M.D. Practitioners use imagination as a means to help patients explore their self-aspects, which in psychosynthesis are called *subpersonalities.* The ultimate goal of psychosynthesis is the development of a differentiated yet integrated self. Although Assagioli's psychological vantage point differs from Linville's, his therapeutic goals mirror her concept of self-complexity.

Because psychosynthesis fosters self-complexity, the question arises as to whether this form of therapy also promotes healing and health. Although no systematic studies have been conducted, one case history is a remarkable testament to the healing potential of psychosynthesis.

Alice Epstein was in her late fifties when she was diagnosed with kidney cancer. Her surgeon removed the kidney, but it was too late—the cancer had already spread to her lungs, where two masses were clearly visible on her X-rays. Her doctor "gave" her three months to live. Her husband looked up her specific prognosis in medical texts and found that only 4 in 1,000 survived her condition. No traditional treatments were even prescribed.

Alice was devastated. Her circumstances shook her to the core and forced her to confront one undeniable reality: Although her medical situation contributed to her despair, she had already felt despair—for years before her diagnosis.

"I had known for a long time that there was a darkness in my soul," she said. "I felt I had dug myself into a deep dark hole. I really sensed that my unhappiness had something to do with my cancer."

Alice talked about her feelings with her husband, Seymour Epstein, a professor of psychology at the University of Massachusetts. Together, the Epsteins searched the mind-body literature and excavated every study and book on cancer and the mind. They found what they felt was confirmation for their evolving belief that Alice's lifelong tendency to "always look out for somebody else, never for myself," and her underlying hopelessness, had contributed to her illness.

What was her despair about? According to Alice and Seymour,

painful childhood experiences had crippled Alice in her capacity to accept love. She had a loving husband and children, but the love never "penetrated" her psychological armor. Being unable to accept love over the course of her adulthood, Alice soon found herself in an existential "black box." After her diagnosis, she simply wanted to "close the box."

Alice and Seymour came to believe that unless she rooted out her despair by literally transforming her personality, she would never accept love, develop genuine faith in her own potential recovery, or get well. To say the least, it was a tall therapeutic order. Both were aware of the skepticism surrounding efforts to change personality, but both believed it was possible, and proceeded to leave no stone unturned in their efforts. The process was helped by Alice's sudden mobilization of a will to live. Seymour recalled a walk in the woods, when a soft snowfall caused Alice to remark that she did not want this to be her last winter. "With passionate anger, she told me, 'I am going to fight this thing.' "

In her transformative efforts, Alice found a therapist who practiced psychosynthesis. The therapist conducted intensive work with Alice, aimed at eliciting her subpersonalities. She used fantasy as a way of delving into the different aspects of her personality— "positive" and "negative"—with the goal of fully exploring and reintegrating them into a unified whole. The Italian psychotherapist Piero Ferrucci, a leading practitioner of psychosynthesis, defined subpersonalities in this way:

We can easily perceive our actual multiplicity by realizing how often we modify our general outlook, changing our model of the universe with the same facility with which we change dress. Thus, life may appear to us at any time as a routine, a dance, an adventure, a nightmare, a riddle, a merry-go-round, etc.

Our varying models of the universe color our perception and influence our way of being. And for each of them we develop a corresponding self-image and a set of body postures and gestures, feelings, behaviors, words, habits, and beliefs. This entire constellation of elements constitutes in itself a kind of miniature personality, or, as we will call it, sub-personality.

Subpersonalities are psychological satellites, coexisting as a multitude of lives within the overall medium of our personality. Each subpersonality has a style and a motivation of its own, often strikingly dissimilar from those of the others. . . .

Each of us is a crowd. There can be the rebel and the intellectual, the seducer and the housewife, the saboteur and the aesthete, the organizer and the bon vivant—each with its own mythology, and all more or less comfortably crowded into one single person.

Alice uncovered six subpersonalities. In their sessions, Alice's therapist guided her to visualize herself "literally taking each subpersonality up the mountain." The purpose was to help her understand each one, what they meant to her, and how they could be rewoven into the fabric of a stronger, more integrated self. "One of my subpersonalities was Mickey," said Alice, referring to the name she had given her. "She represented my intense jealousy. I began to feel that Mickey was trying to kill me." Her initial urge to liquidate Mickey—her competitive, critical, destructive self—eventually gave way to acceptance of her and a deep understanding of her origins in Alice's troubled childhood. Eventually, Alice came to respect Mickey's underlying wish for unconditional love. Little One was the name Alice gave to the personality that contained all her otherwise repressed nastiness and anger. "Little One went up the mountain, and when she got to the top she became a beautiful tiger. That tiger was one of the most wise of all my personalities." The rage that Alice had spent much of her life repressing had emerged in a symbol of courage, wisdom, and power. It was a symbol that would guide Alice in her struggle with life-threatening illness.

Other subpersonalities quickly emerged—Amanda, the builder; Crab, the helpless one; Oriole, the dreamer; and Athena, the guide. But Alice's pivotal subpersonality began its imaginal life as a fearful, needy, dependent two-and-a-half-year-old. She called her "Baby Alice." After taking Baby Alice up the mountain many times, living with her, analyzing dreams about her, and allowing her to interact in fantasy with her other subpersonalities, the infant metamorphosed into a powerful figure possessed of great confidence and energy. In real life, Alice's own childlike innocence had gotten lost when a wholly dependent Baby Alice assumed control over her personality. When adult Alice experienced Baby Alice's heartbreak, she understood why she'd assumed control over her personality. Then the needy infant transformed into a child capable of love and healing.

"Within three weeks, I knew I was changing," said Alice. "I was no longer looking at life as I had. The hopelessness had turned into faith that I was really going to be better."

Soon thereafter, Alice was offered an opportunity to enter an experimental drug program that her doctors considered a last-ditch effort. As part of the final evaluation before this treatment was administered, X rays were taken. The physician was shocked by his finding that one of her lung masses had disappeared and another had shrunk in half. He suggested that she go forward with the experimental program, but Alice and Seymour decided that "a natural healing process is going on here, and we did not want to interfere with it." Postponing treatment, Alice continued her transformative work and had her medical progress carefully monitored. "X ray after X ray showed a smaller and smaller tumor, and after one year the remaining cancer was all gone," recalled Alice.

It has been eight years since Alice's original diagnosis. No medical treatment was ever administered. Her cancer has not returned and she remains healthy.

Alice's interpretation of her cancer experience should not be extrapolated to every cancer patient. Nor are her treatment choices universally applicable. Alice herself believes that the vast majority of cancer patients benefit from combined medical and psychological treatment. Her case, she feels, was an exception to the rule. But Alice's story, which she wrote about in her book *Mind, Fantasy, and Healing,* is instructive. It demonstrates that a therapeutic process of differentiation and integration—namely, psychosynthesis—can have a profound influence on every level of one's being: psychological, physical, and spiritual.

Psychosynthesis is a method that cultivates self-complexity and has demonstrated therapeutic benefits. In Alice's case, it may have spurred a remission of "terminal" cancer, presumably by enhancing her immune system's sensitivity to the tumors growing in her lungs. The potential of mind-body healing with technologies for the development of self-complexity has barely been tapped. But Patricia Linville's work suggests that the time is ripe to make self-complexity an overriding goal of mind-body programs for the prevention and treatment of disease.

Developing self-complexity is itself a multilevel affair. On the level addressed by Dr. Linville, we can enliven our roles, activities, and traits by finding new and creative means of expression. On the level addressed by psychosynthesis, we can find the discrete traits and feelings packaged together in so-called subpersonalities. Linville's self-aspects and Assagioli's subpersonalities have much in common, but they seem to encompass different levels of consciousness. Linville's self-aspects are oriented to here-and-now experience and mental representations of self. Assagioli's subpersonalities are oriented toward past childhood development and emotional and spiritual representations of self. They are by no means mutually exclusive, but they entail different therapeutic approaches. At the end of this chapter, I provide exercises for cultivation of both levels of self-complexity.

THE SEVEN IMMUNE POWER TRAITS AND THE FABRIC OF SELF-COMPLEXITY

As you have followed the program in this book, moving from one Immune Power trait to the next, you have already been working to develop self-complexity. Since each Immune Power trait is a vital self-aspect, each must be differentiated in order to promote your health actively. And each can be integrated in our global personality.

People I have known whom I consider Immune Power Personalities have left me with the undeniable impression that the seven traits represent archetypal self-aspects present in each of us. They just happened to be highly developed in these particular individuals. But Immune Power traits are certainly not the province of a select few. Psychosynthesis demonstrates how people can radically transform their personalities to bring forth hidden, repressed, or otherwise stunted versions of the seven Immune Power traits. In the annals of psychosynthesis, case after case illustrates the flowering of the ACE Factor; the capacity to confide; commitment, control, and challenge; assertiveness; affiliative trust; altruism; and complexity.

These traits appear in subpersonalities groping for means of expression; in archetypes imbedded in the unconscious; in mythic incarnations; in desired roles, activities, or relationships. Often they are trapped in layers of defense or knots of unresolved emotion. One goal of mind-body therapy should be to liberate the seven traits from their hiding places in the personality.

In psychosynthesis, patients explore their subpersonalities until they are transformed. More often than not, Immune Power traits are revealed. People uncover the healthy potentialities—the energy, commitment, self-preservation, creativity, fearlessness, love, and compassion—that were previously masked or buried. But psychosynthesis is far from the only therapy to bring forth Immune Power traits. Many psychotherapies employ methods that achieve similar results. The practices outlined in each chapter of this book enable you to cultivate them on your own.

As I have stated throughout, Immune Power traits are distinct yet overlapping. The threads that connect these seven traits suggest the unifying principle of personality. Robert Lifton's concept of a protean self; Mihaly Csikszentmihalyi's evolving self; Stephen A. Mitchell's multifaceted self; Roberto Assagioli's subpersonalities; and Patricia Linville's self-complexity all share one philosophy: The healthy person has many selves, but one core self that organizes and makes sense of the whole.

The first goal of Immune Power development is therefore to differentiate each trait—to cultivate them completely. The second goal is to integrate each Immune Power trait into the whole of one's personality. Understanding the areas of overlap among these seven traits is one way to encourage their integration. Here are a few examples of overlap among the seven Immune Power traits:

1. *Affiliative Trust and the Capacity to Confide:* The person motivated by affiliative trust will be more able to confide thoughts and feelings to others.
2. *The ACE Factor and the Capacity to Confide:* The person who confides actively expresses emotions, as in the "E" of the ACE Factor.
3. *Hardiness and the ACE Factor:* The individual who attends, connects, and expresses sensations and feelings will have a greater sense of control (one "C" of hardiness) over her body and emotional life. She also may have greater commitment (another "C") to activities rooted in emotional awareness.
4. *Hardiness and Healthy Helping:* The helper has a greater sense of control, because he partakes in service activities that make him feel good and is committed to other human beings or a higher cause.
5. *Affiliative Trust and Healthy Helping:* The motivation to help, based on the trait of altruism, is closely related to unconditional love and affiliative trust.
6. *Assertiveness and All Other Traits:* Assertiveness is necessary in order to (a) confide in others; (b) express emotions actively; (c) meet challenges with a sense of commitment and control; (d) go out into the world and help others effectively; (e) develop healthy relationships rooted in affiliative trust; and (f) develop all the disparate parts of the self, as in self-complexity.
7. *Self-Complexity and All Other Traits:* Being the trait of having many traits, self-complexity subsumes all seven Immune Power traits. In real life, people who exhibit most or all Immune Power traits are certainly complex and highly differentiated *and* integrated personalities.

There are other areas of overlap between Immune Power traits, but these are the most important ones to recognize. You can embrace the distinct qualities of these traits, seeking them in corners of your personality, subpersonalities, activities, roles, and relationships. At the same time, being aware of connections among them strengthens your sense of yourself as an integrated whole. An ineffable awareness at the heart of the personal self unites all these disparate elements.

Over the past ten years, I have met people who have overcome diseases that appeared to be intractible. They had actualized all seven Immune Power traits, each characteristic being manifest in their ways of coping, carrying themselves, and being in the world. Yet, as the stories in this book suggest, each Immune Power Personality was as different from the next as one could imagine. Immune Power traits are not blueprints. They are keys that unlock our individuality.

IMMUNE POWER TRAITS AND THE WAY OF THE SPIRIT

I believe there are archetypal elements to all seven Immune Power traits, as in Jung's primordial images of selfhood. As such, they represent both our deepest and our highest selves. As Carl Jung, Joseph Campbell, Abraham Maslow, Carl Rogers, Roberto Assagioli, and Ken Wilber have all stated in different ways, when we discover and actualize the highest potentialities of our personal selves, we reach toward transcendence. Transcendence is that state of consciousness in which our personal identity becomes one with a higher identity, representing our spiritual origins and our spiritual nature. The contribution of spirit to physical health is controversial, but it is finally being studied and affirmed by many reputable physicians.

I have not devoted a chapter to transcendence because it is not a "proven" Immune Power trait. But my close readings of the literature of transpersonal psychology confirm that self-actualization of the kind advocated here—full development of the personal self—is a necessary path toward a higher Self. Transcendence without self-actualization may not even be possible.

Abraham Maslow wrote about three groups of people: self-actualizers, transcenders, and transcending self-actualizers. As Au-Deane Cowley wrote recently:

> The self-actualizers had strong, effective identities; well integrated personalities; and minimal experience of transcendence. Transcenders had strong contact with the spiritual dimension and frequent transcendent experiences, but their personalities were often underdeveloped. The transcending self-actualizers not only had strong and effective personalities, but, according to Maslow, "are capable of transcending the limitations of personal identity and thus have a deeper sense of eternity and of the sacred."

Maslow believed that people who reach for transcendence without self-actualization probably will not find what they are seeking.

As mentioned in the introduction, Immune Power Personality development moves from level to level of awareness, from "inside" to "outside" and from "low" to "high." In the ultimate transcendent state of awareness, such distinctions no longer exist. But according to Ken Wilber, we can't move to higher levels of consciousness until we achieve integration on each ascending level. In the course of Immune Power development, our attention to each level of our personal selves is another step in an ascent toward a higher awareness.

Self-complexity, which involves cultivation of all seven traits as well as every other significant self-aspect, is the Immune Power trait closest to spirituality. Self-complexity represents complete realization of our inner selves, which in the great mystic traditions are inseparable from God, however one defines the deity.

In chapter 4, I discussed Arthur Ashe as an exemplar of hardiness. Ashe was also highly complex, personifying all seven Immune Power traits. A passage in Ashe's memoir, *Days of Grace,* provides a profound glimpse into the relation between the personal trait of self-complexity and a broader spiritual awareness. Ashe had always been religious, but after he was diagnosed with AIDS, he sought to deepen his spirituality. Ashe began investigating the commonalities among all the major religious and mystical traditions, East and West. Philosopher and theologian Howard Thurman was particularly influential in Ashe's spiritual frame of reference:

> Much has happened in my life, but Dr. Thurman's teaching helps me to maintain control despite these changes. In fact, he insists we remember that the self is not static but constantly changing in accordance with new episodes and facts involving the individual. The self is not a purely ethereal or purely physical entity but one composed of earthly as well as transcendental properties. Thus any journey into the self, any effort at centering down, must take into account new facts and events in the individual's life; all important new "self-facts" must be integrated harmoniously into one's self-image. Such exploration must not be undertaken in willful avoidance of these facts, as if they did not exist. As a devoted pragmatist, I relish the practicality of this teaching, how it respects the concrete aspects of existence even as it facilitates a search for divine grace. In my case, heart disease and AIDS are absolute facts that I must integrate into my sense of my own reality, my self.

Ashe's appreciation of Thurman's teaching, which "respects the concrete aspects of existence as it facilitates a search for divine grace," captures the essence of Immune Power Personality development. The exercises in each chapter emphasize action and reflection, practicality and spirituality, relations with others and relations with the deeper (higher) self. The ordering of these traits is designed to encourage personal growth in the pragmatic areas of everyday life and the ethereal arenas of higher consciousness.

Without our individual identities, there is no state of awareness—no self—that incorporates them all. Without a broader sense of connectedness, there can be no individual identities. The Immune Power Personality, with a rich repertoire of roles, traits, and activities—but also connection to a higher Self—is charged with energy, but also with serenity. The seven traits add up to a harmonious cohabitation of our zestful, loving, grounded, contemplative, feisty, compassionate, spiritual, and contradictory sides. Each seeming opposite, held together in the personality, keeps the whole self in a state of excited equilibrium. That state of balance is a state of grace, one in which body and spirit are united, one in which our ability to heal and repair ourselves is potentially boundless.

EXERCISES IN SELF-COMPLEXITY

Following the work of Patricia Linville, the best way to begin a process of developing self-complexity is to find out about your self-aspects. The following is a combined writing-and-visualizing exercise in four steps, to heighten your awareness of your self-aspects and create strategies for differentiating, reintegrating, and adding self-aspects to your characterological repertoire. I suggest that you practice each step on four consecutive days. Repeat this exercise at regular intervals (such as once every two months) to "keep in touch" with your progress on self-complexity.

EXPLORING AND CULTIVATING SELF-ASPECTS

1. Begin with an exploratory writing exercise to determine your self-aspects and the many traits and characteristics embedded in each one. In her research, Dr. Linville passed out index cards with a multiplicity of features, and asked people to pile them together according to any personally meaningful categories of roles, activities, traits, or other self-aspects. For two examples of the final results from Dr. Linville's subjects, refer back to table 8.1.

Use those examples as a guide. (If you haven't already initiated a journal practice, it would be helpful to start one for this exercise.) In your journal or notebook, create columns like the ones shown in the table, listing significant parts of yourself. They can be active roles, activities, types of relationships, subpersonalities, or personality traits. You don't have to rely on any one of these categories—feel free to mix and match. Under each column, list adjectives that describe qualities you experience and/or exhibit in these self-aspects. When you are finished, count the number and evaluate how many similarities there are, based on commonalities in the list of descriptive terms, from self-aspect to self-aspect.

2. Identify those specific self-aspects that you feel you have neglected. Write in your journal a free-form answer to the question: Why have I neglected this part of myself? Next, practice a simple visualization exercise. After relaxing in a quiet place, imagine the neglected self-aspect as a person—it can be you, someone else, or an unknown figure. Invite that person into your room, and ask him or her how he or she wishes to be treated. Explore this person's needs, desires, feelings. Investigate how you can reintroduce him or her into your inner social circle, so that you and this other person both feel gratified. After this visualization, write about your experience and what it meant to you.

3. Identify those specific self-aspects that you feel are too tightly bound to other self-aspects, either by circumstance or by shared features. Write in your journal a free-form answer to the question: Why is this part of me so bound to this other part of me? There should be no implied criticism in this question or in your approach to the issue. Next, practice a simple visualization, similar to the one in step 2, except this time invite the poorly differentiated self-aspect into your room. Ask him or her how he or she wishes to develop more and how he or she wishes to be different from other parts of you. Explore this person's needs, desires, feelings. Investigate how you can better distinguish and cultivate this person, so that both of you feel gratified. After this visualization, write about your experience and what it meant to you.

4. Identify self-aspects that you did not write down on your initial list. I call these latent or inactive self-aspects. What parts of yourself are so dormant that you did not even think of them? In your journal, create columns for these self-aspects as you did initially. Ask yourself: Which of these self-aspects do I miss most? Which ones do I want to invite back into my inner social circle? Once you have made this determination, practice a visualization similar to the one in step 2. The only difference is that these are the superneglected selves! Find out how you can reintroduce them comfortably, and meaningfully, into your life.

PSYCHOSYNTHESIS: DISCOVERING YOUR SUBPERSONALITIES

Many of our highest (and lowest) traits are present within complex substructures known as subpersonalities. (See "Complexity, Transformation, and Healing" on p. 308 for details.) Piero Ferrucci, a leading practitioner of psychosynthesis, has developed powerful methods for uncovering and transforming subpersonalities. Here are excerpts from his book *What We May Be*, which set forth his method for first recognizing and then transforming subpersonalities.

For Recognition

1. Consider one of your prominent traits, attitudes, or motives.
2. With your eyes closed, become aware of this part of you. Then let an image emerge representing it. It may be a woman, a man, an animal, an elf, an object, yourself in disguise, a monster, or anything else in the universe. Let this image emerge spontaneously. . . .
3. As soon as the image has appeared, give it the chance to reveal itself to you without any interference or judgment on your part. Let it change if it tends to do so spontaneously. Get in touch with the general feeling that emanates from it.
4. Now let this image talk and express itself . . . in particular, find out about its needs . . .
5. Now open your eyes and record in a notebook everything that has happened so far. Then give this subpersonality a name . . . (See the discussion of Alice Epstein on p. 309 for examples.)

For Exploration and Transformation ("Up the Mountain")

1. Choose a subpersonality with whom you are already familiar.
2. Imagine yourself in a valley with this subpersonality. Together, the two of you experience your surroundings. You look around and see the grass, the flowers, the trees, and a mountain. Take

some time to become aware of the sounds of nature around you—the chirping of the birds, the sounds of the leaves in the wind, and the like.

3. Now start walking up the mountain with your subpersonality. As you keep ascending, you can imagine seeing all kinds of scenery, climbing through woods and rocks, walking on wide meadows or near precipices. Keep in touch with the increasing sense of elevation, feel the air becoming purer and more energizing, and listen to the utter silence of the heights.

4. Throughout the ascent, keep in contact with your subpersonality. You may see it going through subtle transformations—such as a variation in mood or facial expression or dress—or even a radical transformation: the subpersonality changing completely into something else.

5. When you reach the top, let the light of the sun shine on the two of you and reveal the very essence of your subpersonality. At this point, let the subpersonality express itself for what it is now, and let it communicate with you.

Do not expect a transformation the first time you try this exercise, though it is possible. Every step of the way, try to stop yourself from judging your subpersonality or, for that matter, your own progress. Allow the drama to unfold, and appreciate the spectacle as an engaged though impartial witness.

INTEGRATING THE SEVEN IMMUNE POWER TRAITS

The seven Immune Power traits can become hidden or ensconced within certain self-aspects or subpersonalities. For instance, assertiveness may be hidden in the underbelly of your nice-guy self. You do not need to reject the nice guy, simply to understand him and the hold he has over your global personality. Then you can put him in his proper place in your gallery of self-aspects.

You can conduct such inquiries as searches for your own latent, inhibited, or undifferentiated Immune Power traits. In your journal, spend time answering these questions:

1. What part of my being—be it a role, activity, relationship, subpersonality,—"contains" my ability to attend, connect, and express my needs and feelings (the ACE Factor)? Are some parts of me more attuned, connected, and expressive than others? If so, which parts?
2. If I do find self-aspects that "contain" the ACE Factor, am I happy with the extent to which ACE is present in my life? Do I need to develop ACE in other parts of my life? If so, which ones?
3. Imagine having the greatest possible ability to attend, connect, and express your needs and emotions. As a result, you experience vibrant good health, a sense of balance and flexibility, and a range of choices in responding to internal and external stressors. In order to achieve that goal, how would I change my life? Inject ACE into more dimensions of my life? Find new roles or activities that help me to develop ACE?

Now substitute all six other Immune Power traits, and conduct the same investigation by answering questions 1 through 3. Use this writing exercise as an adventure in self-discovery. Find out where your healthy potentialities are hidden, and coax them out into the light of consciousness.

APPENDIX

FOLLOWING THE PROGRAM: THE AUTHOR'S EXPERIENCE AND IMMUNE TEST RESULTS

For seven weeks, I followed the program of Immune Power Personality development I recommend in this book. Each week, I concentrated on one Immune Power trait, moving through the program in the order set forth. I kept a running diary of life events and my psychological and physical well-being. I was able to obtain a complete panel of immunological tests, which included counts of my immune cells broken down by each sub-type. I also received so-called "functional" tests, which indicated whether my natural killer cells, granulocytes, and lymphocytes (to name but a few) were vigorous and effective in attacking foreign invaders. I took these tests before I began, during the program, and after completing the program.

I used all the ACE exercises to tune into my state of mind and body, which helped me feel more vibrantly alive. I became aware of pains and conflicts—in work and relationships—that I had too long shelved.

I confided past traumas using Dr. Pennebaker's writing exercise, mainly exploring the sudden death of my father when I was twenty. By week's end, I recognized how unresolved feelings about him still colored my state of mind and heart.

During a week of hardiness training, I enhanced my commitment, control, and challenge through focusing, situational reconstruction, and decisive action. I learned a great deal about how my interpersonal style tended to undermine my sense of control.

The hardiness work led ineluctably to the work of assertiveness. I spent the next week honing my skills, nonaggressively confronting individuals with whom I worked and lived. By following the basic tenets, I was able to initiate much improved communication, which enhanced my sense of control. My commitment and challenge were becoming bolstered as well.

During the week devoted to affiliative trust, I made a conscious effort to attend to people I cared for, to enjoy fully time spent with friends and family. The loving-kindness meditation and visualization produced feelings of warmth and tranquility that helped me make contact with people in a more genuine way throughout the week.

Given my state of mind after cultivating affiliative trust, I could not have been happier to spend time helping others. I concentrated on helping friends (and their friends) who had come to me in the previous six months with medical problems, seeking doctor referrals and research on issues of treatment. I spent hours talking to them and hunting down the right specialist or treatment option. On several occasions I experienced the helper's high described by Allan Luks, accompanied by feelings of psychological and physical well-being.

During the last week devoted to self-complexity, I wrote about my various self-aspects and explored them in visualizations such as those used in psychosynthesis. I also made an effort to spend time each day focusing on each of the other six Immune Power traits. At times these experiences jazzed me up, triggering a desire to experience every facet of myself and the world, along with a frustration that there was too little time to live out so many lives. By and large, however, I completed the program on an exhilarating high.

I took on this challenge during the worst winter I can ever remember. One icy snow storm after another battered New York City, which is a hard place to live during even the most quiescent winters. It was brutally cold, and my daily excursions into the snowy streets seemed to take every ounce of energy I had. During normal winters, I usually get at least two colds. Despite these terrible conditions, I did not suffer one bout with a cold or flu. I remained in excellent health throughout, and have remained in excellent health to this writing—five months later. I have had physical examinations before and after the program, and the only significant finding was a drop in blood pressure from 140/96 to 134/84.

The immunologist who authorized the work-up gave me a printout of my blood cell counts before and after the seven weeks. In addition, he informed me in person of the results of my "functional" tests of immune cell activity.

As it happened, my immune system was in relatively good shape before the program began. My natural killer cell numbers and activity were high. My lymphocytes responded vigorously to laboratory challenges. The ratio of my T-helper to T-suppressor cells was slightly greater than two to one—considered a sign of a strong and properly balanced T-cell system. Only my granulocyte-killing activity was a bit sluggish to begin with. My differential white cell counts—including neutrophils, lymphocytes, and monocytes—were all in the normal range, though slightly below an absolute midrange figure.

What about afterwards? My immunologist told me that everything that was strong remained strong, including the activity of my natural killer cells and lymphocytes. With regard to the functional measures, there was only one significant change. My granulocytes, the only disappointing performers at the start, had undergone a surprising transformation. Before, they killed 30 percent of the target bacteria; now, they were killing 60 percent. In other words, cells that are considered a first line of defense against disease agents had doubled in their killing efficiency. I was particularly pleased by this news because I was aware of recent research on the cancer-killing capabilities of granulocytes.

As intriguing as the change in my granulocytes were increases in the differential counts of several key categories of my immune cells. My neutrophil, lymphocyte, and monocyte counts had gone up markedly. On my laboratory report, I noted the reference range for each of these cell types, which indicates the lowest and highest numbers that can still be considered "normal." In none of these instances had my numbers gone too high, which might have indicated a serious infection that I was doing a poor job of fighting. In fact, in the case of neutrophils and lymphocytes, I had come closer to an absolute middle between the low and high figures in each reference range.

Table A.1 shows the increases in numbers of each cell type, as well as the percentage of these increases from time 1 (before program) to time 2 (one week after completing program). My neutrophils increased by 12.3 percent, my lymphocytes 21 percent, and my monocytes went up 32 percent. Monocytes are considered critical in combating bacteria, viruses, and wayward cancer cells. Recall Gary Schwartz's findings that repressors have lower percentages of monocytes to overall white blood cells. Both my numbers and percentage of monocytes increased (from 8.7 to 9.9 percent of white blood cells). Researchers have also shown that higher monocytes predict fewer infections in a medical population.* Immunological analyses of space shuttle crewmembers showed that the stress of flight reduced monocytes, which in turn seemed to reduce lymphocyte activity.†

Table A.1: Increases in Differential Immune Cell Counts*

	Time 1	Time 2	Ref. Range	% Increase
Neutrophils	3679	4153	1650-8330	+12.3
Lymphocytes	1927	2328	1049-3581	+21
Monocytes	548	722	61-929	+32
Eosinophils	63	73	40-423	+16

*All cell counts are per cubic millimeters. (CU.MM)

---

*A. J. Keiden, et al. (1986): Infective complications of aplastic anemia. *British Journal of Haematology*, 63, pp. 503–506.
†G. R. Taylor, L. S. Neale, J. R. Dardano: Immunological analyses of U.S. Space Shuttle crewmembers. *Aviation Space Environmental Medicine*, 57, pp. 213–217.

For more insight into the possible meaning of my increased cell counts, I contacted the head of the department of clinical immunology at a leading university, a woman I had met previously and whose reputation is impeccable. I told her my numbers and she was intrigued. She said that the increase in my granulocyte killing combined with the increased numbers indicated one of two scenarios. The first was simply a bolstering of my immunological strength for no reason other than my improved state of mind. The other scenario was that I had been challenged by some pathogens—cold or flu viruses, perhaps—and my body was taking action against them. She then asked me the telltale question: "How have you been feeling these past weeks?" "Just fine," I said. "Not even a sniffle."

She completed the second scenario. If I had been challenged by a virus, then my immune system had quite literally risen to the occasion and gotten rid of it so effectively that I hadn't the slightest clue of the invasion. Thus, it was entirely conceivable that I had survived the winter so well because my immune system—strengthened by my developing Immune Power traits—had responded with a delicately balanced and proportional enhancement, just enough to take care of the interlopers but not so much as to cause eruptions of fever and other symptoms.

In either scenario—immune enhancement with or without an offending pathogen—my system had improved, and the program may have been responsible. Of course, it is possible that my immune defenses would have risen to the occasion of an attack even if I hadn't followed the program. However, the fact that I remained physically well in the face of weather conditions that normally make me sick adds weight to the notion that I had successfully bolstered and balanced my immune system.

My experience must be considered merely an anecdote. The truly persuasive evidence that building the seven traits enhances immunity can be found in the systematic studies described throughout this book. But my experience certainly helped to persuade me, and I hope it offers inspiration as you embark on your own Immune Power challenge.

REFERENCES

CHAPTER 1. DEEPER INTO THE MIND-BODY CONNECTION

page 14   The essential findings and breakthroughs in the field of psychoneuroimmunology (PNI) can be found in the classic texts: R. Ader (ed.) (1981). *Psychoneuroimmunology.* Academic Press, New York; and R. Ader, D. L. Felten, and N. Cohen (eds.) (1991). *Psychoneuroimmunology II.* Academic Press, New York.

page 18   A. Hoffman (1905) *Rene Descartes.* F. Frommanns Verlag, Stuttgart. See also R. Descartes (1958). *Descartes' Philosophical Writings,* sel. and tr., Norman Kemp. Modern Library, New York. Quote from Sir William Osler from R. Ornstein and D. Sobel (1988). *The Healing Brain.* Touchstone Books, New York.

page 19   Discussion of Claude Bernard's early contributions to a science of mind and body from: R. Ornstein and D. Sobel (1988). *The Healing Brain.* Touchstone Books, New York; and S. Locke and D. Colligan (1985). *The Healer Within.* E.P. Dutton, New York.

page 19   W. B. Cannon (1939). *The Wisdom of the Body.* Norton, New York; F. Alexander and T. M. French (1948). *Studies in Psychosomatic Medicine.* Ronald Press, New York.

page 21   H. Selye (1956). *The Stress of Life.* McGraw-Hill, New York; H. Selye (1974) *Stress Without Distress.* New American Library, New York.

page 22   George Solomon's early work on personality and arthritis is reviewed in G. F. Solomon (1981). Emotional and personality factors in the onset and course of autoimmune disease, particularly rheumatoid arthritis. In R. Ader (ed.), *Psychoneuroimmunology.* Academic Press, New York. Solomon's early speculations on the linkages between mind and immunity are set forth in G. F. Solomon and R. H. Moos (1964). Emotions, immunity, and disease: A speculative theoretical integration. *Archives of General Psychiatry,* 11, pp. 657–674. His early animal research is described in: A. Amkraut and G. F. Solomon (1972). Stress and murine sarcoma virus (Maloney)-induced tumors. *Cancer Research,* 32, pp. 1428–1433; G. F. Solomon (1969). Stress and antibody response in rats. *International Archives of Allergy,* 35, pp. 97–104; G. F. Solomon, et al. (1968). Early experience and immunity. *Nature,* 220, pp. 821–822; and A. Amkraut and G. F. Solomon (1974). From the symbolic stimulus to the pathophysiological response: Immune mechanisms. *International Journal of Psychiatry in Medicine,* 5, pp. 541–563.

page 24   Robert Ader's original experiments are described in: R. Ader and N. Cohen (1975). Behaviorally conditioned immunosuppression. *Psychosomatic Medicine,* 37, pp. 333–340; R. Ader and N. Cohen (1985). CNS-immune interactions: Conditioning phenomena. *Brain and Behavioral Sciences* 8, pp. 379–426; and R. Ader and N. Cohen (1981). Conditioned immunopharmacologic responses. In R. Ader (ed.), *Psychoneuroimmunology.* Academic Press, New York. Dr. Ader's research on conditioning rats with lupus is detailed in R. Ader and N. Cohen (1982). Behaviorally conditioned immunosuppression and murine systemic lupus erythematosus. *Science* 215, pp. 1534–1536.

page 25   H. O. Besedovsky, E. Sorkin, D. Felix, and H. Haas (1977). Hypothalamic changes during the immune response. *European Journal of Immunology,* 7, pp. 325–328; K. Bulloch and R. Y. Moore (1981). Innervation of the thymus gland by brain stem and spinal cord in mouse and rat. *American Journal of Anatomy,* 162, pp. 315–328.

page 26   D. L. Felten, et al. (1985). Noradrenergic and peptidergic innervation of lymphoid tissue. *Journal of Immunology,* 135, pp. 755s–765s. For a superb overview of research on interactive networks of nerve fibers and cells and immune system organs and cells, see S. Y. Felten and D. L. Felten (1991). Innervation of lymphoid tissue. In R. Ader, D. L. Felten, and N. Cohen (eds.), *Psychoneuroimmunology II.* Academic Press, New York.

page 26   Candace Pert's work on neuropeptides and receptors is reported in: C. B. Pert, G. Pasternak, and S. H. Snyder (1973). Opiate agonists and antagonists discriminated by receptor binding in brain. *Science,* 182 (4119), pp. 1359–1361; C. B. Pert, M. R. Ruff, R. J. Weber, and M. Herkenham (1985). Neuropeptides and their receptors: A psychosomatic network. *Journal of Immunology,* 35(2), pp. 820s–826s; and C. B. Pert (1986). The wisdom of the receptors: Neuropeptides, the emotions, and bodymind. *Advances,* 3:3, pp. 8–16. For thorough discussions and review of two-way communications between the nervous and immune systems, see: D. J. Carr and J. E. Blalock (1991). Neuropeptide hormones and receptors common to the immune and neuroendocrine systems: Bidirectional pathway of intersystem communication; and D. L. Felten, et al. (1991). "Central neural circuits involved in neural-immune interactions." In R. Ader, D. L. Felten, and N. Cohen (eds.), *Psychoneuroimmunology II.* Academic Press, New York.

page 28   Among the animal studies on stress, helplessness, and
            immunity are: M. A. Visintainer, J. R. Volpicelli, and M.
            R. Seligman (1982). Tumor rejection in rats after ines-
            capable or escapable shock. *Science,* 216, pp. 437–439;
            M. Laudenslager, S. Ryan, S. Drugan, R. Hyson, and S.
            Maier (1983). Coping and immunosuppression: Ines-
            capable but not escapable shock suppresses lymphocyte
            proliferation. *Science,* 221, pp. 568–570; S. F. Maier and
            M. L. Laudenslager (1988). Inescapable shock, shock
            controllability, and mitogen stimulated lymphocyte pro-
            liferation. *Brain, Behavior, and Immunity,* 2, pp. 87–91;
            and B. Bohus and J. M. Koolhaas (1991). Psychoimmu-
            nology of social factors in rodents and other
            subprimate vertebrates. In R. Ader, D. L. Felten, and N.
            Cohen (eds.), *Psychoneuroimmunology II.* Academic Press,
            New York. Lawrence LeShan's body of research on
            cancer patients is described in his books: L. LeShan
            (1977). *You Can Fight for Your Life.* M. Evans, New York;
            and L. LeShan (1989). *Cancer As a Turning Point.* E.P.
            Dutton, New York.

page 29   The study of exam stress, loneliness, and immunity is
            described in J. K. Kiecolt-Glaser, et al. (1984). Psychoso-
            cial modifiers of immunocompetence in medical stu-
            dents. *Psychosomatic Medicine,* 46, pp. 7–14. See also J. S.
            House, K. R. Landis, and D. Umberson (1988). Social
            relationships and health. *Science,* 241, pp. 540–545.

page 29   S. E. Locke, et al. (1984). Life change stress, psychiatric
            symptoms and natural killer cell activity. *Psychosomatic
            Medicine,* 46(5), pp. 441–453.

page 30   Suzanne Ouellette explains her challenge to prevailing
            notions of stress and health in the book she coau-
            thored, S. R. Maddi and S. C. Kobasa (1984). *The Hardy
            Executive: Health Under Stress.* Dow Jones–Irwin,
            Homewood, IL.

page 34   Lydia Temoshok's research on psychological and immu-
            nological factors in melanoma (skin cancer) is de-
            scribed in: L. Temoshok and B. H. Fox (1984). Coping

styles and other psychosocial factors related to medical status and to prognosis in patients with cutaneous malignant melanoma. In B. H. Fox and B. H. Newberry (eds.), *Impact of Psychoendocrine Systems in Cancer and Immunity.* C. J. Hogrefe, Toronto; L. Temoshok, B. W. Heller, R. W. Sagabiel, M. S. Blois, D. M. Sweet, R. J. DiClemente, and M. L. Gold (1985). The relationship of psychosocial factors to prognostic indicators in cutaneous malignant melanoma. *Journal of Psychosomatic Medicine,* 29, pp. 139–154; L. Temoshok (1985). Biopsychosocial studies on cutaneous malignant melanoma: Psychosocial factors associated with prognostic indicators, progression, psychophysiology, and tumor-host response. *Social Science and Medicine,* 20(8), pp. 833–840; and L. Temoshok and H. Dreher (1992). *The Type C Connection: The Behavioral Links to Cancer and Your Health.* Random House, New York.

page 38　　The footnote on the role of immunological factors in coronary heart disease refers to a spate of recent studies over the past ten years. These studies are reviewed in a recent article, L. G. Lange and G. F. Schreiner (1994). Immune mechanisms of cardiac disease. *New England Journal of Medicine,* 330(16), pp. 1129–1135.

page 38　　The immune system primer is based on essential tenets of immunology established over the past half-century. See: O. G. Bier, et al. (1981). *Fundamentals of Immunology.* Springer-Verlag, New York; and B. Benacerraf and E. R. Unanue (1979). *Textbook of Immunology.* Williams and Wilkins, Baltimore. Two fine popular works on the immune system are: S. Mizel and P. Jaret (1985). *In Self Defense.* Harcourt Brace Jovanovich, New York; and J. Davis (1989). *Defending the Body: Unraveling the Mysteries of Immunology.* Atheneum, New York.

page 44　　Research identifying and characterizing immune substances that are structurally similar to neuropeptides and neuropeptides that are structurally similar to immune substances is summarized in D. J. Carr and J. E. Blalock (1991). Neuropeptide hormones and receptors common to the immune and neuroendocrine systems: Bidirectional pathway of intersystem communication. In R. Ader, D. L. Felten, and N. Cohen (eds), *Psychoneuroimmunology II*. Academic Press, New York.

page 44 George Solomon's analogies between our psychological and immunological systems can be found in his article, G. F. Solomon (1985). The emerging field of psychoneuroimmunology: Hypotheses, supporting evidence, and new directions. *Advances*, 2, pp. 6–19.

page 46 D. Spiegel, J. Bloom, H. C. Kraemer, et al. (1989). Effect of psychosocial treatment on survival of patients with metastatic breast cancer. *The Lancet*, 2, pp. 888–891; D. Spiegel (1991). A psychosocial intervention and survival time of patients with metastatic breast cancer. *Advances*, 7:3, pp. 10–19. See also M. H. Antoni, L. Baggett, G. Ironson, et al. (1990). Cognitive-behavioral stress management intervention buffers distress responses and immunologic changes following notification of HIV-1 seropositivity. *Journal of Consulting and Clinical Psychology*, 59, pp. 906–915.

page 46 F. I. Fawzy, M. E. Kemeny, et al. (1990). A structured psychiatric intervention for cancer patients. II. Changes over time in immunological measures. *Archives of General Psychiatry*, 47, pp. 729–735; F. I. Fawzy, M. O. Fawzy, et al. (1993). Malignant melanoma: Effects of an early structured psychiatric intervention, coping, and affective state on recurrence and survival six years later. *Archives of General Psychiatry*, 50, pp. 681–689.

page 47 D. M. Ornish, S. E. Brown, L. W. Scherwitz, et al. (1990). Can lifestyle changes reverse coronary atherosclerosis? The Lifestyle Heart Trial. *The Lancet*, 336, pp. 129–133. See also D. M. Ornish (1991). *Dr. Dean Ornish's Program for Reversing Heart Disease*. Random House, New York.

CHAPTER 2. THE ACE FACTOR

page 50   Gary Schwartz's "systems" approach to health and illness, which accounts for multiple factors including personality, has been set forth in a series of papers, including: G. E. Schwartz (1979). Disregulation and systems
theory: a biobehavioral framework for biofeedback and
behavioral medicine. In N. Birbaumer and H. D.
Kimmel (eds.), *Biofeedback and Self-Regulation*. Erlbaum,
Hillsdale, NJ; G. E. Schwartz (1984). Psychobiology of
health: A new synthesis. In B. L. Hammonds and C. J.
Scheirer (eds.), *Psychology and Health: Master Lecture Series*, vol. 3, pp. 145–195. American Psychological Association, Washington, DC; and G. E. Schwartz (1990).
Psychobiology of Repression and Health: A systems approach. In J. L. Singer (ed.), *Repression and Dissociation:
Implications for Personality Theory, Psychopathology, and
Health*. University of Chicago Press, Chicago.

page 52   Gary Schwartz's early study of "grief muscles" and the
effects of antidepressants on psychiatric patients and
controls was reported in an interview with the author in
March 1993.

page 63   D. A. Weinberger, G. E. Schwartz, and R. J. Davidson
(1979). Low-anxious, high-anxious, and repressive coping styles: Psychometric patterns and behavioral and
physiological responses to stress. *Journal of Abnormal Psychology*, 88, pp. 369–380.

page 64   The discussion of Schwartz's research on repression
and heart disease, including his studies of hypertension, is derived from G. E. Schwartz (1983). Disregulation theory and disease: Applications to the repression/
cerebral disconnection/cardiovascular disorder hypothesis. *International Review of Applied Psychology*, 32, pp.
95–118.

page 66   Schwartz's key study of psychological factors, opioid
peptides, and immunity is reported in L. Jamner, G. E.
Schwartz, and H. Leigh (1988). The relationship be-

tween repressive and defensive coping styles and monocyte, eosinophile, and serum glucose levels: Support for the opioid peptide hypothesis of repression. *Psychosomatic Medicine,* 50, pp. 567–575.

page 69   L. D. Jamner and G. E. Schwartz (1986): Self-deception predicts self-report and endurance of pain. *Psychosomatic Medicine,* 48, pp. 211–223.

page 70   Y. Shavit, G. W. Terman, F. C. Martin, et al. (1985). Stress, opioid peptides, the immune system, and cancer. *The Journal of Immunology,* 135:2, pp. 834s–837s. See also Y. Shavit, J. Lewis, G. Terman, et al. (1984). Opioid peptides mediate the suppressive effect of stress on natural killer cell cytotoxicity. *Science,* 223, pp. 188–190.

page 70   The complex effects of endorphins on immunity, as addressed in the text and footnote, are described in the following studies and review papers: N. E. Kay, J. Allen, and J. E. Morley (1984). Endorphins stimulate normal human peripheral blood lymphocyte natural killer activity. *Life Sciences,* 35, pp. 53–59; J. E. Morley, N. E. Kay, G. F. Solomon, and N. P. Plotnikoff (1987). Neuropeptides: Conductors of the immune orchestra. *Life Sciences,* 41, pp. 527–544; C. Heijnen (1987). Modulation of the immune response by POMC-derived peptides. I. Influence on proliferation of human lymphocytes. *Brain, Behavior, and Immunity,* 1, pp. 284–291; and Y. Shavit (1991). Stress-induced immune modulation in animals: Opiates and endogenous opioid peptides. In R. Ader, D. L. Felten, and N. Cohen (eds.), *Psychoneuroimmunology II.* Academic Press, New York.

page 71   The various biochemical imbalances evident among repressors are detailed and Schwartz's research with Willian Polonski on imagery, immunity, and asthma is described in G. E. Schwartz (1990). Psychobiology of repression and health: A systems approach. In J. L. Singer (ed.), *Repression and Dissociation: Implications for Personality Theory, Psychopathology, and Health.* University of Chicago Press, Chicago. Studies on the important role of monocytes in preventing disease include: A. J. Keiden, et al. (1986). Infective complications of aplastic anemia. *British Journal of Haematology*, 63, pp. 503–506; G. R. Taylor, L. S. Neale, J. R. Dardano. Immunological analyses of U.S. Space Shuttle crewmembers. *Aviation Space Environmental Medicine*, 57, pp. 213–217; S. D. Somers, W. J. Johnson, and D. O. Adams (1986). Destruction of tumor cells by macrophages: Mechanisms of recognition and lysis and their regulation. In R. B. Herberman (ed.), *Cancer Immunology: Innovative Approaches to Therapy*. Martinus Nijhoff, Boston; and A. A. Mathe and P. H. Knapp (1971). Emotional and adrenal reactions to stress in bronchial asthma. *Psychosomatic Medicine*, 33, pp. 323–340.

page 72   G. F. Solomon (1981). Emotional and personality factors in the onset and course of autoimmune disease, particularly rheumatoid arthritis. In R. Ader (ed.), *Psychoneuroimmunology*. Academic Press, New York; L. Abramson, D. C. McClelland, D. Brown, and S. Kelner (1991). Alexithymic characteristics and metabolic control in diabetic and healthy adults. *The Journal of Nervous and Mental Disease*, 179(8), pp. 490–494; S. Greer and T. Morris (1975). Psychological attributes of women who develop breast cancer: A controlled study. *Journal of Psychosomatic Research*, 19, pp. 147–153; A. W. Kneier and L. Temoshok (1984). Repressive coping reactions in patients with malignant melanoma as compared to cardiovascular disease patients. *Journal of Psychosomatic Medicine*, 28(2), pp. 145–155; L. Temoshok (1985). Biopsychosocial studies on cutaneous malignant melanoma: Psychosocial factors associated with prognostic indicators, progression, psychophysiology, and tumor-host response. *Social Science and Medicine*, 20(8), pp. 833–840.

page 73   M. R. Jensen (1987). Psychobiological factors predicting the course of cancer. *Journal of Personality*, 55(2), pp. 317–342.

page 74   D. Spiegel, J. Bloom, H. C. Kraemer, et al. (1989). Effect of psychosocial treatment on survival of patients with metastatic breast cancer. *The Lancet,* 2, pp. 888–891.

page 74   J. K. Kiecolt-Glaser, R. Glaser, D. Williger, et al. (1985). Psychosocial enhancement of immunocompetence in a geriatric population. *Health Psychology,* 4, pp. 25–41; J. K. Kiecolt-Glaser, R. Glaser, E. Strain, et al. (1986). Modulation of cellular immunity in medical students. *Journal of Behavioral Medicine,* 9, pp. 5–21; T. Moore (1993). *Care of the Soul.* HarperCollins, New York.

page 75   K. Duff (1993). *The Alchemy of Illness.* Pantheon, New York.

page 75   Gary Schwartz discusses his approach to mind-body therapy in G. E. Schwartz (1988). From behavior therapy to cognitive therapy to systems therapy. In D. B. Fishman, et al. (eds.), *Paradigms in Behavior Therapy: Present and Promise.* Springer, New York.

page 77   Schwartz's therapy for repressors, and his concept of repression as a talent, is discussed in G. E. Schwartz (1990). Psychobiology of repression and health: A systems approach. In J. L. Singer (ed.), *Repression and Dissociation: Implications for Personality Theory, Psychopathology, and Health.* University of Chicago Press, Chicago (also source for quote on page 83).

page 81   J. Kabat-Zinn (1991). *Full Catastrophe Living: Using the Wisdom of Your Body and Mind to Face Stress, Pain, and Illness.* Delacorte, New York.

page 84   Gary Schwartz's research on cerebral disconnection among repressors is reviewed in G. E. Schwartz (1990). Psychobiology of repression and health: A systems approach. In J. L. Singer (ed.), *Repression and Dissociation: Implications for Personality Theory, Psychopathology, and Health.* University of Chicago Press, Chicago. See also: B. E. Wexler, S. Warrenberg, G. E. Schwartz, and L. D. Jamner (1992). EEG and EMG responses to emotion-evoking stimuli processed without conscious awareness. *Neuropsychologia,* 30(12), pp. 1065–1079; and G. A.

Bonanno, P. J. Davis, J. L. Singer, and G. E. Schwartz (1991). The repressor personality and avoidant information processing: A dichotic listening study. *Journal of Research in Personality,* 25(4), pp. 386–401. The concept of cerebral disconnection was first suggested to Schwartz by an early paper, D. Galin (1974): Implications of left-right cerebral lateralization for psychiatry: A neurophysiological context for unconscious processes. *Archives of General Psychiatry,* 9, pp. 412–418.

page 91   The "sweeping the body" meditation is adapted from S. Levine (1987). *Healing into Life and Death.* Anchor Press/Doubleday, Garden City, NY.

page 92   "Listening to Your Symptoms" is exerpted from M. L. Rossman (1989). *Healing Yourself.* Pocket Books, New York.

CHAPTER 3. THE CAPACITY TO CONFIDE

page 96   J. W. Pennebaker (1990): *Opening Up: The Healing Power of Confiding in Others.* William Morrow and Company, New York.

page 99   J. W. Pennebaker and S. Beall (1986). Confronting a traumatic event: Toward an understanding of inhibition and disease. *Journal of Abnormal Psychology,* 95, pp. 274–281.

page 101   Pennebaker's studies on confession and healing among various populations are discussed in J. W. Pennebaker (1989). Confession, Inhibition, and Disease. *Advances in Experimental Social Psychology,* 22, pp. 212–244. Pennebaker's research on holocaust survivors is detailed in J. W. Pennebaker, S. D. Barger, H. Tiebout (1989). Disclosure of traumas and health among holocaust survivors. *Psychosomatic Medicine,* 51, pp. 577–589.

page 102   Pennebaker's studies on spoken confessions are summarized in J. W. Pennebaker, C. Hughes, and R. C. O'Heeron (1987). The psychophysiology of confession:

Linking inhibitory and psychosomatic processes. *Journal of Personality and Social Psychology*, 52, pp. 781–793.

page 103   Martha's story and her quote is included in J. W. Pennebaker, J. K. Kiecolt-Glaser, and R. Glaser (1988). Disclosure of traumas and immune function: Health implications for psychotherapy. *Journal of Consulting and Clinical Psychology*, 56, pp. 239–245.

page 104   The immunological benefits of confiding were revealed in Pennebaker's study with Janice Kiecolt-Glaser and Ronald Glaser. J. W. Pennebaker, J. K. Kiecolt-Glaser, and R. Glaser (1988). Disclosure of traumas and immune function: Health implications for psychotherapy. *Journal of Consulting and Clinical Psychology*, 56, pp. 239–245.

page 107   The study at the State University of New York at Stony Brook: M. A. Greenberg and A. A. Stone (1992). Writing about disclosed versus undisclosed traumas: Immediate and long-term effects on mood and health. *Journal of Personality and Social Psychology*, 63, pp. 75–84. The University of Miami study: B. A. Esterling, M. Antoni, M. Kumar, and N. Schneiderman (1990). Emotional repression, stress disclosure responses, and Epstein-Barr viral capsid antigen titers. *Psychosomatic Medicine*, 52, pp. 397–410.

page 108   Pennebaker's CARMEN machine and LIWC methods, research, and findings are fully described in J. W. Pennebaker (1993). Putting stress into words: Health, linguistic, and therapeutic implications. *Behavioral Research and Therapy*, 31(6), pp. 539–548.

page 110   Pennebaker's study of confiding among unemployed individuals is described in S. Spera, E. Buhrfeind, and J. W. Pennebaker (1993). Expressive writing and coping with job loss (in press).

page 113   J. W. Pennebaker, M. Colder, and L. K. Sharp (1990): Accelerating the coping process. *Journal of Personality and Social Psychology*, 58, pp. 528–537.

page 115   Pennebaker's collaboration with Anne Krantz on movement and writing: A. M. Krantz (1993). Dancing out trauma: The effects of psychophysiological expression on health (submitted for publication).

page 117 Laura's story and quote: J. W. Pennebaker (1990): *Opening Up: The Healing Power of Confiding in Others.* William Morrow and Company, New York.

CHAPTER 4. HARDINESS

page 126 Discussion of Ouellette's critical review of stress research is based on and the quote is from S. R. Maddi and S. C. Kobasa (1984). *The Hardy Executive: Health Under Stress.* Dow Jones–Irwin, Homewood, IL.

page 130 Ouellette's tale of a low-hardy executive is from R. Ornstein and D. Sobel (1988). *The Healing Brain.* Touchstone Books, New York.

page 131 Chuck's story is from S. R. Maddi and S. C. Kobasa (1984): *The Hardy Executive: Health Under Stress.* Dow Jones–Irwin, Homewood, IL.

page 132 S. C. Kobasa (1979): Stressful life events, personality and health: An inquiry into hardiness. *Journal of Personality and Social Psychology,* 37, pp. 1–11.

page 132 S. C. Kobasa, S. Maddi, and S. Kahn (1982). Hardiness and health: A prospective study. *Journal of Personality and Social Psychology,* 42, pp. 168–177.

page 133 S. C. Kobasa, S. R. Maddi, M. C. Puccetti, and M. A. Zola (1985). Effectiveness of hardiness, exercise, and social support as resources against illness. *Journal of Psychosomatic Research,* 29, pp. 525–533.

page 135 The cases of Andy and Bill are derived from S. R. Maddi and S. C. Kobasa (1984). *The Hardy Executive: Health Under Stress.* Dow Jones–Irwin, Homewood, IL.

page 137 G. F. Solomon, M. E. Kemeny, and L. Temoshok (1991). Psychoneuroimmunologic aspects of human immunodeficiency virus infection. In R. Ader, D. L. Felton, and N. Cohen (eds.), *Psychoneuroimmunology II.* Academic Press, New York; L. Temoshok, D. M. Sweet,

S. Jenkins, et al. (1988). Psychoneuroimmunologic studies of men with AIDS and ARC. Paper presented at the Fourth International Conference on AIDS, Stockholm, Sweden, June 12–16, 1988; G. F. Solomon and L. Temoshok (1990). A psychoneuroimmunologic perspective on AIDS research: Questions, preliminary findings, and suggestions. In L. Temoshok and A. Baum (eds.) *Psychosocial Perspectives on AIDS.* Lawrence Erlbaum Associates, Hillsdale, NJ; H. Dreher (1988). The healthy elderly and long-term survivors of AIDS: Psychoimmune connections. A conversation with George F. Solomon, M.D. *Advances,* 5:1, pp. 6–14. Dr. Temoshok has completed another study of psychological factors in fifteen AIDS patients, in which she found that patients who scored higher on Ouellette's hardiness measure lived significantly longer than those who did not. This statistical relationship approached (though did not reach) significance when initial CD4 counts were taken into account. L. Temoshok, A. O'Leary, and S. R. Jenkins (1990). Survival time in men with AIDS: Relationships with psychological coping and autonomic arousal. Paper presented at the Sixth International Conference on AIDS, San Francisco, June 20–24, 1990.

page 138   M. H. Antoni, L. Baggett, G. Ironson, et al. (1990). Cognitive-behavioral stress management intervention buffers distress responses and immunologic changes following notification of HIV-1 seropositivity. *Journal of Consulting and Clinical Psychology,* 59, pp. 906–915; H. Dreher (1994). Using the psyche in the fight against AIDS. *Natural Health* (January/February).

page 139   M. A. Okun, A. J. Zautra, and S. E. Robinson (1988). Hardiness and health among women with rheumatoid arthritis. *Personality and Individual Differences,* 9(1), pp. 101–107.

page 139   E. J. Langer and J. Rodin (1976). The effects of choice and enhanced responsibility for the aged: A field experiment in an institutional setting. *Journal of Personality and Social Psychology*, 34, pp. 191–198.

page 141 Discussion of various populations and hardiness is in S. C. Ouellette (1993): Inquiries into hardiness. In L. Goldberger and S. Breznitz (eds.), *Handbook of Stress: Theoretical and Clinical Aspects*, 2nd ed. Free Press, New York. See also P. T. Bartone (1989). Predictors of stress-related illness in city bus drivers. *Journal of Occupational Medicine*, 31, pp. 857–863. The quote is from C. Wood (1987): The buffer of hardiness: An interview with Suzanne C. Ouellette Kobasa. *Advances*, 4(1), pp. 37–45.

page 143 S. C. Kobasa (1982.) Commitment and coping in stress resistance among lawyers. *Journal of Personality and Social Psychology*, 42(4), pp. 707–717.

page 150 The discussion of blood pressure effects of hardiness and the cases of Arthur and Edgar are drawn from S. R. Maddi and S. C. Kobasa (1984). *The Hardy Executive: Health Under Stress*. Dow Jones–Irwin, Homewood, IL.

page 153 E. Gendlin (1978). *Focusing*. Everest House, New York.

page 162 Studies on meditation and control included in: W. L. Mikulas (1990). Meditation, self control, and personal growth; and D. Shapiro (1990). Meditation, self-control, and control by a benevolent other: Issues of content and context. In M. G. T. Kwee (ed.), *Psychotherapy, Meditation, and Health: A Cognitive-Behavioral Perspective*. East-West Publications, London/The Hague; and L. A. Hjelle (1974). Transcendental Meditation and psychological health. *Perceptual and Motor Skills*, 39, p. 623–628.

page 162 J. Kabat-Zinn (1991). *Full Catastrophe Living: Using the Wisdom of Your Body and Mind to Face Stress, Pain, and Illness*. Delacorte, New York.

page 164 The quote is from C. Wood (1987). The buffer of hardiness: An interview with Suzanne C. Ouellette Kobasa. *Advances*, 4(1), pp. 37–45.

page 165 This short version of the hardiness questionnaire first appeared in S. C. Kobasa (1984). How much stress can you survive? *American Health* (September).

CHAPTER 5. ASSERTIVENESS

page 168   G. F. Solomon and R. H. Moos (1964). Emotions, immunity, and disease: A speculative theoretical integration. *Archives of General Psychiatry*, 11, pp. 657–674. Solomon's study of healthy characteristics of people susceptible to rheumatoid arthritis who nevertheless resist the disease is one of the finest and perhaps the earliest explorations of Immune Power traits: G. F. Solomon and R. H. Moos (1965). The relationship of personality to the presence of rheumatoid factor in asymptomatic relatives of patients with rheumatoid arthritis. *Psychosomatic Medicine*, 27, pp. 350–360.

page 169   S. Locke and D. Colligan (1985). *The Healer Within*. E.P. Dutton, New York. Among Solomon's vital contributions to psychoneuroimmunology is his historical overview of the field, which has led him to chart new directions. He regularly publishes papers that set forth his unique sociocultural and scientific perspectives on the emerging medicine of mind and body. The most recent such paper is G. F. Solomon (1993). Whither psychoneuroimmunology? A new era of immunology, of psychosomatic medicine, and of neuroscience. *Brain, Behavior, and Immunity*, 7, pp. 352–366.

page 170   G. F. Solomon, L. Temoshok, A. O'Leary, and J. Zich (1987). An intensive psychoimmunologic study of long-surviving persons with AIDS. *Annals of the New York Academy of Sciences*, 496, pp. 647–655.

page 171   The quote is adapted from H. Dreher (1988). The healthy elderly and long-term survivors of AIDS: Psychoimmune connections. A conversation with George F. Solomon, M.D. *Advances*, 5:1, pp. 6–14.

page 171   G. F. Solomon, M. E. Kemeny, and L. Temoshok (1991). Psychoneuroimmunologic aspects of human immunodeficiency virus infection. In R. Ader, D. L. Felton, and N. Cohen (eds.), *Psychoneuroimmunology II*. Academic Press, New York; L. Temoshok, D. M.

Sweet, S. Jenkins, et al. (1988). Psychoneuroimmunologic studies of men with AIDS and ARC. Paper presented at the Fourth International Conference on AIDS, Stockholm, Sweden, June 12–16, 1988; G. F. Solomon and L. Temoshok (1990). A psychoneuroimmunologic perspective on AIDS research: Questions, preliminary findings, and suggestions. In L. Temoshok and A. Baum (eds.), *Psychosocial Perspectives on AIDS*. Lawrence Erlbaum Associates, Hillsdale, NJ; H. Dreher (1988). The healthy elderly and long-term survivors of AIDS: Psychoimmune connections. A conversation with George F. Solomon, M.D. *Advances*, 5:1, pp. 6–14; S. Sontag (1977). *Illness As Metaphor.* Farrar Straus Giroux, New York.

page 174   Solomon's recent study of HIV-positive patients with CD4 T-cell counts below fifty: G. F. Solomon, et al. (1993). Prolonged asymptomatic states in HIV seropositive persons with fewer than 50 CD4+ T-cells/mm^3: Preliminary psychoimmunologic findings. *Journal of Acquired Immune Deficiency Syndromes*, 6(10), pp. 1173–1174.

page 176   G. F. Solomon and R. H. Moos (1965): The relationship of personality to the presence of rheumatoid factor in asymptomatic relatives of patients with rheumatoid arthritis. *Psychosomatic Medicine*, 27, pp. 350–360.

page 177   A. A. Amkraut and G. F. Solomon (1972). Stress and murine sarcoma virus (Moloney)-induced tumors. *Cancer Research*, 32, pp. 1428–1433.

page 179   R. H. Moos and G. F. Solomon (1965): Psychologic comparisons between women with rheumatoid arthritis and their non-arthritic sisters: I. Personality test and interview rating data. *Psychosomatic Medicine*, 27, pp. 135–149; R. H. Moos and G. F. Solomon (1965): Psychologic comparisons between women with rheumatoid arthritis and their non-arthritic sisters. II. Content analysis of interviews. *Psychosomatic Medicine*, 27, pp. 150–164; R. H. Moos and G. F. Solomon (1966). Social and personal factors in rheumatoid arthritis: Pathogenic considerations. *Clinical Medicine,* 73, pp. 19–23.

page 182   G. F. Solomon (1981). Emotional and personality factors in the onset and course of autoimmune disease, particularly rheumatoid arthritis. In R. Ader (ed.), *Psychoneuroimmunology.* Academic Press, New York.

page 183   B. D. Naliboff, D. Benton, G. F. Solomon, et al. (1991). Immunological changes in young and old adults during brief laboratory stress. *Psychosomatic Medicine,* 53, pp. 121–132.

page 184   Solomon's more recent pilot studies on assertiveness and immunity were reported to the author in an interview in September 1993.

page 185   K. M. Rost, et al. (1991). Change in metabolic control and functional status after hospitalization: Impact of patient activation intervention in diabetic patients. *Diabetes Care,* 14, pp. 881–889. The quote from Tom Ferguson is from: T. Ferguson (1993): Working with your doctor. In D. Goleman and J. Gurin (eds.), *Mind-Body Medicine: How to Use Your Mind for Better Health.* Consumer Reports Books, New York. The Tufts study is reported in S. H. Kaplan, S. S. Greenfield, and J. E. Ware (1989). Assessing the effects of physician-patient interactions on the outcomes of chronic disease. *Medical Care,* 27(Suppl.3), pp. S110–S127.

page 186   Greer's oft-cited study of psychological coping and survival in breast cancer was first reported at five years after the patients' diagnosis in S. Greer, T. Morris, and K. W. Pettingale (1979). Psychological response to breast cancer: Effect on outcome. *The Lancet,* 2, pp. 785–787. The ten-year follow-up was reported in S. Greer, K. W. Pettingale, T. Morris, and J. Haybittle (1985). Mental attitudes to cancer: An additional prognostic factor. *The Lancet,* 1, p. 750. The most recent follow-up, at fifteen years, was reported in S. Greer, T. Morris, K. W. Pettingale, and J. Haybittle (1990). *The Lancet,* 1, pp. 49–50.

page 186   Solomon's research on the healthy elderly reported in G. F. Solomon, et al. (1988). Psychoimmunologic and endorphin function in the aged. *Annals of the New York Academy of Sciences,* 521, pp. 43–58.

page 201   L. Temoshok and H. Dreher (1992). *The Type C Connection: The Behavioral Links to Cancer and Your Health.* Random House, New York.

page 201   The discussion is based on and the chart (p. 205) comes from E. A. Charlesworth and R. G. Nathan (1985). *Stress Management: A Comprehensive Guide to Wellness.* Ballantine Books, New York.

page 204   The "Rights Fantasy" is adapted from A. J. Lange and P. Jakubowski (1976). *Responsible Assertive Behavior.* Research Press, Champagne, IL.

page 207   The steps to verbal assertiveness is adapted from H. G. Lerner (1985). *The Dance of Anger.* Harper and Row, New York.

CHAPTER 6. THE POWER OF LOVE VS. THE LOVE OF POWER

page 212   B. Siegel (1986). *Love, Medicine, and Miracles.* Harper and Row, New York.

page 213   M. Friedman and R. H. Rosenman (1974). *Type A Behavior and Your Heart.* Ballantine, New York.

page 214   Quote from J. Z. Borysenko (1985). Healing motives: An interview with David C. McClelland. *Advances,* 2(2), pp. 29–41. The originator of Thematic Apperception tests was Dr. Henry Murray. See H. A. Murray (1938). *Explorations in Personality,* Oxford, New York.

page 215   McClelland wrote extensively about his pioneering research on motivation and behavior in such books as D. C. McClelland (1961). *The Achieving Society.* Van Nostrand, Princeton, NJ; D. C. McClelland (1971). *The Drinking Man.* Free Press, New York; and D. C. McClelland (1985). *Human Motivation.* Scott Foresman, Glenview, IL.

page 217   M. Friedman and R. H. Rosenman (1974). *Type A Behavior and Your Heart.* Ballantine, New York.

page 218   D. C. McClelland (1979). Inhibited power motivation and high blood pressure in men. *Journal of Abnormal Psychology,* 88, pp. 182–190.

page 219   D. C. McClelland, E. Floor, R. J. Davidson, and S. Saron (1980). Stressed power motivation, sympathetic activation, immune function, and illness. *Journal of Human Stress,* 6(2), pp. 11–19; D. C. McClelland and J. B. Jemmott (1980). Power motivation, stress, and physical illness. *Journal of Human Stress,* 6(4), pp. 6–15; D. C. McClelland, G. Ross, and V. Patel (1985). The effect of an academic examination on salivary norepinephrine and immunoglobulin levels. *Journal of Human Stress,* 11, pp. 52–59.

page 220   Quote from J. Z. Borysenko (1985). Healing motives: An interview with David C. McClelland. *Advances,* 2(2), pp. 29–41.

page 221   J. B. Jemmott, J. Z. Borysenko, M. Borysenko, D. C. McClelland, R. Chapman, D. Meyer, and H. Benson (1983). Academic stress, power motivation, and decrease in salivary immunoglobulin A secretion rate. *The Lancet,* 1, pp. 1400–1402.

page 221   McClelland's meta-analysis of studies of IgA antibodies, showing their validity as a measure of immune functioning, was reported in J. B. Jemmott and D. C. McClelland (1989). Secretory IgA as a measure of resistance to infectious disease: Comments on Stone, Cox, Valdimarsdottir, and Neale. *Behavioral Medicine,* (Summer), pp. 63–71.

page 223   J. B. Jemmott, C. Hellman, D. C. McClelland, et al. (1990). Motivational syndromes associated with natural killer cell activity. *Journal of Behavioral Medicine,* 13(I), pp. 53–73.

page 223   McClelland's Mother Teresa studies are reported in: D. C. McClelland and C. Kirshnit (1988). The effect of motivational arousal through films on salivary immunoglobulin A. *Psychology and Health,* 2, pp. 31–52; and D. C. McClelland (1986): Some reflections on the two psychologies of love. *Journal of Personality,* 54, pp. 334–353.

page 227   The development of research on affiliative trust is detailed in: D. C. McClelland (1989). Motivational factors in health and disease. *American Psychologist,* 44(4), pp. 675–683; and J. R. McKay (1992). Affiliative Trust-Mistrust. In C. P. Smith, J. W. Atkinson, and D. C. McClelland (eds.), *Motivation and Personality: Handbook of Thematic Content Analysis.* Cambridge University Press, New York.

page 227   James McKay's studies of affiliative trust, mistrust and various immune functions are fully detailed in J. R. McKay (1991). Assessing aspects of object relations associated with immune function: Development of the Affiliative Trust-Mistrust coding system. *Psychological Assessment,* 3(4), pp. 641–647.

page 229   The prospective findings of McClelland, Carole Franz, and colleagues are reported in D. C. McClelland (1989). Motivational factors in health and disease. *American Psychologist,* 44(4), pp. 675–683. James McKay's recently completed study on affiliative trust and NK cells in depressed patients: J. R. McKay, L. Luborsky, J. P. Barber, and R. Kabasakalian-McKay (1994). Affiliative Trust-Mistrust and natural killer cells in patients with major depression. University of Pennsylvania, Department of Psychiatry (submitted for publication).

page 230   Redford Williams (1989). *The Trusting Heart.* Times Books, New York; R. B. Shekelle, M. Gale, A. M. Ostfeld, and O. Paul (1983). Hostility, risk of coronary heart disease, and mortality. *Psychosomatic Medicine,* 45, pp. 109–114.

page 231   McClelland's study of the healer Karmu and McClelland's results are reported in J. Z. Borysenko (1985): Healing motives: An interview with David C. McClelland. *Advances,* 2(2), pp. 29–41.

page 236   McClelland's research and findings on behavioral medicine programs are detailed in C. J. C. Hellman, M. Budd, J. Borysenko, D. C. McClelland, and H. Benson (1990). A study of the effectiveness of two group behavioral medicine interventions for patients with psychoso-matic complaints. *Behavioral Medicine* (Winter), pp. 165–173. McClelland further elaborates on the motivational changes experienced by participants in these groups in D. C. McClelland (1989). *Motivational factors in health and disease. American Psychologist,* 44(4), pp. 675–683. He reported unpublished data regarding the changes in affiliative trust among program participants in an interview with the author in February 1993.

page 238   H. Benson and M. Z. Klipper (1976). *The Relaxation Response.* Avon Books, New York; H. Benson and E. N. Stuart (1992). *The Wellness Book: The Comprehensive Guide to Maintaining Health and Treating Stress-Related Illness.* Birch Lane Press, New York.

page 239   F. I. Fawzy, M. E. Kemeny, et al. (1990). A structured psychiatric intervention for cancer patients: II. Changes over time in immunological measures. *Archives of General Psychiatry,* 47, pp. 729–735; F. I. Fawzy, M. O. Fawzy, et al. (1993). Malignant melanoma: Effects of an early structured psychiatric intervention, coping, and affective state on recurrence and survival six years later. *Archives of General Psychiatry,* 50, pp. 681–689; M. H. Antoni, L. Baggett, G. Ironson, et al. (1990). Cognitive-behavioral stress management intervention buffers distress responses and immunologic changes following notification of HIV-1 seropositivity. *Journal of Consulting and Clinical Psychology,* 59, pp. 906–915. See also M. H. Antoni (1993): Stress management: Strategies that work. In D. Goleman and J. Gurin (eds.), *Mind-Body Medicine: How to Use Your Mind for Better Health.* Consumer Reports Books, New York.

page 244   J. Kabat-Zinn (1994): *Wherever You Go, There You Are.* Hyperion Books, New York.

page 244   The results of David McClelland's collaboration with Joel Weinberger in studying oneness motivation and health among patients in Jon Kabat-Zinn's Stress Reduction Clinic remain unpublished. They were reported to the author in an interview with Weinberger in May 1993.

page 246   Dr. Kelner's study of a "oneness" visualization and its effect on immunity is described in J. R. McKay (1992). *Affiliative Trust-Mistrust.* In C. P. Smith, J. W. Atkinson, and D. C. McClelland (eds.), *Motivation and Personality: Handbook of Thematic Content Analysis.* Cambridge University Press, New York. The quote is from J. Kabat-Zinn (1991). *Full Catastrophe Living: Using the Wisdom of Your Body and Mind to Face Stress, Pain, and Illness.* Delacorte, New York.

page 249   The quote is from T. Moore (1993). *Care of the Soul.* HarperCollins, New York.

page 249   The quote is from K. Menninger (1963). *The Vital Balance.* Viking Press, New York.

page 251   The quote and meditation are excerpted from J. Kornfield (1993). *A Path with Heart.* Bantam Books, New York.

CHAPTER 7. HEALTHY HELPING

page 256   Allan Luks tells of his involvement in research on healthy helping and details his survey in his book, A. Luks (1992). *The Healing Power of Doing Good.* Fawcett Columbine, New York.

page 256   Although Luks's statistical findings are described in his book, further detail is provided by biostatistician Howard Andrews: H. F. Andrews (1990). Helping and health: The relationship between volunteer activity and health-related outcomes. *Advances,* 7(1), pp. 25–34. (The graphs are from this source).

page 263   The Luks quote is from R. Flippin (1992). Good Luks: A champion of volunteerism insists helping is healthy. *American Health* (November).

page 264   Panksepp's studies of puppies taken from their mothers: J. Panksepp, et al. (1978). The biology of social attachments: Opiates alleviate separation distress. *Biological Psychiatry,* 13(5), pp. 607–618.

page 264   Panksepp's study of the social behavior of rats: J.
Panksepp, N. Najam, and F. Soares (1979). Morphine
reduces social cohesion in rats. *Pharmacology Biochemistry
& Behavior*, 11, pp. 131–134. His research on guinea
pigs and their contact with their mothers is reported in
B. H. Herman and J. Panksepp (1978). Effects of morphine and naloxone on separation distress and approach attachment: Evidence for opiate mediation of
social affect. *Pharmacology Biochemistry & Behavior*, 9, pp.
213–220. The study in which mothers treated with an
opiate-antagonist were less likely to retrieve their pups:
J. Panksepp, et al. (1980). Endogenous opioids and social behavior. *Neuroscience and Biobehavioral Reviews*,
4(4), pp. 473–487. Panksepp's concepts of the neurobiology of bonding were articulated in J. Panksepp
(1989). Altruism, neurobiology. In *Yearbook of Neurobiology*. Birkhauser, Boston.

page 265   M. A. Fiatarone, et al. (1989). The effect of exercise on
natural killer cell activity in young and old subjects.
Journal of Gerontology, 44, pp. M37–45; M. A. Fiaratone,
et al. (1988). Endogenous opioids and the exercise-
induced augmentation of natural killer cell activity.
Journal of Laboratory and Clinical Medicine, 112,
pp. 544–552.

page 267   P. Moen, D. Dempster-McClain, and R. M. Williams
(1989). Social integration and longevity: An event history analysis of women's roles and resilience. *American
Sociological Review*, 54, pp. 635–647.

page 268   P. Moen, D. Dempster-McClain, and R. M. Williams
(1992). Successful aging: A life course perspective on
women's multiple roles and health. *American Journal of
Sociology*, 97(6), pp. 1612–1638; P. Moen, D. Dempster-
McClain, and R. M. Williams (1993): Women's roles
and well-being in later adulthood: A life course perspective (submitted for publication).

page 269   J. S. House, K. R. Landis, and D. Umberson (1988). Social relationships and health. *Science*, 241, pp. 540–545.

page 271   The empathy studies of Drs. Martin Hoffman, Carolyn
           Zahn-Waxler, Leslie Brothers, and Marion Radke-
           Yarrow are detailed in D. Goleman. Researchers trace
           empathy's roots to infancy. *New York Times,* March 28,
           1989. The work of Drs. Hoffman and Zahn-Waxler is
           also described in M. Hunt (1987). *The Compassionate
           Beast: What Science Is Discovering About the Human Side of
           Humankind.* William Morrow & Company, New York.

page 274   The quote is from Ram Dass and P. Gorman (1986).
           How Can I Help? Alfred A. Knopf, New York.

page 275   A. Huxley (1945). *The Perennial Philosophy.* Harper &
           Brothers, New York.

page 275   Marie's story is excerpted from Ram Dass and P.
           Gorman (1986). *How Can I Help?* Alfred A. Knopf, New
           York.

page 278   The quote is from K. Wilber (1992). *Grace and Grit: Spir-
           ituality and Healing in the Life and Death of Treya Killam
           Wilber.* Shambhala, Boston.

page 280   Blanche's story and the survey findings on helping and
           self-esteem are from A. Luks (1992). *The Healing Power
           of Doing Good.* Fawcett Columbine, New York.

page 281   The Kelner study is reported in J. R. McKay (1992).
           Affiliative Trust-Mistrust. In C. P. Smith, J. W. Atkinson,
           and D. C. McClelland (eds.), *Motivation and Personality:
           Handbook of Thematic Content Analysis.* Cambridge Uni-
           versity Press, New York.

page 286   The discussion and quote on "tonglen" practice are de-
           rived from K. Wilber (1992). *Grace and Grit: Spirituality
           and Healing in the Life and Death of Treya Killam Wilber.*
           Shambhala, Boston.

CHAPTER 8. SELF-COMPLEXITY

page 289   Dr. Linville's concept of self-complexity is set forth in P.
           W. Linville (1985). Self-complexity and affective ex-
           tremity: Don't put all of your eggs in one cognitive bas-
           ket. *Social Cognition,* 3(1), pp. 94–120.

page 290 Linville's initial research on the complexity of people's views of other groups is detailed in P. W. Linville, G. W. Fischer, and P. Salovey (1989). Perceived distributions of the characteristics of in-group and out-group members: Empirical evidence and a computer simulation. *Journal of Personality and Social Psychology*, 57(2), pp. 165–188.

page 292 P. W. Linville (1985). Self-complexity and affective extremity: Don't put all of your eggs in one cognitive basket. *Social Cognition*, 3(1), pp. 94–120.

page 293 Table 8.1 is from P. W. Linville (1987). Self-complexity as a cognitive buffer against stress-related illness and depression. *Journal of Personality and Social Psychology*, 52(4), pp. 663–676. Reprinted with permission of Dr. Linville.

page 295 P. W. Linville (1987): Self-complexity as a cognitive buffer against stress-related illness and depression. *Journal of Personality and Social Psychology*, 52(4), pp. 663–676.

page 297 P. W. Linville (1993). Self-complexity and multiple self-esteems. Unpublished manuscript. Duke University, North Carolina.

page 299 P. Moen, D. Dempster-McClain, and R. M. Williams (1989): Social integration and longevity: An event history analysis of women's roles and resilience. *American Sociological Review*, 54, pp. 635–647; P. Moen, D. Dempster-McClain, and R. M. Williams (1992). Successful aging: A life course perspective on women's multiple roles and health. *American Journal of Sociology*, 97(6), pp. 1612–1638. (The quote is from the latter).

page 302 From the perspective of cognitive psychology, Linville reviews a remarkable body of research on the dynamic self in P. W. Linville and D. E. Carlston (1993). Social cognition of the self. In P. G. Devine, D. L. Hamilton, and T. M. Ostrom (eds.), *Social Cognition: Contributions to Classical Issues in Social Psychology*. Springer-Verlag, New York.

page 302   R. J. Lifton (1993). *The Protean Self: Human Resilience in an Age of Fragmentation.* Basic Books, New York.

page 303   The discussion and quote are from S. A. Mitchell (1993). *Hope and Dread in Psychoanalysis.* Basic Books, New York.

page 306   The discussion and quote are from M. Csikszentmihalyi (1993). *The Evolving Self: A Psychology for the Third Millennium.* HarperCollins, New York.

page 309   R. Assagioli (1965). *Psychosynthesis.* Viking Compass, New York.

page 309   Alice Epstein tells her story in A. Epstein (1989). *Mind, Fantasy, and Healing.* Delacorte, New York.

page 310   The quote is from P. Ferrucci (1982). *What We May Be: Techniques for Psychological and Spiritual Growth Through Psychosynthesis.* Jeremy P. Tarcher/Perigee Books, Los Angeles.

page 317   The quote is from A. S. Cowley (1993). Transpersonal social work: A theory for the 1990's. *Social Work,* 38(5), pp. 527–534.

page 318   A. Ashe, with A. Rampersad (1993). *Days of Grace.* Alfred A. Knopf, New York.

page 321   Psychosynthesis exercises are adapted from P. Ferrucci (1982). *What We May Be: Techniques for Psychological and Spiritual Growth Through Psychosynthesis.* Jeremy P. Tarcher/Perigee Books, Los Angeles.

INDEX

Abramson, Lauren, 72
Acceptance of reality, 170
Ace Factor (attend, connect, express),
    48–95, 192, 314
  and capacity to confide, 114, 119, 315
  defined, 51–52
  discovery of, 48–52
  and endorphins, 71
  enhancing, 10, 59–60, 75–91
  exercises for, 91–94, 324
  and hardiness, 315
  record template, **95**
  research on, 2–3, 60–75
Achievement, 212, 213, 215
Achterberg, Jeanne, 92
ACTH, 21
Action plan, 159
Active copers, 138
Actors, 142
Adaption, 45
Ader, Robert, 24–25, 169
Adrenal glands, 21
Adrenaline, 21, 106, 219
Adult Children of Alcoholics, 117
Affiliation motives, 212, 220–26, 325

Affiliative trust, 314
  and capacity to confide, 315
  defined, 227–31
  enhancing, 234–51
  exercises in, 251–54
  and healers, 231–34
  and helping, 315
  and oneness motive, 246–47
  visualization exercise for, 253–54
Aggressiveness, 201–2
"Aha" experience, 84–88
AIDS, 6–8, 15, 37, 137–38, 147–48, 170–76,
    187, 194–95, 197–99
Alchemy of Illness, The, (Duff), 75
Alcoholics Anonymous, 117
Alexander, Franz, 20–22
Alexander technique, 192
Alexithymia, 72
Alienation, 153
Allergies, 8, 15, 37, 67, 72, 75, 266
  defined, 39
Altruism, 170, 255–87, 314
  guidelines for, 259
  how to awaken, 274–79
  how to exercise, 286–87

Altruism *(continued)*
  meditation for, 286–87
  muscle analogy, 271, 274
  research on, 3–4, 255–74
  unhealthy, 284–86
  writing practice, 287
Alzheimer's disease, 259
American Health, 263
Amkraut, Alfred, 23, 169, 177
Anatomy of an Illness, The (Cousins), 270
Andrews, Howard, 256–60
Anger, 33, 34, 99, 103, 111–12, 179, 187–88, 200–01
  transformational vs. regressive coping and, 150–53
Anthrax, 18
Antibodies, 40–41, 220
Antidepressant medication, 52–53
Antigen-antibody bond, 41
Antigens, 25, 39–40, 43
Antihypertensive medication, 89
Antibiotics, 19
Antoni, Michael, 46, 138, 239
Anxiety, 32–33, 53, 61–63, 112, 241
Aristotle, 17–18
Arthritis, 8, 15, 37, 258
Ashe, Arthur, 147–48, 317–18
Assagioli, Dr. Roberto, 309, 314, 316
Assertive action, 187–88
Assertiveness, 35, 45–46, 168–210, 314
  defined, 201–2
  guide to, 199–210
  importance of, 189
  and other traits, 315–16
  planning and visualizing, 209–10
  rating, **205**
  research on, 168–86
  rules for effective, 207–8
  and search for meaning, 196–99
  self-training guidelines, 201–10
  and social support, 195–96
  test, 182
  training, 193
Asthma, 8, 21, 37, 72, 75–76, 266, 258
Atherosclerosis, 240
Attention, 45, 81–82, 90
Authentic selves, 302
Autoimmune disorder, 23–25, 37, 39, 175, 178, 189, 236, 266
Autonomic nervous system, 106, 108–10

Awfulizing, 156–57
AZT, 198

Back pain, 15, 258, 297
Bacterial disease, 18, 39
Balance, 19–20, 71, 81, 91, 250, 291, 295
Behavioral medicine, 31, 34–35, 235–36
Behavior therapy, 15
Bellow, Saul, 48
Benson, Dr. Herbert, 235–36, 238–40, 241, 282
Bernard, Claude, 19
Besedovsky, Hugo, 25
Bhagavatam, Srimad, 278
Big Brothers/Big Sisters, 256
Biochemical pathways, 175
Biofeedback, 15, 46, 54–55, 59, 73, 76, 79–80, 162
Biological response modifiers, 44
Biologicals, 44
Blood pressure, ·150, 326
Blood sugar (serum glucose), 19, 21, 69–71, **68**, 72–73, 185
B-lymphocytes (B-cells), 40–41, 43, 220
Body-based therapies, 192
Bodymind "system" model, 55–56
"Body scan" medication, 85
Bone marrow, 26
Borysenko, Joan, 156, 235–36
Brain, 20–28, 31–32, 44–45, 265–66
  and immune system, 14–15, 20–28
  left and right, 84–85
Breast cancer, 46, 73–74, 161, 186
Bronfenbrenner, 299
Brothers, Dr. Leslie, 273
Budd, Dr. Matthew, 236, 239
Buddhism, 163, 244, 275, 286
  loving-kindness meditation, 251–52
Buffers, 187, 296
Bulimia, 98
Bulloch, Karen, 25–26
Burnout prevention, 285

Callen, Michael, 6–8, 197–99
Campbell, Joseph, 316
Cancer, 8, 15, 37, 175, 189
  and ACE Factor, 72–75
  and assertiveness, 178
  and authentic self, 302
  and expression of emotion, 34
  and group therapy, 74

guided imagery for, 157–58
and hardiness, 134
and helplessness, 28
and psychotherapy, 118
and self-complexity, 308–13
and stress, 23
Cancer-cell, 39–40, 43–44
Cancer-specific antigens, 39–40
Cannon, Walter B., 19–20, 22, 91
Cardiovascular system, 186, 219, 235
Care of the Soul (Moore), 248–49
CARMEN machine, 108–10
Cartesian dualism, 18
Catecholamines, 21, 71
Catharsis, 101, 122
Catholic church, 119
Causal words, 108–9
CD4 cells. *See* T-helper cells
Cell-mediated immunity, 40–41, 43
Cell products, 44
Challenge, 3, 141–42, 163, 314
defined, 128–29
Charlesworth, Edward A., 201, 203
Cholesterol, 240, 243
Christianity, 275
Chronic fatigue, 8, 37, 75, 189
Chronic pain, 37, 75, 261, 266
City University of New York (CUNY), 126, 146
Cognitive-behavioral treatments, 46
Cognitive insights, 108–9, 119–20, 122
Cognitive psychology, 289
Cognitive restructuring, 15, 46, 235, 236, 238, 241–42
Cognitive therapies, 46
Cohen, Nicholas, 24
Colds, 233, 258, 266, 297
Colligan, Douglas, 169
Commitment, 3, 33, 142, 143, 162–63, 314
defined, 128
Communication, 45, 90
Community Research Initiative on AIDS, 198
Compassion, 286
Compensatory self-improvement, 161–62
Competitiveness, 217
Complexity, 314
and evolution, 306–8
and healing, 308–13
See also Self-complexity
Computer studies, 108–10

Conditioning, 24–25
Confession, 97, 315
culture of, 119–20
and health, 99–107
movement and writing, 123–24
spoken, 122–23
written, 120–22
Confiding, capacity for, 96–124, 314
and ACE factor, 114, 119
guidelines for, 120–24
psychotherapy as aid to, 117–18
research on, 3, 99–116
Connections, 90
Control, 3, 140, 161–64, 188, 314
and aging, 187–88
defined, 128–29
and helping, 269–70
vs. power motive, 216
Conversion disorders, 20
Cooperation, 265–66
Coping abilities, 236, 239
and aging, 186–87
and AIDS, 138, 170, 174–76
and health, 28–34, 43, 177, 188
and social support, 135–36
transformational vs. regressive, 151–53
Coping categories, 62–63, 66–69
Coronary bypass surgery, 240
Corticosteroids, 21, 71, 219
Cortisol, 21
Cousins, Norman, 12, 270–71, 274
Cowley, Au-Deane, 317
Crick, Francis, 308
Csikszentmihalyi, Mihaly, 306–7, 314
Cytokines, 44

Dance of Anger, The (Lerner), 207
Darwin, Charles, 52, 265
Dass, Ram, 274–77
Days of Grace (Ashe), 317
Decisive action, 158–60
Deep breathing, 31, 235
Defense, 45
Defensive High Anxious, 62–63, 66–67, **68**
Delusion of consciousness, 274
Demoralization, 32, 33
Dempster-McClain, Donna, 267
Depression, 33, 153, 179, 188, 280
and grief muscles, 52–53
and immune function, 29–30, 32
and self-complexity, **293,** 297–98

Descartes, René, 18
"Detached concern," 142
Diabetes, 72–73, 75, 185
Diabetes Care, 185
Differentiation, 305–8, 315
Disconnected people, 55, 59–60
Distress, 2, 32, 34, 187
"Don't Put All of Your Eggs in One
    Cognitive Basket" (Linville), 295
Duff, Kat, 75

Ego mastery, 176
Einstein, Albert, 255, 274
Elderly, 186–88
Electromyelograph (EMG), 52
El Salvador study, 144
Emotional aspect of healing mind, 34–35
Emotions, 21, 27, 34–37, 46, 52–54, 72–73,
    105, 238
  linked to immunity, 21, 169–70
"Emotions, Immunity, and Disease"
    (Solomon and Moos), 168
Empathy, 271–74
Endocrine system, 14, 21
Endorphins, 27, 69–71, 73, 106, 264–66,
    280
Eosinophiles, 67, **68, 327**
Epstein, Alice, 309–13
Epstein, Seymour, 309–10
Esterling, Brian, 71*n*.
Evolving Self, The (Csikszentmihalyi), 306
Exercise, 133–37, 192, 236, 243, 264, 266
Exploring and cultivating self-aspects
    exercise, 319–21
Expression of emotion, 45, 59–60, 67, 189
Expressive action, 87–91, 199

Faith healing, 234
Family history, 134
Family support, 135–37
Fatigue, 32
Fawzy, Dr. Fawzy I., 46, 239
Fear, 34, 53
Feedback, 50–51, 54–56, 159–60
Feel-good sensation, and helping, 257–58
Felten, David, 26
Ferguson, Dr. Tom, 185
Ferrucci, Piero, 310, 321
Fighting spirit, 186
"Fight-or-flight" response, 20–22, 64,
    183–84, 219, 238

Flexibility, 82, 145, 305
Focusing, 153–55
Food and Drug Administration (FDA), 52
Francis, Martha, 109
Frankl, Viktor, 126
Franz, Carol, 229
Freud, Sigmund, 20, 22, 60–61, 96, 199
Friedman, Meyer, 213, 217–18
Full Catastrophe Living (Kabat-Zinn), 81,
    246

Galen, 18
Gastrointestinal disturbances, 236
Gendlin, Eugene, 153–54
Genetic inheritance, 35–36, 134
Germ theory of disease, 18–20
Givens, 161
Glaser, Ronald, 29, 104–6, 259
Goeble, Blanche, 280
Goleman, Daniel, 272
Gorman, Paul, 274–77
Granulocytes, 42, 324, 326–28
Greenfield, Sheldon, 185
Greer, Dr. Steven, 73, 186
Grief, 33–34, 52–53, 99, 103, 252–53,
    300–1
Group therapy, 15, 46, 235, 239
Growth factors, 44
Guided imagery, 15, 46
  and ACE factor, 76, 79–80
  and affiliative trust, 235
  and best-case scenarios, 157
  Listening to Your Symptoms
    exercise, 92–94
  Rights Fantasy exercise, 203–6

Hardiness, 45, 125–67, 315, 325
  and assertiveness, 200
  defined, 30, 126–29
  and mind-body medicine, 162–64
  questionnaire, 165–67
  research on, 3, 129–48
  and self-complexity, 300
  training, 148–62
  writing exercise, 164–65
Hardiness Institute, 149
Hardy Executive, The (Ouellette and
    Maddi), 131, 135, 151
Harmony, 19, 55
Harvard Community Health Plan
    (HCHP), 236

Headaches, 15, 56–60, 236, 258
Head First (Cousins), 270
Healers, 231–34
Healer Within, The (Locke and Colligan), 169
"Healing and the Mind" (TV series), 16
Healing Brain, The (Ornstein and Sobel), 130
Healing emotions, 34
Healing personality, 45
Healing Power of Doing Good, The (Luks), 261
Healing Yourself (Rossman), 92
Health
　and affiliative trust, 229–30
　and altruism, 256–61, **260, 261**
　and confession, 100–1
　and hardiness, 134–37
　and personality, 33–38
　-promoting traits, 37, 188–89
　and self-complexity, **293,** 295–300
Heart disease, 15, 22, 37, 38*n*, 47, 64–65, 137, 219, 230, 240–43
Heidegger, Martin, 126
Hellman, Caroline, 236
Helper's high, 4, 261–63, 279–82, 325
Helping, 45
　as addiction, 264–66
　and affiliative trust, 315
　and hardiness, 315
　and health, 256–63, **260,** 267–70
　healthy, defined, 282–85
　and meditation, 281
　and strangers, 258–59, 260, **261,** 283
Helplessness, 28–29, 32, 73, 153
Hercules, labors of, 288–89
Herpes, 8
High disclosers, 106–7
High-risk pregnancies, 146
Hilker, Dr. Robert, 130
Hinayana path, 286
Hinduism, 275, 278
Hippocrates, 17, 18
HIV-positive people, 46, 137–38, 147–76, 229, 239. *See also* AIDS
HIV virus, 8, 41–42
Hoffman, Dr. Martin L., 271–72
Holmes-Rahe test, 132
Homeostasis, 19–20
Hopelessness, 32–33
Hormonal messengers, 21

Horniak, Nancy, 85–87
Hostility, 217, 230, 241–43
House, Dr. James, 29, 269
How Can I Help? (Ram Dass and Gorman), 274–77
Humoral arm, 40, 43
Huxley, Aldous, 275
Hydra, 288–89
Hypertension (high blood pressure), 21, 64–65, 75, 87–91, 136, 150, 185, 218–19
Hyperthyroidism, 21
Hypnosis, 15, 46, 162, 163, 235
Hypothalamus, 21, 23, 25

Illinois Bell Telephone study, 130, 149–50
Illness as Metaphor (Sontag), 172
Imagery and Healing (Achterberg), 92
Immune cells
　and ACE Factor, 66–69
　and AIDS patients, **173**
　and assertiveness, 172
　and capacity to confide, 104–6
　defined, 38–40
　and endorphins, 70*n*
　and hardiness, 172
　and Immune Power Personality program, 326–28, **327**
　nerve connections to, 26–27
　products, 44
　sites, 38
Immune chemicals, 44
Immune competence, 178
Immune Power Personality
　and assertiveness, 196–97
　defined, 2, 37–38, 46
　developing, 8–11
　first studies on, 176–86
　mind and immune system analogies, 45
Immune Power traits, 2, 37–38, 45
　and AIDS, 6–8
　developing, 9, 44–47, 191–99
　integrating exercise, 323
　overlapping of, 313–16
　researchers on, 2–5
　and self-complexity, 313–16
　and way of spirit, 316–19
　See also specific traits
Immune response, 22, 24–25, 41–44
Immune system
　and affiliative trust, 228–30

Immune system *(continued)*
  analogies between psychological system
    and, 44–46
  and assertiveness, 175–76
  biology of, 38–44
  and brain, 23–28, 44, 169–70
  and confession, 104–7
  defined, 13–14, 38–39
  and distress, 32–33
  and endorphins, 70–71
  and exercise, 266
  and hardiness, 137–40
  and helping or altruism, 266
  and Immune Power Personality
    program, 324–28
  and inhibited power motive, 219–21
  and nervous and endocrine system,
    14–15, 21
  personality traits and, 37–38, 171–76,
    188–89
  and stress response, 22
Immunoglobulin A (IgA), 40, 220–28,
  233–34
  and helping, 281–82
  and love, 223–26
  and oneness motive, 246
  and resistance to illness, 221–23, **222,**
    225
Immunologic memory, 41
Impatience, 217
Infectious diseases, 72, 175, 189, 223
Influenza, 37, 297
Inhibition, 97–98, 107–8
Institute for the Advancement of Health,
  256
Integration, 306–7, 308, 314, 317
  exercise, 323
Interferons, 44
Interleukins, 43–44
Ironson, Dr. Gail, 239
Islam, 275
Isolation, 32
"I" statements, 202, 207

Jakubowski, Patricia, 204
James, William, 17, 36
Jamner, Larry, 66–67, 69, 71–73
Jemmott, John, III, 223
Jensen, Mogens R., 73
Johnson, Magic, 7

Judaism, 275
Jung, Carl, 271, 316

Kabat-Zinn, Jon, 81, 85, 163, 244, 245–47,
  284
Kansas Area Organization on Aging, 257
Kaplan, Sherrie, 185
Kaposi's sarcoma, 174
Karmu (Edgar Warner), 231–34
Kelner, Dr. Steven P., 246, 281
Kiecolt-Glaser, Janice, 29, 74, 104–5, 106,
  259
Killer (cytotoxic) T-cells, 42, 171, 173
Knapp, P. H., 72
Koch, Robert, 18–19
Kornfeld, Jack, 252
Krantz, Anne M., 115–16, 123

"Labeling" sensations, 155
Lange, Arthur J., 204
Langer, Ellen, 140
Lawyers, 143
Leigh, Dr. Hoyle, 65–66
Lerner, Harriet Goldhor, 207
LeShan, Lawrence, 10–11, 28, 118, 302
Letting-go experience, 103, 107, 112–16
Letting-go of results, and helping, 284–85
Levine, Stephen, 91
Life events, stressful
  and hardiness, 145–46
  situational reconstruction for, 155–58
  and transformational vs. regressive
    coping, 150–51
Lifton, Robert J., 302–3, 306, 314, 315
Linville, Patricia, 4, 10, 289–306, 308, 313,
  314, 319–29
"Listening to your Symptoms," 92–94
LIWC (Linguistic Inquiry and Word
  Counts), 109, 110
Locke, Dr. Steven, 29–30, 169
Loneliness, 249
Longevity, 269, 298–99
Love, 211–15, 254
  motive, enhancing, 234–37, 247
  research on, 3, 223–31
  unconditional, 231
Love, Medicine and Miracles (Siegel), 212
Loving-kindness meditation, 251–53
Low disclosers, 106
Luks, Allan, 4–5, 255–67, 269–71, 279–80,
  282, 284–85, 325

Lupus erythematosus, 8, 24, 37, 39, 72, 258
Lymph nodes, 26, 41
Lymphocytes, 40, 43, 44, 73, 324, 326–27, **327**

McClelland, David, 3, 33, 72, 212–39, 244, 246–49, 250–51, 281
McCleod, Carolyn, 244
McKay, James R., 227–30
Macrophage, 42–44
Maddi, Dr. Salvador R., 128–29, 131–34, 149–51, 153–54, 158–62, 164
"Magic bullet," 19
Mahayana path, 286, 287
Manifest Anxiety Scale (MAS), 61–62
Man's Search for Meaning (Frankl), 126
Marlow-Crowne Social Desirability Scale (M-C), 61–62
Martin-Baro, Ignacio, 143–45
Maslow, Abraham, 17, 189, 316–17
Massage, 192
Mathe, A. A., 72
May, Rollo, 168
Meaning and purpose, 170, 189, 196–99
Medical science, concentration on sickness, 16–17
Meditation, 15, 31, 46, 192
    and ACE factor, 76, 79–80
    and affiliative trust, 235, 238, 241
    and hardiness, 162–63
    /helping connection, 281
    loving-kindness, 251–52
    Tonglen, for compassion, 286–87
Melanoma (skin cancer), 46–47, 239
Melnechuk, Ted, 38
Memory, 45
    blocked, 114
Memory cells, 41
Menninger, Karl, 249–50
Messenger molecules, 43–44, 71
Migraine headaches, 56–60, 75, 85
Milieu interior, 19
Mind, Fantasy, and Healing (Epstein), 312
Mind, role of, in health, 1, 28–33
Mind-body connection
    analogies of, 44–46
    continuing mysteries of, 15–16
    defined, 12–13
    development of, 48–49
    and Hydra model, 289

and mainstream medicine, 13–14
and NK cells, 43
research proving, 14–15
Mind/Body Groups, 236–40
Mind-body medicine
    defined, 31
    and hardiness, 162–64
    history of, 17–33
    and life-threatening illnesses, 46–47
    methods of, 15
    new research, 1–2, 5–6
Mind-body therapies
    and affiliative trust, 235–37
    changing personality through, 247
    key to effective, 76
Mindfulness, 81, 85, 91
    and affiliative trust, 238, 241, 244–46
    defined, 244
    and hardiness, 163
    and oneness, 247
Mind-immune dialogue, 27–28
Mistrust, 230, 236
Mitchell, Stephen A., 303–4, 314
Mitogen, 104
Moen, Phyllis, 267–70, 299
Molecular biology, 27
Monocytes, 326–27, **327**
    and ACE Factor, 66–67, **68,** 71–72
Mood
    and self-complexity, 294–95
    transforming, 236–43
Moore, Thomas, 75, 248–49
Moos, Rudolf, 168, 176, 179
Mother, and endorphins, 265
Motive patterns
    ability to change, 246–47
    changing, through relaxation, 237–43
    and immunity, 219–27
    and relationships, 248–51
Movement experiment, 115
    exercise, 123–24
Moyers, Bill, 16
Multiple personality disorder (MDP), 305–6
Multiple sclerosis (MS), 262
Murray, Dr. Henry, 147, 214

Nathan, Ronald G., 201, 203
Natural killer (NK) cells
    and affiliative trust, 230, 239
    and age, 186

Natural killer (NK) cells *(continued)*
  assertiveness and, 184–86
  and brain chemicals, 44
  defined, 29, 43
  and endorphins, 70
  healthy coping and, 174, 174*n*
  and helping and exercise compared,
    266
  and Immune Power Personality
    program, 324, 326
  and progressive muscle relaxation, 74
  and relaxed affiliative motives, 223,
    224
  stress and, 29–30, 183–84
Needs, being in touch with, 188, 192
Negative emotions
  attending to, 34, 92
  and immune function, 67
  writing about, 108–9, 121
Nerve networks, 26
Nervous system, 14, 21
Neural messengers, 21
Neurobiology
  of bonding and altruism, 264–66
  of empathy, 273–74
Neurodermatitis, 21
Neuropeptide receptors, 27
Neuropeptides, 26–27, 44
Neurotransmitters, 15, 44
Neutrophils, 326–27, **327**
New York Times, 272
Nietzsche, Friedrich, 126
"No," field-testing, 208–9
Nonjudgmental responses, 122
Nonspecific immune cells, 43
Noradrenalin, 219
Nursing home residents, 140

Object relations, 228
Obsessiveness training, 111
Okun, Morris A., 139
Oneness motive, 244–48
  defined, 245
  and helping, 281–82
Optimism, 35
Options, 88–90
Organ transplants, 39
Ornish Dr. Dean, 47
Ornstein, Robert, 130
Ortega Y Gasset, José, 125
Osler, Sir William, 18, 28

Ouellette, Suzanne Kobasa, 3, 5, 30,
  125–46, 149–52, 154, 161, 163–65,
  172, 187, 216, 300

Pain relief, and helping, 266
Palpitations, 236
Panic, 32, 33
Panksepp, Jaak, 264–66
Parental teaching, 258
Paris, Howard, 240–42
Passivity, 35, 184–85, 201–2
Pasteur, Louis, 18–19
Pathology, emphasis on, 16–17, 235
Path with Heart, A (Kornfeld), 252
Pauling, Linus, 307–8
Payne, Peggy, 261
Pennebaker, James W., 3, 96–121, 258–59,
  324
Pennebaker method, 107–11, 113–17
Pent-up rage, 32–33
Peptic ulcers, 21
Perennial Philosophy, The (Huxley), 275,
  278–79
Personal contact, 282–83
Personality
  altruistic, 270–74
  ability to change traits, 36–37, 149,
    189–90, 246–47
  and AIDS survivors, 170–76
  and health, 33–38
  inheritance and, 35
  and response to stress, 127–28
  and rheumatoid arthritis, 179–82
Personality templates, 35–37
Personality tests, 66
Perspective and understanding, 155, 156
Pert, Candace, 15, 26–27
Pessimism, 153
Pessoa, Fernando, 288
PET (positron emission tomography), 84
PHA, 104–5
Philadelphia (film), 198
Piaget, Jean, 271
Pilot Club International, 257
Pituitary gland, 21
Plasma cells, 40–41
Plasmapheresis, 190
Pleasure and play, 189, 199
Pneumocystis Carinii pneumonia (PCP),
  174
Polonski, William, 72

Polygraph, 97
"Positive emotions", 16
    importance of expressing, 34
    writing, 108–9
Positive thoughts, 239
Power motives, 212–13, 216–23
    de-stressing, 251
    inhibited, 217–20, 221
    and NK cells, **224**
    and relationships and balance, 250
Prayer, 238
Prescriptions, for self-care, 192
Prior exposure, 45
Proactive coping, 34, 152–53
Problem-solving, 37
Progressive muscle relaxation, 74, 238, 241
"Propaganda of hopelessness," 7
Protean self, 302–3, 306, 315
Protean Self, The (Lifton), 302
Psychoimmunology, 25
Psychological states
    influence of, on immune functions,
        28–33
    that promote health, 33–38
Psychological system, vs. immune system,
    44–46
Psychology Today, 98
Psychoneuroimmunology (PNI), 183, 270
    and AIDS, 170–74, **173**
    breakthrough of, 22–28, 44
    and confession, 104–7
    defined, 14–15
    early pioneers of, 3
    field founded, 168–71
    and hardiness, 134–35
    and love, 215
"Psychosocial Factors in AIDS"
        conference, 197
Psychosomatic medicine, 20–21
Psychosomatic seven, 21
Psychosynthesis, 309–13, 314
    exercise, 321–22
Psychotherapy, 15, 35–36, 46, 117–19, 193
Pyle, Howard, 96
Radke-Yarrow, Dr. Marion, 273–74
Rationality, 33
Raynaud's disease, 85
Receptors, 26, 27, 44
Record keeping, 80, 83–84
    template, **95**
Recovery movement, 119

Reduced stress concept, 16
Regressive coping, vs. transformational
    coping, 150–53
Reichian treatments, 192
Relatedness, 249
Relationships, 37, 212, 248–51
Relaxation, 16, 46, 55
    and ACE factor, 76
    and affiliative trust, 235–43
    and coping, 31, 153
    and diabetes, 73
    response, 235, 238–40
Religious training, 258
Repression
    and ACE Factor, 60–65
    defined, 51
    development of, in childhood, 77–78
    diseases linked with, 72–74
    Freud on, 60–61
    and heart disease, 64–65
    and immunity, 66–69
    measurement of, 61–64
    undoing, 78–79
Repressive coping and copers (repressors)
    and blood sugar, 69–71
    defined, 51, 58, 61–65
    diseases linked with, 72–74
    and endorphins, 69–71
    healing, 58–60
    and immune system, 66–67, **68**
    and left-right brain disconnect, 84–85
Resignation, 35
"Resistance resources," 30
Responsibility, 38, 140
Rheumatoid arthritis (RA), 21–23, 39, 169
    and ACE Factor, 72, 85
    and assertiveness, 176–80, 190–91
    and hardiness, 134, 139
    and personality, 179–84
Rheumatoid factor, 176
Right brain, 84–85, 92
Rights
    believing in, 203–6
    Fantasy exercise, 203–6
    recognizing legitimate, 202–3
Rodin, Judith, 140
Rogers, Carl, 316
Rosenman, Ray, 213, 217
Rossman, Dr. Martin L., 92
Ruff, Michael, 26

"Safe sex" concept, 197
St. Gregory the Great, 211
Sartre, Jean-Paul, 126
Scavenger cells (phagocytes), 42–43
Schwartz, Gary E., 2–3, 48–88, 92, 106,
    145, 192, 327
Scleroderma, 189
Self
  balance between multiple and unitary,
    305–8
  psychosynthesis and, 309–13
  temporal vs. spatial metaphor of, 303–4
SELF, becoming part of bigger, 275
Self-actualization, 189, 316
Self-aspects
  defined, 4, 289
  distinctness, 294
  exercise to explore and cultivate,
    319–21
  self-esteem of each, 297–98
  vs. subpersonalities, 313
Self-awareness, 192
Self-care, 192, 239
Self-complexity, 45, 288–314, 325
  defined, 10, 289–90
  dynamics of, 301–8
  exercises in, 319–22
  measuring, 292–95
  overlap with other traits, 315
  research on, 4, 291–300
  therapy to develop, 308–13
  and transcendence, 316–19
Self-esteem
  and assertiveness, 202–3
  and helping, 280, 284
  and self-complexity, 297–98
  and situational reconstruction, 157–58
Self-hypnosis, 31, 46
Self-regulation, early theories on, 20
Selye, Hans, 21–22
Set point, 61
Sexual trauma, 98, 103, 117–18, 181
Shavit, Yehuda, 70
Siegel, Bernie, 212
Simonton-Atchley, Stephanie, 157, 253
Sitting meditation, 86
Situational reconstruction, 155–58
Sjogren's syndrome, 85
Sleep disorders, 236
Sobel, David, 130
Social contact, and endorphins, 264–65

Social support, 46, 236
  and affiliative trust, 238–39
  developing, for health, 248–50
  getting what you need, 194–96
  and hardiness and health, 133–37
  and stress, 29
Societal factors, 258
Solano, Luigi, 138
Solomon, Dr. George F., 3, 9, 22–25,
    44–45, 72, 137–38, 168–200, 208
Sontag, Susan, 172
Spatial metaphor of self, 303
Specific etiology theory, 18–19
Spera, Stefanie, 110
Spiegel, Dr. David, 46, 74
Spirituality
  awakening, 278–79
  and health, 244
  and self, 275
  and self-complexity, 315–19
Spleen, 26, 41
Spoken confessions, guidelines for, 122–23
Sports Illustrated, 147
Spouse, loss of, 136–37
Stomachaches, 258
Stone, Arthur, 229n.
Strangers, helping, 258–60, 283
Stress
  ability to cope, and immune system, 1,
    5–6, 28–33
  and affiliative trust, 244–45
  avoiding, vs. coping with, 16, 125–27
  buffers for, 187
  and corporate executives, 129–33
  defined, 21
  vs. distress, 2, 32
  early theories of, 19–22
  good, and NK cells, 265–66
  and hardiness, 143
  and IgA, 222
  -illness link, and coping skills, 30–31
  and immunity studies in mice, 177–78
  and inhibition, 97–98
  locating sources of, 154–55
  management, 236, 239
  "message," 21
  model, positive attitudes and, 5–6
  personality and response to, 127–28,
    143
  response, defined, 21–22
  and self-complexity, 289–90, 296–97

and transformational vs. regressive coping, 151–53
Stressed power motive syndrome (SPMS), **224**
Stress hormones
and ACE factor, 71
and confession, 106
defined, 22
and immune system, 64, 71
and power motive, 219–20
Stuart, Eileen, 241–42
Subpersonalities, 308–13, 314
exercises, 321–22
Success, 294–95
Supernormals, 53–54, 84
Support, asking for, 189
Support groups, 46
Supportive/Expressive Therapy, 74
Suppressor (CD8) T-cells, 171, 326
and affiliative trust, 228–29
defined, 42
and personality, 172, **173**
Survival of the fittest, 265
vs. of most compassionate, 266
Surviving AIDS (Callen), 198
Surwit, Richard, 73
"Sweeping the body," 82
exercise, 91–82
Symptoms, as feedback signals, 50–51
Systems approach, 50–51

Talking out trauma, 102
Taoism, 275
T-cells (T-lymphocytes), 220
and age, 180
biological action of, 41–42
and confessions, 104–5, **105**, 106–7
defined, 25–26, 40
and hardiness, 139
and Immune Power Personality program, 326
subcategories of, 41
See also Killer T-cells; Suppressor T-cells; T-helpers
Tecumseh Community Health Study, 269
Temoshok, Lydia, 34, 73, 137–38, 170–72, 201
Temporal metaphor of self, 303
Temporomandibular joint syndrome (TMJ), 75
Teresa, Mother, 225–27, 231

Terrain concept, 19–20
Texas Instruments, 110
T-helper (CD4) cells, 46, 326
and affiliative trust, 228–29, 239
and AIDS, **173**, 174
and assertiveness, 172
defined, 41–43, 174
and hardiness, 138
Thematic Apperception Test (TAT), 214–15, 217–18, 236
Thomas, Dylan, 6, 7
Three Cs (control, commitment and challenge), 3, 300
defined, 126, 128–29
See also Hardiness
Three Faces of Eve, The (film), 305
Thurman, Dr. Howard, 318
Thymus gland, 25–26, 38, 41
Time and space, for confession, 122–23
Time-management exercise, 111
Tolerance, 45
Tonglen, 286
Toxoplasmosis, 147–48
Tranquility, 33
Transcendence, 316–17
Transcendental Meditation (TM), 54
Transcenders, 317
Transcending self-actualizers, 316–17
Transformational coping, 150–53
Trauma
confession of, and health, 99–107, 119–20
and going with flow, 112–16, 121
how to create written confession of, 120–22
and movement, 115–16
physiology of writing about, 107–10
and psychotherapy, 117–18
and self-complexity, 300–1
of unemployment, 110–12
True High Anxious, 62–63
and immune system, 66–67, **68**
True Low Anxious, 62–63
and immune system, 66–67, **68**
Trust, 45, 228
and confession, 122
See also Affiliative trust
Tuberculosis, 18
Tumor necrosis factor (TNF), 43
Type A behavior, 22, 217–19

Type A Behavior and Your Heart (Friedman and Rosenman), 213, 217
Type B personality, 201
Type C Connection, The (Temoshok and Dreher), 201

Uhlmann, Carmen, 108
Ulcerative colitis, 21, 193
Ulcers, 75, 136, 185
Unemployment, 110–12
Unstressed affiliation motive syndrome (UAS), **224**
"Up the Mountain" exercise, 322

Vaccine, 18–19
Vagus nerve, 26
Vajrayana path, 286
Vasoconstriction, 56
Verbal assertiveness, 206–8
Viruses, 37, 39
Virus-killing cells (virucidal), 43, 171, **173**
Visualization
  for affiliative trust, 253–54
  and hardiness, 162, 163
Volunteers, 257–59, 263, 267–70

Watson, James, 308
Ways to Wellness, 236
Weinberger, Daniel, 60–64
Weinberger, Joel, 244–45
Weintraub, Judy, 262, 284
Western Electric study, 230

What We May Be (Ferrucci), 321
White blood cells, 22, 27, 40, 326, 327
Wilber, Ken, 278–79, 286, 316–17
Williams, Dr. Redford, 230
Williams, Robin M., Jr., 267
Will to live, 186
Women, 299–300
Women's Roles and Well-Being Project, 267–70, 299
Woodward, Joanne, 305
Worst-case scenarios, 156–57
Writing
  and altruism, 287
  and assertiveness, 210
  bodily changes while, 107–10
  and confession, 101–4, 106–7
  exercise, 324
  and going with the flow, 112–16, 121
  hardiness exercise, 164–65
  and movement, 115–16, 123–24
  Pennebaker method of, 107–10, 113–16
  vs. talking about trauma, 116–18
  and unemployment, 110–12
Written confessions, guidelines for, 120–22

Yale Behavioral Medicine Clinic (YBMC), 56, 65–66, 87
Yoga, 31, 235, 238, 241
Yogi, Maharishi Mahesh, 54
"You" statements, 202

Zahn-Waxler, Dr. Carolyn, 272–73